Pediatric Neuroimaging

Hongsheng Liu • Xiaoan Zhang
Editors

Pediatric Neuroimaging

Cases and Illustrations

PEOPLE'S MEDICAL PUBLISHING HOUSE

Springer

Editors
Hongsheng Liu
Department of Radiology
Guangzhou Women and Children's Medical Center
Guangzhou, Guangdong, China

Xiaoan Zhang
Department of Radiology
The Third Affiliated Hospital of Zhengzhou
University Institute of Neuroscience, Zhengzhou
University
Zhengzhou, Henan, China

ISBN 978-981-16-7927-8 ISBN 978-981-16-7928-5 (eBook)
https://doi.org/10.1007/978-981-16-7928-5

Jointly published with People's Medical Publishing House, PR of China

This Springer imprint is published by the registered company Springer Nature Singapore Pte Ltd.
The registered company address is: 152 Beach Road, #21-01/04 Gateway East, Singapore 189721, Singapore

Contents

Contributors

Bin Ai, MM Department of Radiology, Guangzhou Women and Children's Medical Center, Guangzhou City, Guangdong, China

Jing Chen, MM Department of Medical Imaging, Tianjin Children's Hospital (Children's Hospital of Tianjin University), Tianjin, P.R. China

Department of Radiology, Tianjin Children's Hospital (Children's Hospital of Tianjin University), Tianjin, P.R. China

Wangchun Dai, MM Department of Radiology, Guangzhou Women and Children's Medical Center, Guangzhou City, Guangdong, China

Wen He, MM Division of Diagnostic, Guangzhou Women and Children's Medical Center, Guanzhou, Guangdong, China

Xin Li, BD Tianjin Second People's Hospital (Tianjin Institute of Hepatology), Tianjin, P.R. China

Xinzi Li, MM Department of Radiology, Tianjin Children's Hospital (Children's Hospital of Tianjin University), Tianjin, P.R. China

Hongsheng Liu, MD, PhD Guangzhou Women and Children's Medical Center, Guangzhou City, Guangdong, China

Jungang Liu, MM Department of Radiology, Xiamen Children's Hospital, Children's Hospital of Fudan University, Xiamen, Fujian, China

Zhenqing Liu, MM Division of Diagnostic, Guangzhou Women and Children's Medical Center, Guanzhou, Guangdong, China

Yuanting Lu, MM Division of Diagnostic, Guangzhou Women and Children's Medical Center, Guanzhou, Guangdong, China

Honglei Shang, MM Department of Radiology, The Third Affiliated Hospital of Zhengzhou University, Zhengzhou, Henan, China

Jingshi Wang, MM Department of Medical Imaging, Dalian Women and Children's Medical (Group), Dalian, Liaoning, China

Shuai Wang, MM Division of Diagnostic, Guangzhou Women and Children's Medical Center, Guanzhou, Guangdong, China

Hong Yu, BD Department of Medical Imaging, Dalian Women and Children's Medical (Group), Dalian, Liaoning, China

Mengjie Zhang, MM Department of Radiology, Tianjin Children's Hospital (Children's Hospital of Tianjin University), Tianjin, P.R. China

Xiaoan Zhang, MD, PhD Department of Radiology, The Third Affiliated Hospital of Zhengzhou University, Institute of Neuroscience, Zhengzhou University, Zhengzhou, Henan, China

Xin Zhao, MM Department of Radiology, The Third Affiliated Hospital of Zhengzhou University, Institute of Neuroscience, Zhengzhou University, Zhengzhou, Henan, China

Guifen Zheng, MM Department of Radiology, Tianjin Children's Hospital (Children's Hospital of Tianjin University), Tianjin, P.R. China

Zidong Zhou, MM Division of Diagnostic, Guangzhou Women and Children's Medical Center, Guanzhou, Guangdong, China

Congenital Malformations of the Brain

1

Jungang Liu

Brain malformation is a common finding in the neuroimaging evaluation of children who presented with developmental delay, mental retardation, or epilepsy.

There are various manifestations of the central nervous system, which are related to the involved developmental stages in utero. The earlier the occurrence, the more serious. These malformations may occur solitary or in combination. For example, the development of corpus callosum malformation, once occurred, needs to pay attention to the combined gray matter heterotopia and/or other abnormalities.

In recent years, significant progress in neuroimaging techniques, development of genetic sequencing, allow us to advance the correct definition/classification of congenital brain abnormalities and has resulted in a better understanding of their pathogenesis.

Neuroimaging is very important to diagnose congenital brain malformations, and MRI is the ideal method. Conventional MRI sequences allow detailed evaluation of the brain anatomy. Advanced MRI sequences provide microstructural and functional information that can reveal pathogenesis. For example, DTI provides detailed qualitative and quantitative information about the microstructure and organization of the white matter tracts. So MRI may allow the definition of subphenotypes within a group of congenital brain malformations and establish correlations between the neuroimaging phenotype and genotype.

Case 1.1 Anomalies of Corpus Callosum

Clinical Presentation

A 2-year-old boy presents with headache and low intelligence.

J. Liu (✉)
Department of Radiology, Xiamen Children's Hospital, Children's Hospital of Fudan University, Xiamen, Fujian, China

Imaging Findings

A. Axial T1WI shows the parallel bodies of the lateral ventricles, separated from the interhemispheric fissure by Probst bundles and the medial hemispheric cortex (Fig. 1.1a).
B. Axial T2WI shows the signal intensity of the Probst bundles is consist with white matter (Fig. 1.1b).
C. DTI shows the Probst bundles (white arrow) extending anterior to posterior (Fig. 1.1c).
D. Sagittal T1WI shows agenesis of the corpus callosum with the medial hemispheric sulci radiating into the third ventricle (Fig. 1.1d).

Discussion

Agenesis of corpus callosum (ACC) includes complete or partial absence of corpus callosum, is one of the most common congenital cerebral malformations [1]. It can be seen at any age and is mostly found in early childhood. It is more prevalent among males than females. When the corpus callosum is absent, the axons of both hemispheres cannot cross the midline, but run longitudinally along the medial edge of the lateral ventricle. These nerve bundles are called Probst bundles, which are the characteristics of the absence of corpus callosum.

ACC is an abnormality of prosencephalic midline development, and there are more than 200 congenital syndromes associated with ACC [2]. Isolated ACC may asymptomatic. When accompanied by other malformations, patients with ACC usually present with visual impairment, convulsions, mental retardation, or hypothalamic dysfunction [3, 4].

MRI is the first choice for agenesis of the corpus callosum. Axial imagings will show the lateral ventricles like a Formula One car viewed from above. Coronal imaging at the level of the frontal horns shows the characteristic appearance because of CCA and eversion of bilateral cingulate gyri into the frontal horns. Along the surface of lateral ventricles, Probst bundles may be present. Sagittal imaging shows that the cingulate gyrus is everted, the sulcus on the inner side of the cerebral hemisphere extends directly to the third ventricle, the third ventricle extends upward into the interhemispheric

H. Liu, X. Zhang (eds.), *Pediatric Neuroimaging*, https://doi.org/10.1007/978-981-16-7928-5_1

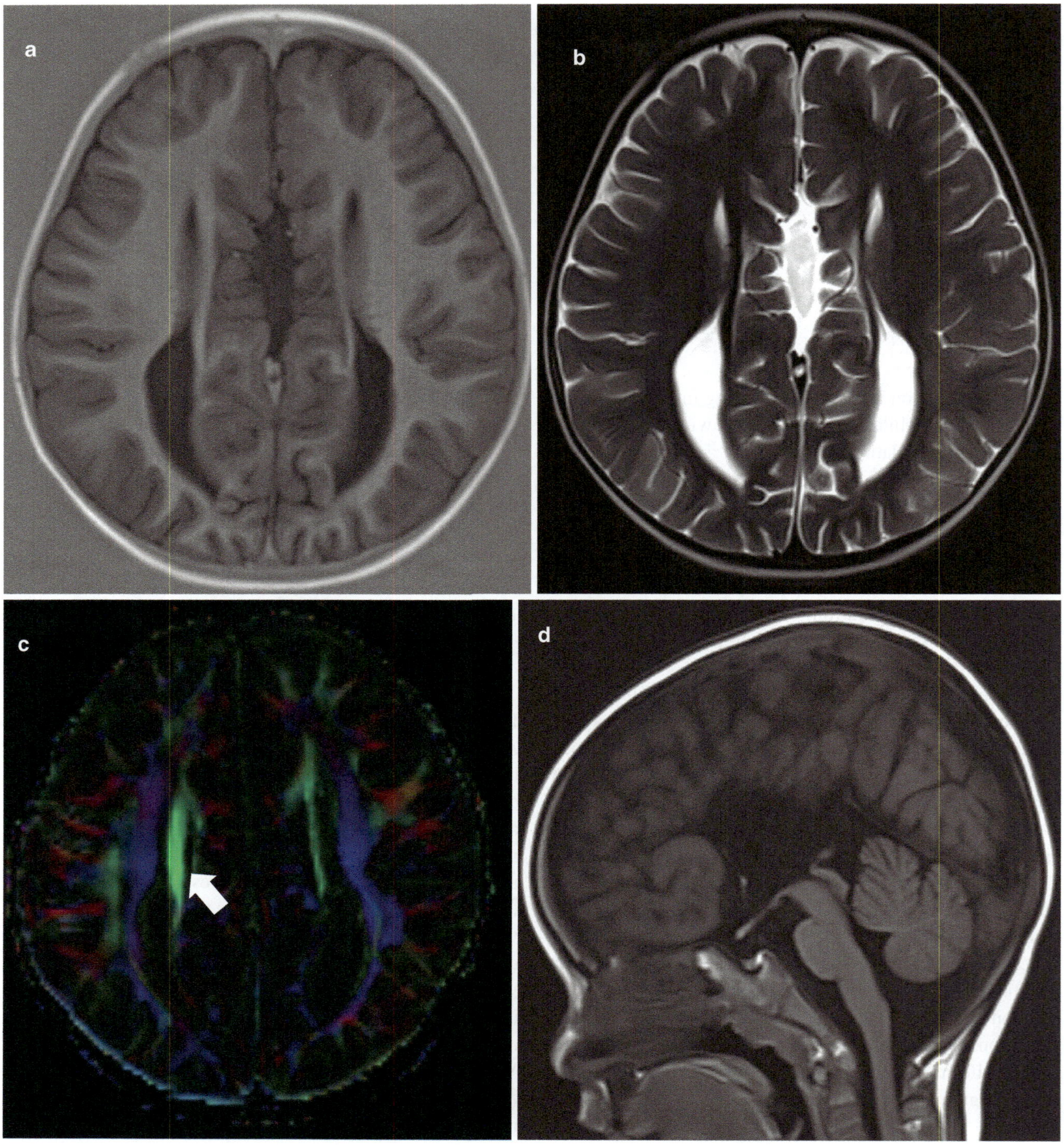

Fig. 1.1 Anomalies of corpus callosum

fissure, and the sulcus on the inner side of the cerebral hemisphere is arranged radially around the inner wall of the third ventricle. Corpus callosum malformation is often associated with interhemispheric fissure cyst and lipoma.

This disease is mainly differentiated from congenital hydrocephalus and destructive disease of corpus callosum in children. Severe hydrocephalus can lead to the thinning of corpus callosum, but the structure of corpus callosum is complete. Destructive lesions of the corpus callosum, may be due to periventricular leukomalacia, trauma, and surgery. Periventricular leukomalacia may have perinatal injury in preterm infants. The corpus callosum is thinning, and bilateral ventricles enlarged irregularly.

Case 1.2 Callosal Lipoma

Clinical Presentation

An 8-year-old girl presented with headaches.

Imaging Findings

A. Sagittal T1WI shows the corpus callosum is hypoplastic with no anterior genu, rostrum, and splenium, a mass of high signal intensity immediately superior to the corpus callosum (white arrow) (Fig.1.2a).

B. After contrast administration, sagittal T1WI with fat-suppressed shows the high signal intensity has been suppressed with no enhanced. (Fig. 1.2b).

Discussion

Interhemispheric lipomas are commonly called "callosal lipomas" or "lipomas of the corpus callosum," because they are situated adjacent to the corpus, and are always associated with hypogenesis or agenesis of the corpus callosum.

These malformations can be large and lobulated in appearance (most typically seen in the anterior callosal region), or thin and curvilinear (typically seen in the posterior callosal region, curving around the most posterior part of the corpus). Encephaloceles and cutaneous lipomas can be associated, as well, usually in the frontal region. In fact, several midline developmental disorders appear to have lipomas of the interhemispheric fissure as a part of the syndrome. Many of these are associated with midline facial clefts, basilar cephaloceles, and retinal dysplasia, a condition known as midline craniofacial dysraphism or frontonasal dysplasia [5]. When interhemispheric lipomas and callosal anomalies are associated with median cleft lip or palate and cutaneous polyps of the face, a diagnosis of Pai syndrome can be made.

The most common location is the deep interhemispheric fissure (dorsal to the corpus callosum, 40–50%), followed by the quadrigeminal plate/supravermian cisterns (20–30%), the suprasellar/interpeduncular cisterns (10–20%), the cerebellopontine angle cisterns (~10%), and the Sylvian cisterns (~5%) [6]. Occasionally, lipomas are found on the surface of the cerebrum. In such situations, blood vessels course through the lipoma and the underlying cortex is dysgenetic with poorly defined cortical lamination, fusion of the molecular layer, disrupted basal lamina, prominent astrocytosis, and abnormal synaptic profiles [7].

The MRI appearance of a lipoma is that of a hyperintense mass on T1WI sequences, becoming hypointense on conventional spinecho T2WI as the TE increases and when fat suppression is applied Interhemispheric lipomas may appear large and lobulated or thin and curvilinear. Lobulated interhemispheric lipomas tend to be located more anteriorly, may wrap around the anterior and posterior ends of the corpus callosum, and sometimes extend through the choroidal fissure and into the stroma of the choroid plexuses of the lateral ventricles, Curvilinear lipomas are thin and typically extend posteriorly behind the corpus, sometimes wrapping around and coursing into the velum interpositum. The adjacent corpus callosum is essentially always hypogenetic, with lipoma extending around the posterior portion of the corpus; no callosal fibers are seen dorsal or posterior to the lipoma.

Case 1.3 Encephaloceles

Clinical Presentation

A 1.5-year-old boy presented to the department of Oto-Rhino-Laryngology for mouth breathing when he was sleeping.

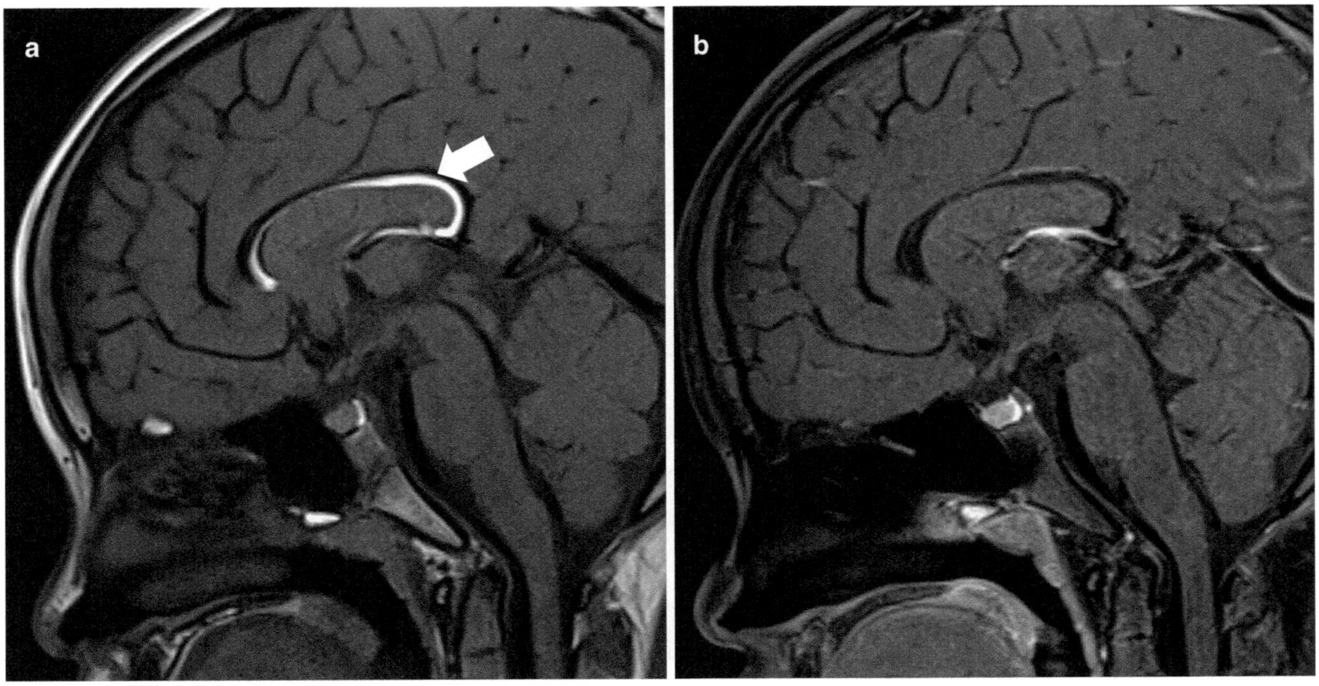

Fig. 1.2 Callosal lipoma

Imaging Findings

A. Sagittal T1WI shows intrasphenoidal meningocele comprised of extension of the floor of the 3rd. ventricle herniating into the sphenoid sinus through a defect in the floor of the sella tursica (white arrow) (Fig. 1.3a).
B. Sagittal T2WI shows cerebrospinal fluid flow (white arrow) demonstrating signal intensity flow voids (Fig. 1.3b).
C. Sagittal CT reformatted imagings shows the large bony defect (white arrow) involving the sphenoid body (Fig. 1.3c).
D. Coronal CT reformatted imagings shows absent of the sphenoid body (white arrow) (Fig. 1.3d).

Discussion

The term cephalocele refers to a defect in the skull and dura with an extracranial extension of intracranial structures. Cephaloceles are divided into two types [8]. Meningoencephaloceles are herniations of CSF, brain tissue, and meninges through the skull defect. Meningocele refers to herniation of the meninges and CSF only.

The cause of congenital cephaloceles has not been fully determined. Some argue that cephaloceles result from a failure of neurulation (failure of primary neural tube closure) [9].

Cephaloceles are named for the location of the bone defects, which include (a) occipito-cervical (involving the occipital bone, foramen magnum, and posterior arches of upper cervical vertebrae), (b) occipital, (c) parietal, (d) frontal, (e) temporal (along the superior surface of the petrous ridge), (f) frontoethmoidal (between nasal bones and ethmoid bone), (g) sphenomaxillary (through orbital fissures

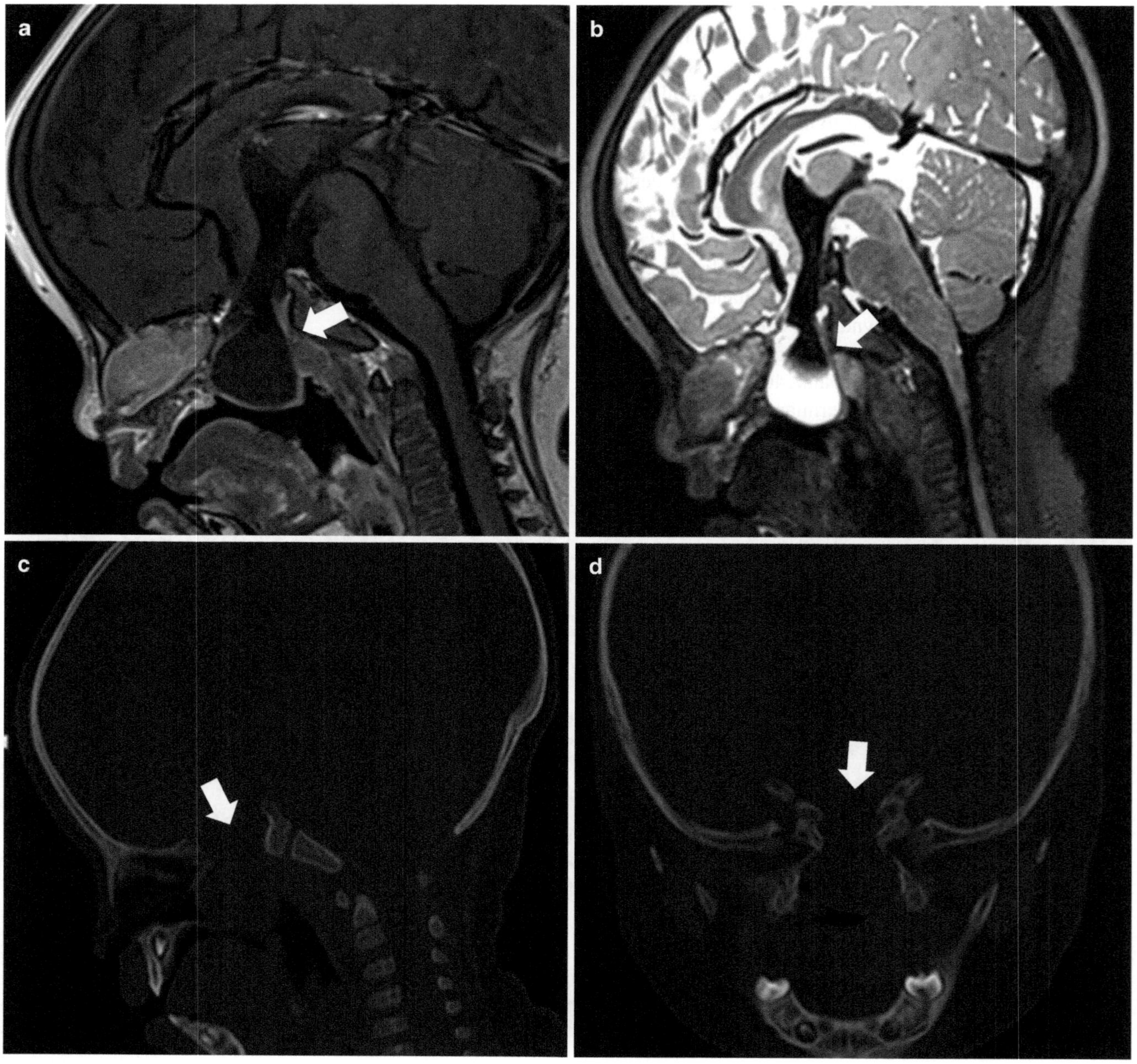

Fig. 1.3 Encephaloceles

into pterygopalatine fossa), (h) spheno-orbital (through defect in sphenoid bone or optic canal/orbital fissure into orbit), (i) nasopharyngeal (through ethmoid, sphenoid, or basiocciput into nasal cavity or pharynx), and (j) lateral (along coronal or lambdoid sutures).

Among above, the occipital bone is the most common location. The neurodevelopmental outcome is related to the size of the cephalocele, the amount of tissue present in the sac, and the presence of associated anomalies (up to 50%) [10]. CT better depicts the bony defects, MRI will show the contents in the cephalocele, and demonstrate associated cerebellar cortical dysplasia, venous sinus anomalies, dorsal interhemispheric cysts, callosal anomalies, gray matter heterotopia, tonsillar and brainstem ectopia, or Dandy–Walker malformations, all of which have higher frequencies in patients with cephaloceles [11, 12].

Case 1.4 Pachygyria

Clinical Presentation

A 2-year-old girl present with developmental delay and epilepsy.

Imaging Findings

A. Axial T1WI shows thickened cortex with relatively few and large gyri and sulci in the frontal, temporal lobes (white arrow) (Fig. 1.4a).
B. Axial T2WI shows white matter volume decreased significantly (Fig. 1.4b).
C. Sagittal T1WI shows the formation of occipital lobe is relatively normal (Fig. 1.4c).

Discussion

Pachygyria defined as the presence of a few broad, flat gyri with thickened cortex and may be used the term "incomplete lissencephaly" [13]. These definitions adopt the concepts of Hennekam and Barththat proper use of the terms agyria and pachygyria requires a thick cortex and that these malformations result from an arrest of neuronal migration. Both agyria and pachygyria are likely caused by abnormal regulation of microtubule activities [14]. Incomplete lissencephaly, in which areas of pachygyria are present together with areas of agyria or areas of normal brain, is much more common than complete lissencephaly. Areas of pachygyria also have a thickened cortex, but broad gyri and shallow sulci are present.

It is important to distinguish pachygyria from polymicrogyria, the sulci seen in pachygyria are normal, early forming sulci that can be identified and named by those experienced in neuroanatomy; the sulci in polymicrogyria are abnormal and do not correspond to those described in neuroanatomy texts. In addition, the cortex of pachygyria has smooth inner and outer surfaces, whereas that of polymicrogyria will be seen to have irregularities due to the microgyri and microsulci [15].

Case 1.5 Schizencephaly

Clinical Presentation

A 9-year-old girl present with weak left leg, unsteady gait, poor balance in the past 7 years.

Imaging Findings

A. Axial T1WI shows a large open lip schizencephaly at the right hemisphere (Fig. 1.5a).
B. Axial T2WI shows the lesion communicating with the right lateral ventricle (Fig. 1.5b).
C. Sagittal T1WI shows the lesion separated the right hemisphere (Fig. 1.5c).
D. Axial 3D T1WI shows irregular gray matter extending from the cortex to the ventricular surface (white arrow) (Fig. 1.5d).

Discussion

Schizencephaly, sometimes called agenetic porencephaly, is the term used to describe gray-matter lined clefts that extend through the entire cerebral mantle, from the ependymal lining of the lateral ventricles to the pial covering of the cortex [16]. It may occur in association with multiple etiologies of genetic, toxic, vascular, and infectious events.

Schizencephaly is a rare malformation, with a population prevalence of approximately 1.5 per 100,000 population. It is associated with young parental age. One-third of affected patients have a non-CNS abnormality, more than half of which may be classified as secondary to vascular disruption, including gastroschisis, bowel atresias, and amniotic band syndrome [17].

Patients with schizencephaly typically present with seizures, hemiparesis, or variable developmental delay. Children with unilateral schizencephaly present with hemiparesis and mild mental delay. Children with bilateral cleft are tetraparesis with severe mental deficits.

On pathologic exam, the gray matter lining schizencephalic clefts is dysmorphic and does not exhibit normal cortical lamination [18]. The clefts can be unilateral or bilateral and are most commonly located near the precentral or postcentral gyri. The frontal or parietal lobes, or both, were most commonly occurred. MRI not only demonstrates the cleft, but also the presence of adjoining heterotopic gray matter, as well as gyral anomalies of the insular regions.

The septum pellucidum is absent in approximately 70% of patients, and is almost always absent when the clefts are bilateral and frontal; The optic nerve hypoplasia, in conjunction with a high incidence of absence of the septum pellucidum, results in the classification of many affected patients in the category of septo-optic dysplasia.

Case 1.6 Holoprosencephaly

Clinical Presentation

A 4-year-old girl present with epilepsy.

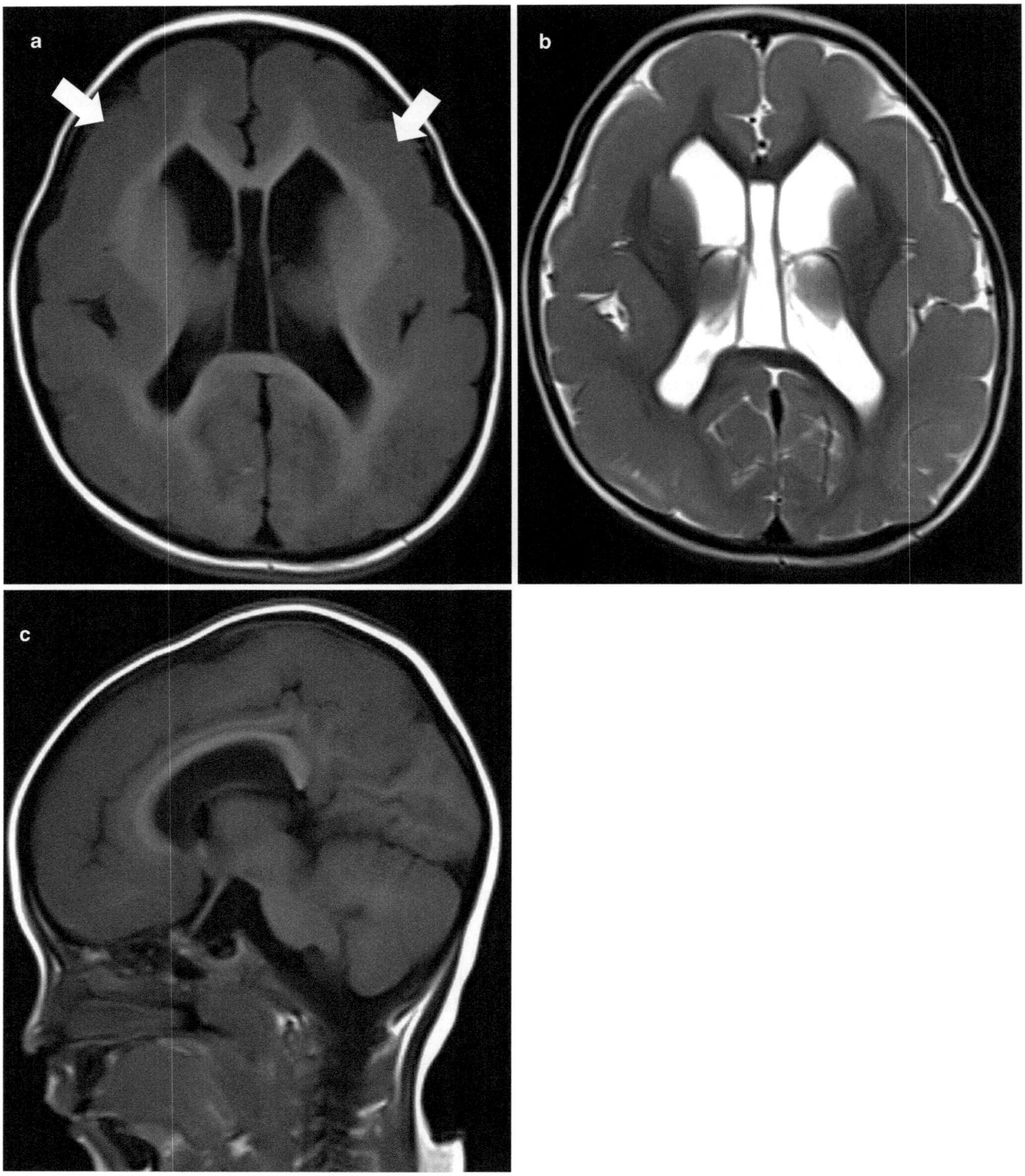

Fig. 1.4 Pachygyria

Imaging Findings

A. Axial T1WI shows bilateral frontal and parietal lobe fused (white arrow), without a interhemispheric fissure (Fig. 1.6a).

B. Axial T2WI shows the anterior middlepart of the interhemispheric fissure is missing (Fig. 1.6b).

C. Sagittal T1WI shows the remaining of a callosal splenium and genu (white arrow head) without callosal body (Fig. 1.6c).

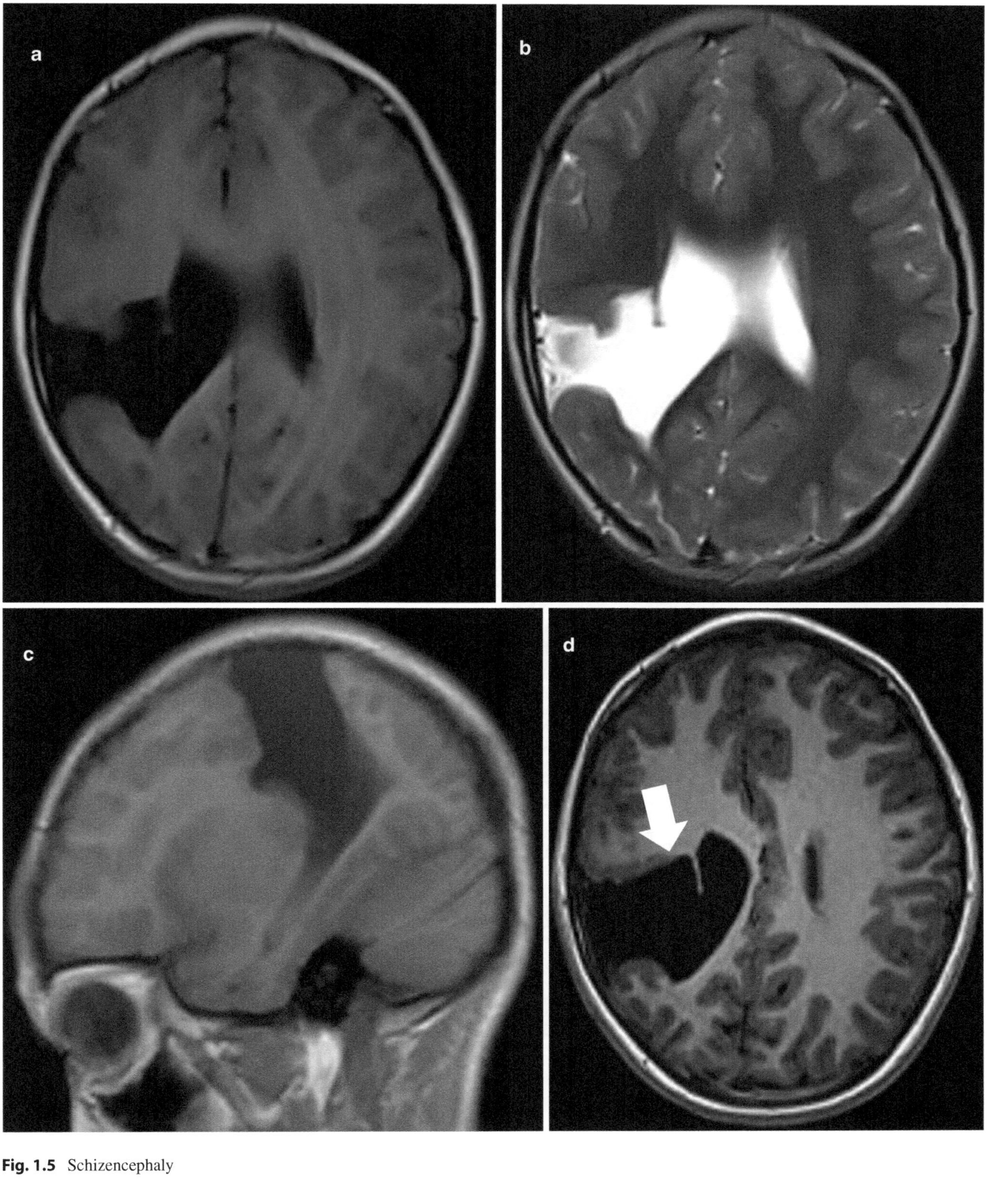

Fig. 1.5 Schizencephaly

Discussion

The holoprosencephalies are a group of disorders that are characterized by a failure of prosencephalic cleavage [19]; alobar holoprosencephaly is the most severe form, and septo-optic dysplasia is the mildest form. These anomalies are associated with several genetic syndromes such as Smith–Lemli–Opitz, Meckel–Gruber, trisomy 13 and 18 [20]. Midline structures often are abnormal and can present with proboscis, trigonocephaly, cyclopia, hypotelorism, and facial clefts.

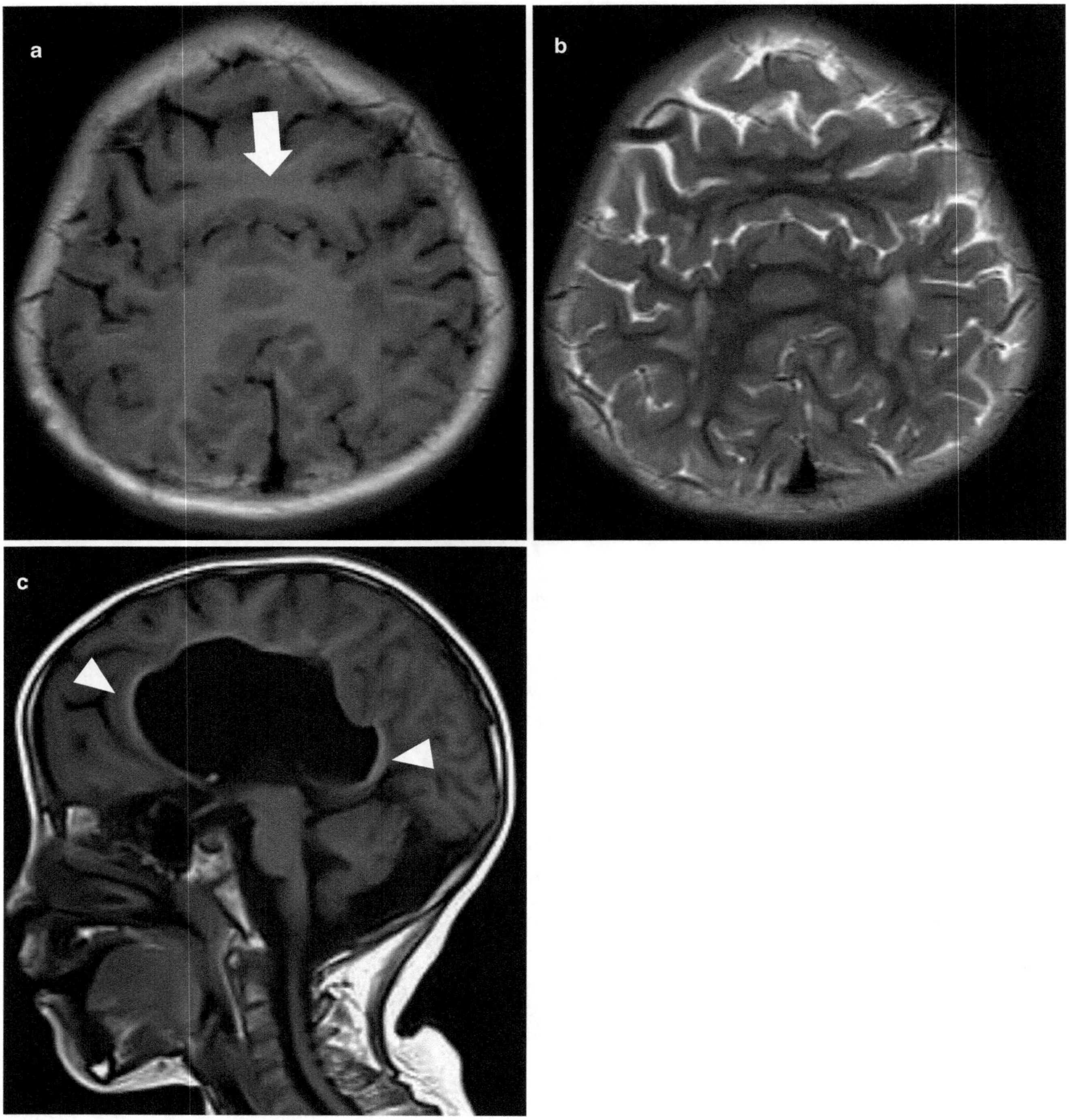

Fig. 1.6 Holoprosencephaly

Alobar holoprosencephaly is complete failure of division of the promesencephalic vesicle. The corpus callosum, falx, and interhemispheric fissure are absent. The cerebrum, halami, and basal ganglia are fused, and a monoventricle is identified behind the fused cerebrum. With semilobar and lobar forms, a posterior interhemispheric fissure is present, with absence of the genu of the corpus callosum. Lobar holoprosencephaly may have a normally formed thalamus and callosal splenium. The anterior frontal lobes are fused and the frontal lobes typically are hypoplastic. The septum pellucidum and anterior falx are absent. Syntelencephaly is a middle interhemispheric variant in which the anterior parietal lobe or posterior frontal lobes are contiguous across the midline [21].

Septo-optic dysplasia may be diagnosis by an absent septum pellucidum, the ventricles are dilated, and the roof of frontal horns is flattened. Bilateral optic nerves are thinning. Schizencephaly, heterotopias, and callosal dysgenesis often are associated with this sporadic anomaly and are better seen by MRI [22].

Case 1.7 Chiari Malformation

Clinical Presentation

An 8-year-old girl present with occipital or posterior cervical headaches, especially when straining or coughing.

Imaging Findings

A. Sagittal T2WI shows the cerebellar tonsil is enlarged, compressed, and extends more than 1.5 cm below the bottom of the foramen magnum (white arrow). The upper cervical spinal cord is compressed between the odontoid and the cerebellar tonsil (Fig. 1.7a).
B. Sagittal T1WI of cervical spine shows cervical hydromyelia (white arrow head) (Fig. 1.7b).

Discussion

Chiari malformation is a group of hindbrain malformations, and Chiari I is the most common type, which occurs in approximately 1 in 1000 births [23]. There is a slight female predominance of cases (1.3–1) [24].

The Chiari I malformation is defined by cerebellar tonsils downward displacement of cerebellar tonsils below the foramen magnum greater than 6 mm [25]. In symptomatic patients, the low-lying tonsils disrupt CSF flow across the foramen magnum, which predisposes to syringomyelia in the thoracic or cervical spinal cord.

Many patients with Chiari I malformations are asymptomatic; but some others may present with suboccipital headaches, neck pain, ataxia, dysmetria, nystagmus, and dysequilibrium because of brainstem or cerebellar compression [26].

The imaging features of Chiari I malformation should be differentiated with Chiari II malformation. In Chiari I malformation, the cerebellar tonsils are downward herniation resulting in compression of cervicomedullary brainstem; the cerebrospinal fluid flow impeded, Syringomyelia can be seen in 30–70% patients [27], but the Brain usually normal. Chiari II malformation demonstrates downward herniation of dysplastic lower brainstem and cerebellar vermis, commonly associated with Callosal dysgenesis, neuronal migration anomalies, and hydrocephalus [28].

Case 1.8 Joubert Syndrome

Clinical Presentation

A 5-year-old girl presented with mental retardation and hypotonia.

Imaging Findings

A. Sagittal T1WI shows the dysplastic, small cerebellar vermis that lies abnormally high (white arrow). The isthmus is abnormally narrow (Fig. 1.8a).
B. Axial T1WI shows the triangular fourth ventricle, resulting from absence of the inferior vermis (white arrow) (Fig. 1.8b)
C. Axial T1WI shows the "molar tooth" appearance of the midbrain secondary to the narrow isthmus and the enlarged superior cerebellar peduncles (white arrow) (Fig. 1.8c).

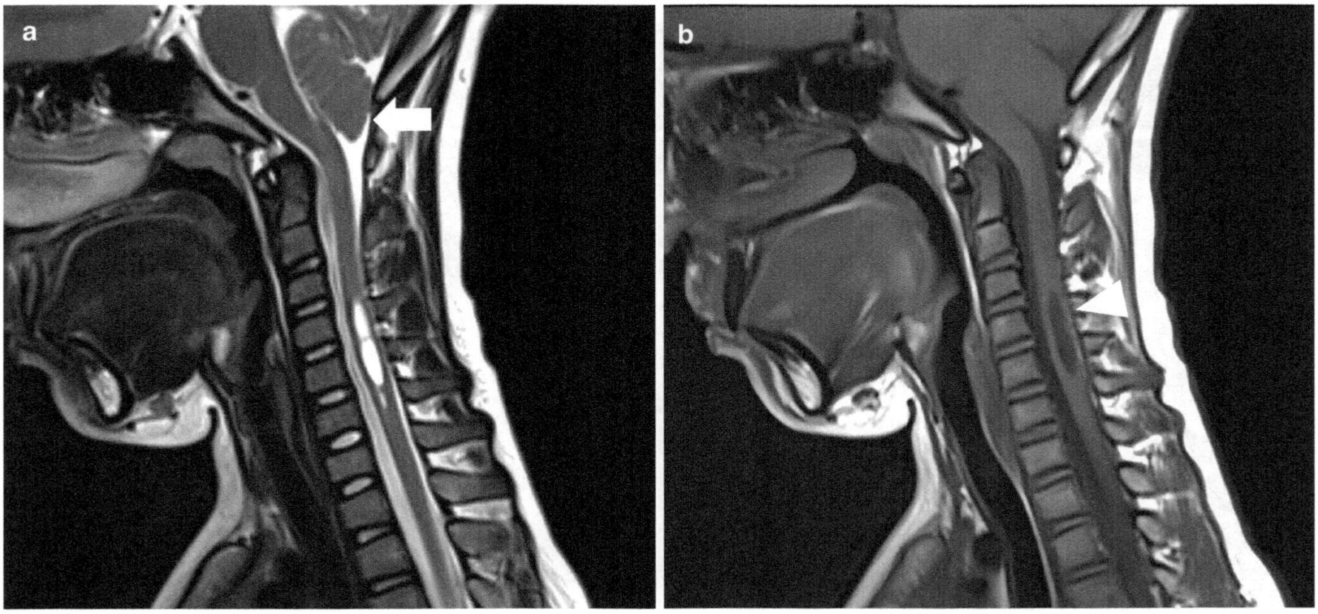

Fig. 1.7 Chiari I malformation

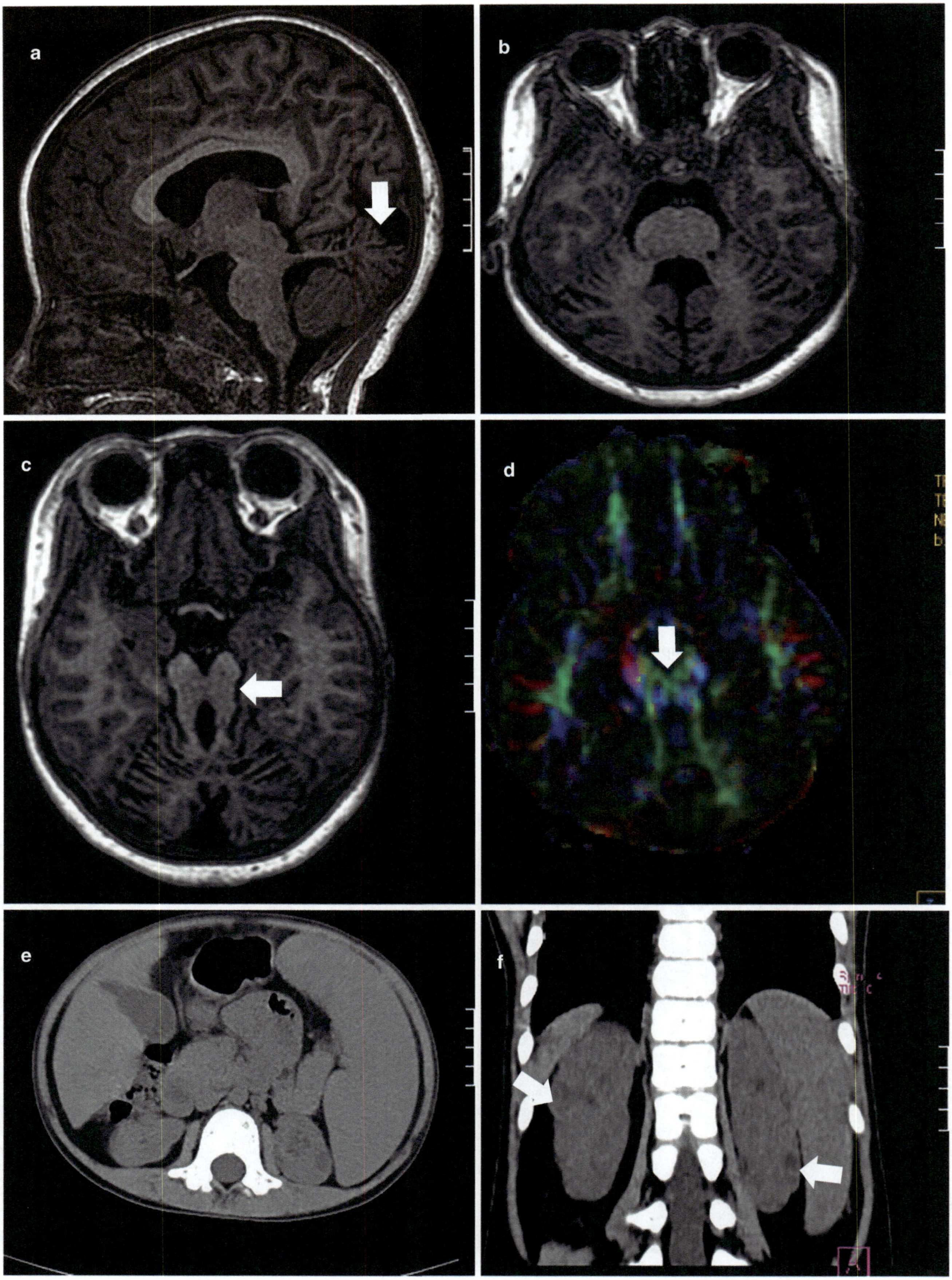

Fig. 1.8 Joubert syndrome

D. DTI confirms the absence of decussation of the superior cerebellar peduncles (white arrow) (Fig. 1.8d).
E. Axial CT shows hepatomegaly, splenomegaly (Fig. 1.8e).
F. Coronal CT shows multiple renal cysts (white arrow) (Fig. 1.8f).

Discussion

Joubert syndrome and related disorders (JSRD), formerly were named several different syndromes, including classic Joubert syndrome, COACH (Cerebellar vermis hypoplasia, Oligophrenia, Ataxia, Ocular Coloboma, Hepatic fibrosis) syndrome, CORS (Cerebro-Oculo-Renal Syndrome), and Oculo-Facial-Digital Syndrome Type VI (OFD-VI syndrome) [29].

Recent studies have shown that all of these syndromes seem to be the result of mutations to genes encoding ciliary proteins [30], which are important in a wide range of functions, including ciliogenesis, body axis formation, renal function, brain development, and ocular development. Therefore, mutations that affect these structures cause a wide range of disorders. So these are called, as a group, Joubert syndrome and related disorders (JSRD). Patients with all JSRD may present with episodic hyperpnea, abnormal eye movements, ataxia, and mental retardation, and the "molar tooth sign" on brain MRI.

The "molar tooth sign" is the characteristic imaging feature, consisting of elongated, thickened, and horizontally oriented superior cerebellar peduncles; a deep interpeduncular fossa. The superior cerebellar peduncles do not cross in the dorsal midbrain, DTI confirms the absence of decussation of the superior cerebellar peduncles [31]. The vermis is hypoplasia, situated abnormally high, and the fastigium of the fourth ventricle is at the upper pons or at the pontomesencephalic junction. The small size of the dysmorphic vermis results in atriangular-shaped mid-fourth ventricle and a "bat-wing" shaped superior fourth ventricle on axial images. Inferiorly, below the small vermis, the two cerebellar hemispheres come into apposition in the midline.

Detection of "molar tooth sign" should strongly suggest the diagnosis of JSRD, and should initiate a fully imaging examination for associated findings such as supratentorial anomalies (polymicrogyria or other cortical malformations), nephronophthisis, ocular (colobomas, retinal dystrophy), hepatic (congenital hepatic fibrosis), and skeletal (various forms of polydactyly). The ultimate diagnosis will depend on whether other anomalies are found and, ultimately perhaps, on the genetic analysis.

Case 1.9 Dandy–Walker Malformation

Clinical Presentation

A 6-year-old girl presented to the hospital because of an enlarged head circumference.

Imaging Findings

A. Axial T2WI shows cystic dilation of the 4th ventricle (white arrow), and enlarged posterior fossa (Fig. 1.9a).
B. Sagittal T1WI shows partial agenesis of the vermis (white arrow), with upward displacement of the transverse sinuses, tentorium, and torcula (Fig. 1.9b).

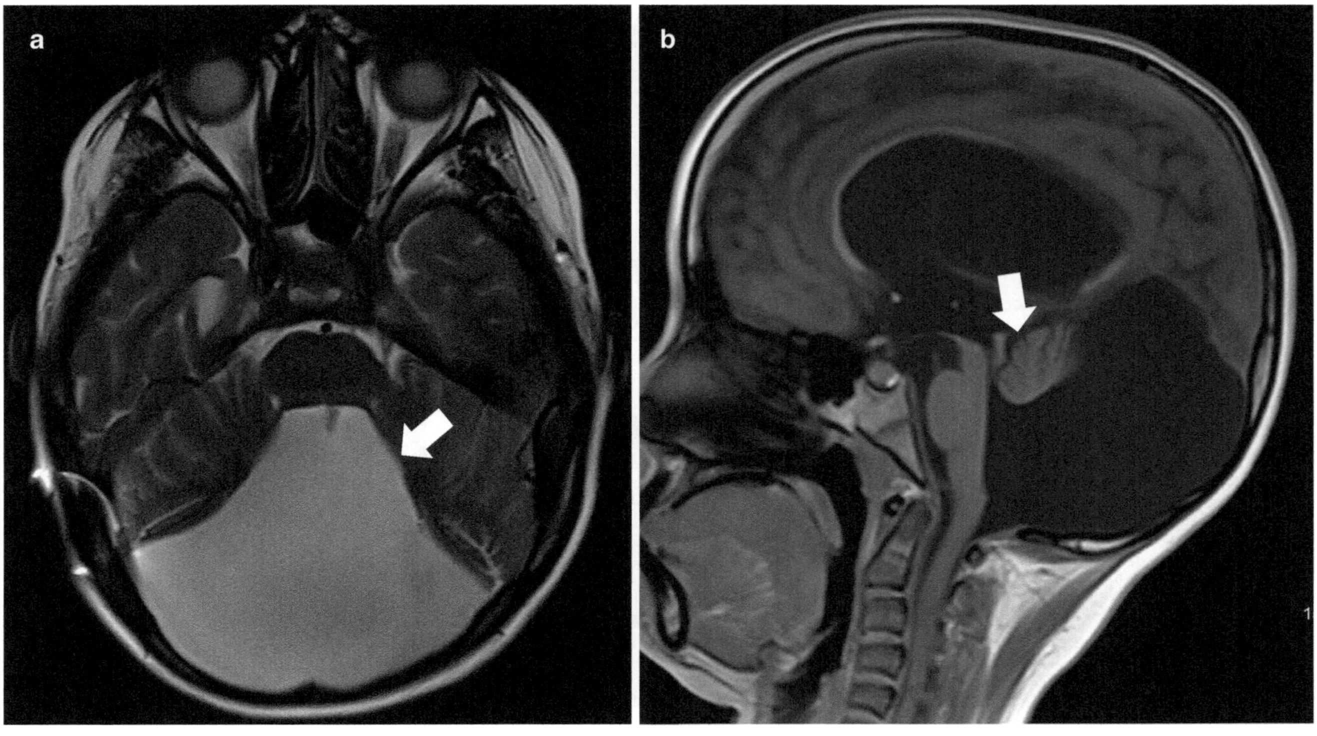

Fig. 1.9 Dandy–Walker malformation

Discussion

The Dandy–Walker malformation was defined as consisting of a cystic enlargement of the fourth ventricle associated with agenesis or more frequently hypoplasia of the vermis [32]. But the severity of the vermian hypoplasia, the size of the fourth ventricle, and the elevation of the tentorium, are quite different, thus generate considerable confusion and controversy in classic Dandy–Walker malformation, cerebellar hypoplasia, Blake's pouch cyst, mega cisterna magna, and retrocerebellar arachnoid cysts. Now, these diseases are considered to be a group of disorders related to a development arrest in the hindbrain [33].

The classic Dandy–Walker malformation demonstrates complete or partial agenesis of the vermis, cystic dilation of the fourth ventricle, and enlarged posterior fossa, with upward displacement of the transverse sinuses, tentorium, and torcula. The disease commonly associated with hydrocephalus, callosal anomalies, polymicrogyria, gray matter heterotopias, and occipital cephaloceles, and can occur in Walker–Warburg syndrome, Meckel–Gruber syndrome, and many other syndromes.

In cerebellar hypoplasia, the vermis hypoplasia and rotation are usually present and is a key feature to differentiate from other cystic malformations. The fourth ventricle, although enlarged, is not large enough to produce enlargement of the posterior fossa; however,

In Blake pouch cyst, the cerebellum and posterior fossa is typically normal in size. A cyst locates in a retrocerebellar or infraretrocerebellar position, which is communicated to the fourth ventricle. The cyst displaced the choroid plexus inferior to the vermis along the anterosuperior aspect of the cyst.

Mega cisterna magna is an enlarged cisterna magna with a normal vermis, a normal fourth ventricle. Hydrocephalus, is not common [34].

Posterior fossa arachnoid cysts may be located inferior or posterior to the vermis, cranial to the vermis, anterior or lateral to the cerebellar hemispheres, or anterior to the brainstem. Arachnoid cysts may produce mass effect on the cerebellum and vermis, which may cause obstruction of the fourth ventricular, hydrocephalus, and/or remodeling or thinning of the overlying occipital bone.

Case 1.10 Blake Pouch Cysts

Clinical Presentation

A boy of 6-day-old presented with an abnormal finding of posterior cranial fossa in uterus.

Imaging Findings

A. Axial T2WI shows a cyst in the posterior fossa, which communicates with the fourth ventricle (white arrow) (Fig. 1.10a).
B. Sagittal T1WI C+ shows the choroid plexus of the fourth ventricle extends inferiorly along the superior wall of the cyst (Fig. 1.10b).

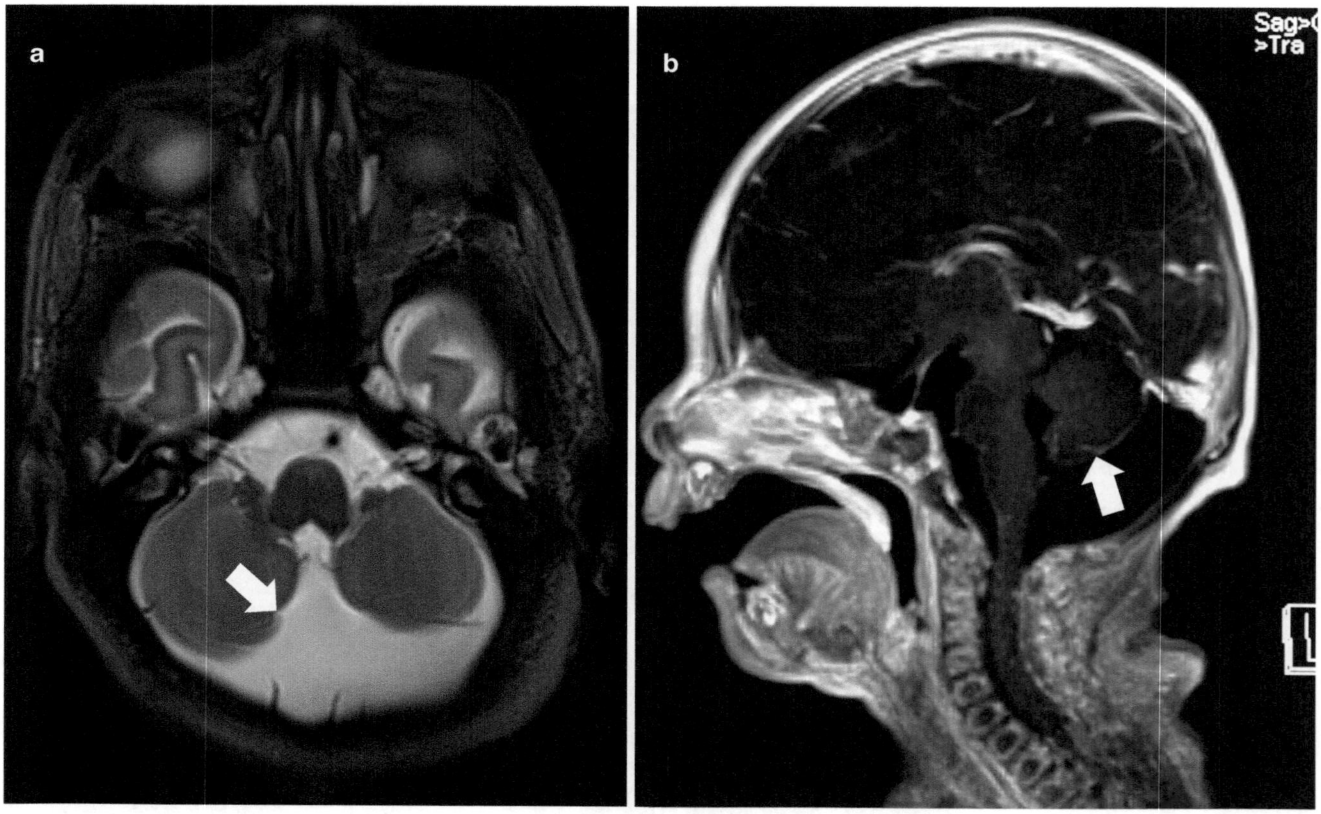

Fig. 1.10 Blake pouch cysts

Discussion

Blake pouch cysts (BPC), first described as a separate condition by Tortori-Donati et al. in 1996 [35]. In normal embryogenesis the Blake pouch is a transient structure, usually communicates with the subarachnoid space by 18 weeks gestation to form the foramen of Magendie. In case of nonperforation, the Blake pouch persists, continuous with the fourth ventricle, but lack of communication with the subarachnoid space [36].

On imaging, the Blake pouch is seen as a CSF collection posterior and inferior to the fourth ventricle. The fourth ventricle may be enlarged resulting in a large posterior fossa. With tetra-ventricular hydrocephalus. The cerebellum usually appears normal, the vermis is normal and not rotated. The choroid plexus of the fourth ventricle usually extends inferiorly along the superior wall of the persistent Blake pouch, which can be seen in enhanced MRI [37].

Case 1.11 Rhombencephalosynapsis

Clinical Presentation

A 6-year-old girl with a history of developmental delay, infantile spasms, refractory partial-complex epilepsy, and autistic features.

Imaging Findings

A. Axial T2WI shows continuity of the cerebellar hemispheres, dentate nuclei, without an intervening vermis. The 4th ventricle is keyhole-shaped (white arrow) (Fig. 1.11a).
B. Sagittal T1WI shows the vermis is absent, the fourth ventricle is narrow, and associated with a deformity corpus callosum (white arrow) (Fig. 1.11b).

Discussion

Rhombencephalosynapsis, originally described by Obersteiner in 1914, is characterized by absence or severe hypoplasia of the vermis and fused cerebellar hemispheres, dentate nuclei, and superior cerebellar peduncles [38]. Most patients are nonsyndromic [39], but is also a key feature of Gómez–López-Hernández syndrome, and may be seen in patients with VACTERL association (vertebral anomalies, anal atresia, cardiovascular anomalies, tracheoesophageal fistula, renal anomalies, and limb defects).

The most common clinical manifestations include ataxia, abnormal eye movements, and delayed motor development. Patients with more severe patient, associated holoprosencephaly, or VACTERL features have more severe neurodevelopmental impairment [40].

The MRI imaging findings are cerebellar folia appear horizontal and continuous across the midline without intervening vermis on coronal images, the normal vermian folial is absent on the midline sagittal image, and the narrowing of the posterior aspect of the fourth ventricle on axial images, resulting in a keyhole-shaped. The superior cerebellar peduncles and dentate nuclei are also fused, and associated anomalies include hydrocephalus, mostly due to aqueductal stenosis and forebrain abnormalities including absent olfactory bulbs, dysgenesis of the corpus callosum, absent septum pellucidum, and bilateral lambdoid suture synostoses [41].

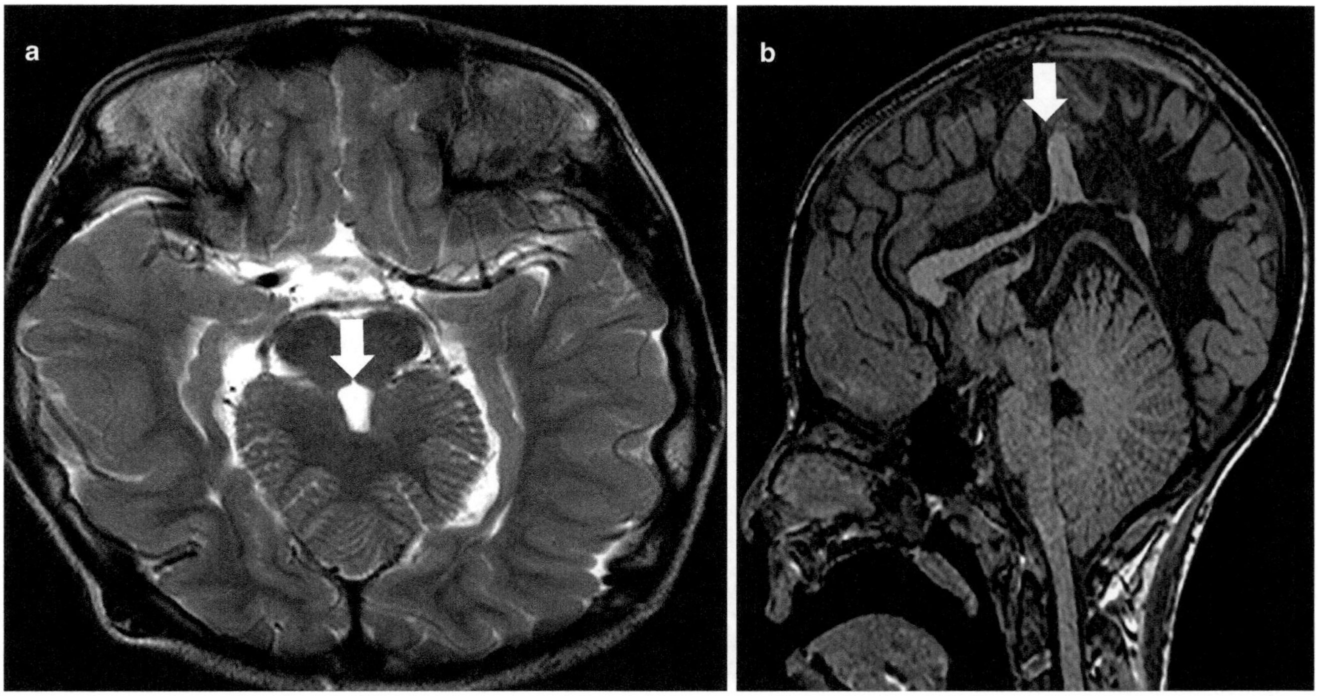

Fig. 1.11 Rhombencephalosynapsis

Case 1.12 Septo-Optic Dysplasia

Clinical Presentation

A girl of 7-month-old presented with visual impairment.

Imaging Findings

A. Axial T1WI shows the septum pellucidum is absent, bilateral frontal horns of the lateral ventricles fused like a box (white arrow) (Fig. 1.12a).
B. Axial T1WI shows bilateral optic nerves are thinning (white arrow) (Fig. 1.12b).

Discussion

Septo-optic dysplasia (SOD), also known as de Morsier syndrome, is considered along the continuum of malformation of ventral forebrain differentiation. Most cases are sporadic. The estimated incidences are 1 in 10,000 ~ 50,000 live births [42]. Both sexes are equally affected. Most cases are detected in infancy, the patients often manifest as short stature, visual impairment, nystagmus, and endocrine dysfunction [43].

The characteristic imaging features are absence of the septum pellucidum and variable hypoplasia of the optic nerves and/or chiasm. In the coronal plane, absence of the septal leaves results in downward displacement of the fornices into the third ventricle, the frontal horns of the lateral ventricles appear as "point down or box-like" [44]. The neurohypophysis is often ectopic or may be absent, in which case the pituitary stalk may be interrupted. SOD is associated with multiple malformations, such as schizencephaly, neuronal migration anomalies, and neural tube defects. Hypoplasia of the brainstem and cerebellum has also been reported in SOD [45].

Case 1.13.1 Tuberous Sclerosis

Clinical Presentation

A 13-year-old girl with a history of developmental delay, infantile spasms, refractory partial-complex epilepsy, and autistic features.

Imaging Findings

A. Axial T2WI shows multiple subependymal nodules (white arrow) with hypointensity (Fig. 1.13a).
B. Axial T1WI shows multiple subependymal nodules (white arrow) with hyperintensity (Fig. 1.13b).
C. Axial T2WI-FLAIR reveals multiple cortical hyperintense lesions in cortex and subcortical white matter (white arrow) (Fig. 1.13c).
D. Coronal T2WI shows multiple cysts in bilateral kidneys (white arrow) (Fig. 1.13d).

Discussion

Tuberous sclerosis complex (TSC) is an autosomal dominant disorder with *TSC1* or the *TSC2* gene mutations [46]. The estimated incidence is 1 in 6000. TSC is a multisystem disorder characterized by hamartomas occurred most commonly in the brain, skin, kidneys, and eyes. D. M. Bourneville first described

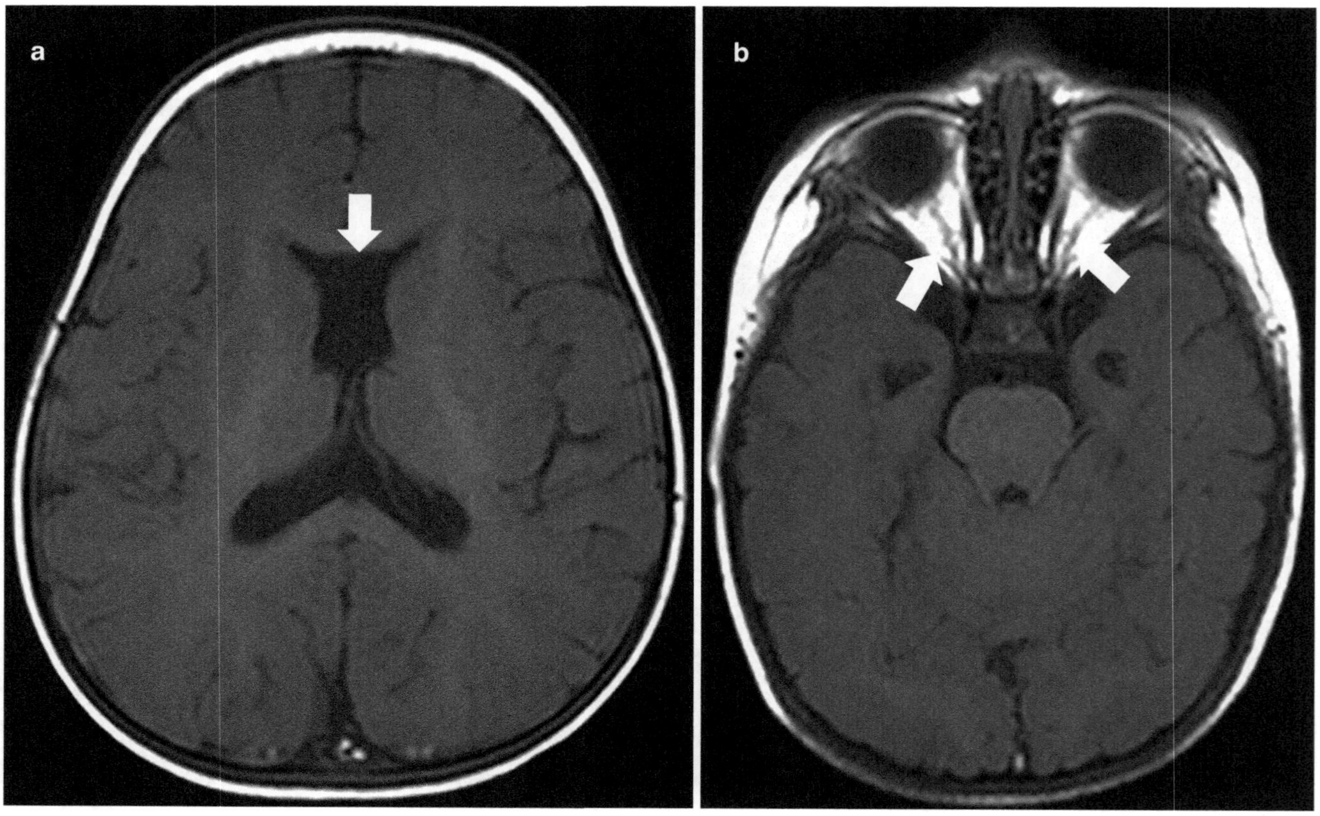

Fig. 1.12 Septo-optic dysplasia

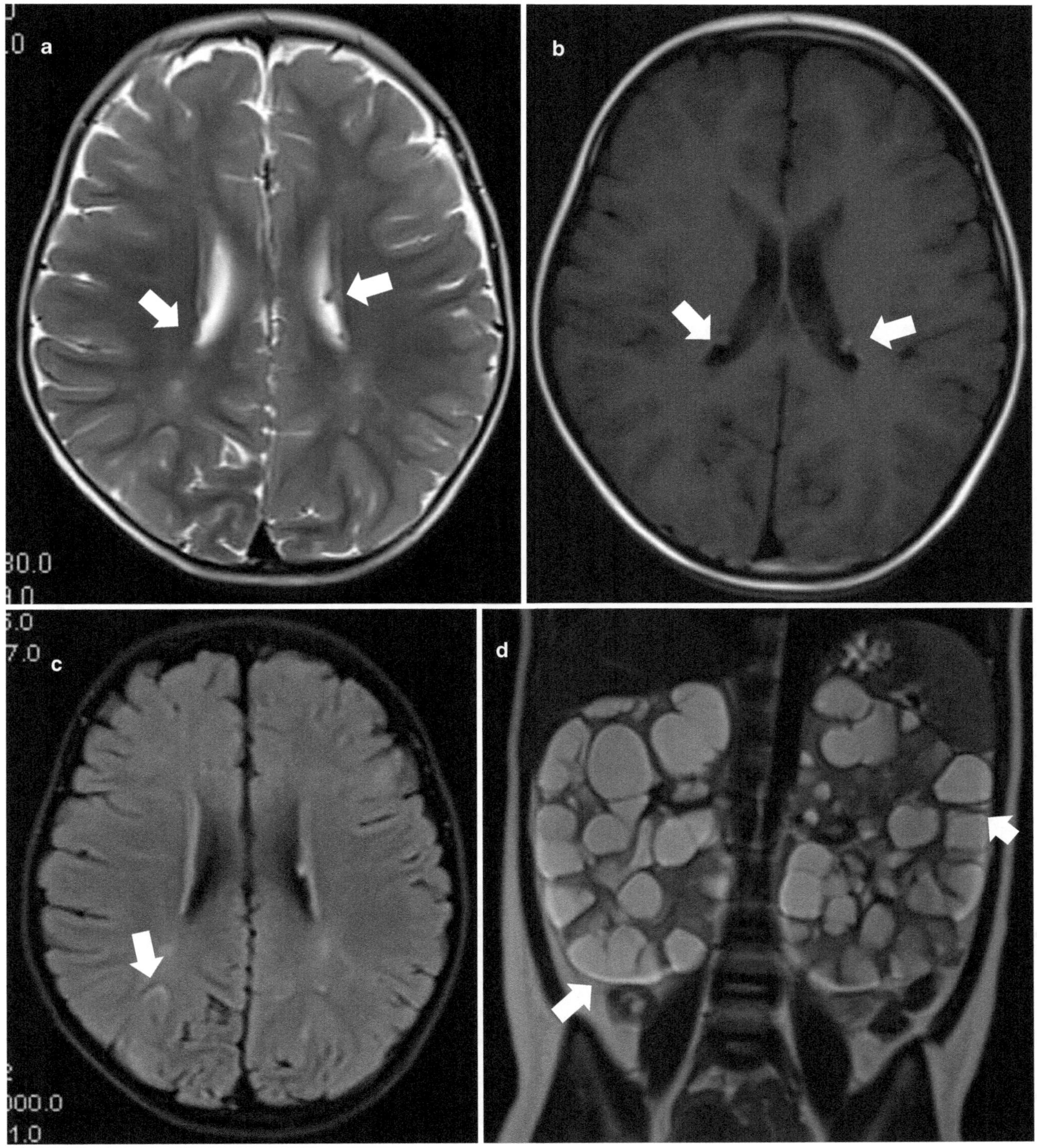

Fig. 1.13 Tuberous sclerosis

the neurologic manifestations, and lately Vogt described the "classic triad" of symptoms: seizures, mental retardation, and adenoma sebaceum (angiofibromas), but not more than 30% of patients have these three manifestations [47].

Most patients develop seizure disorders and often show within the first year of life. And many of them present with developmental delay and behavioral disorders, including autism spectrum disorders [48].

The most common imaging features in TSC include subependymal hamartomas (nodules), cerebral tubers, and subependymal giant cell tumors. The most common features are subependymal hamartomas (or nodules), and most located along the ventricular surface of the caudate nucleus, are slightly T1WI hyperintensity and T2WI hypointensity on MRI, and calcifications can be seen on CT. On MRI, FLAIR images are the most sensitive sequences in detection of cerebral tubers, which appear as enlarged gyri with hyperintensity. And the underlying white matter may show hyperintensity, extending from the cerebral tubers to the lateral ventricular surface. Subependymal giant cell astrocytoma is an enlarging subependymal nodule, most commonly located near the foramen of Monro.

In non-CNS Manifestations, Renal angiomyolipomas are a major feature in TSC. Others include renal, cardiac rhabdomyomas, and rhabdomyosarcomas.

Case 1.13.2 Sturge–Weber Syndrome

Clinical Presentation

An 8 months girl was born with facial nevus flammeus.

Imaging Findings

A. Axial T2WI shows abnormal hypointensity in the right frontal lobe (white arrow) (Fig. 1.14a).
B. Axial T1WI shows the boundary between the gray matter and withe matter blurring (white arrow) (Fig. 1.14b).

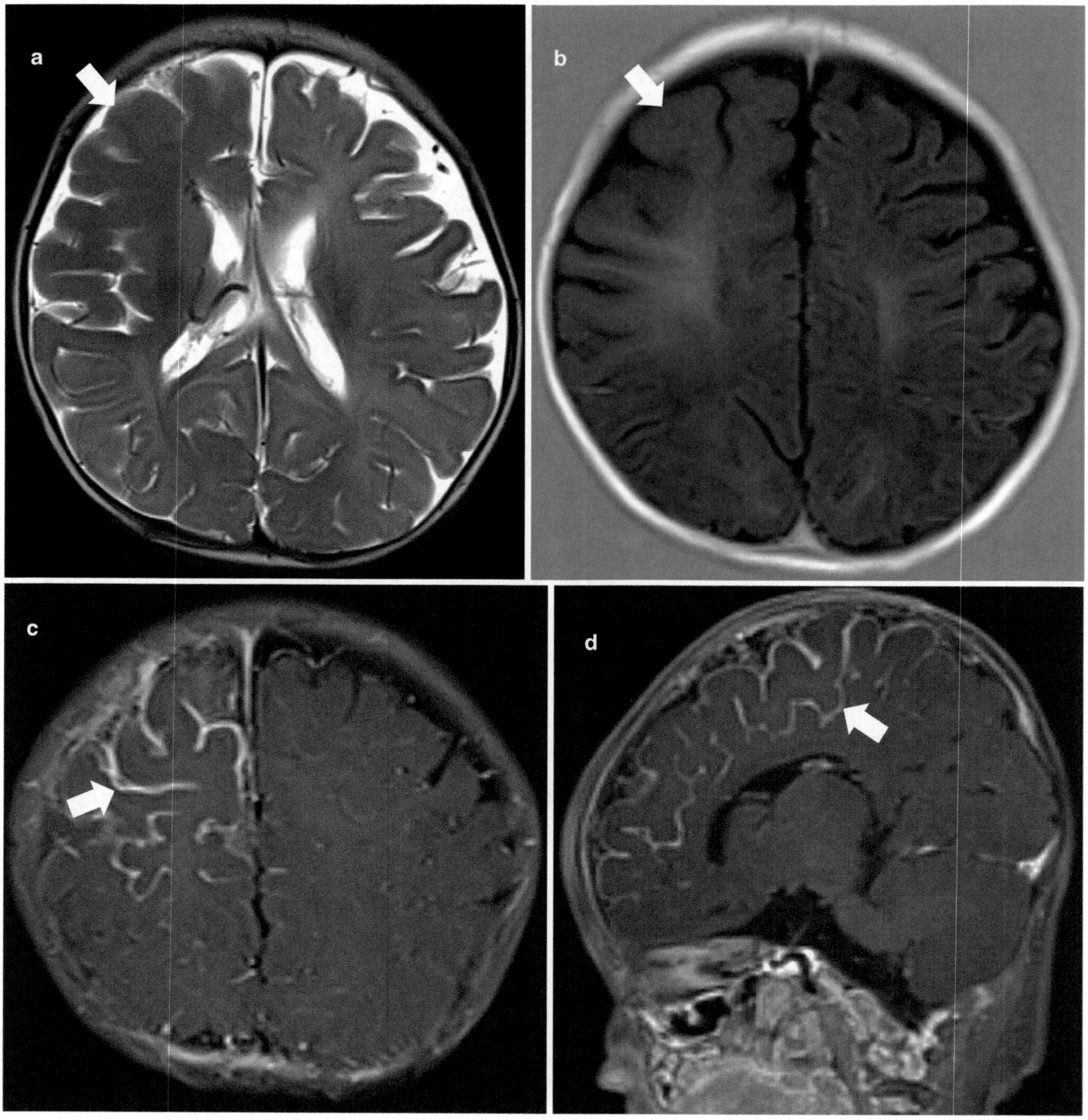

Fig. 1.14 Sturge–Weber syndrome

C. Axial enhanced T1WI showed meningeal enhancement (white arrow) involving the frontal lobe (Fig. 1.14c).
D. Sagittal enhanced T1WI showed meningeal enhancement (white arrow) involving the frontal lobe and parietal lobe (Fig. 1.14d).

Discussion

Sturge–Weber syndrome, also known as encephalotrigeminal angiomatosis, is a phakomatosis characterized by a facial "port wine stain" in the territory of the trigeminal nerve, ipsilateral angiomatosis of the choroid of the eye, and the leptomeninges [49].

Seizures are the most common symptoms, usually initially occur in the first year of life, and they may have hemiparesis, status epilepticus, and developmental delay [50].

Imaging findings include leptomeningeal angiomatosis, enlargement of the choroid plexus, parenchymal atrophy, calvarial changes, and calcification. Contrast-enhanced MRI is the most accurate sequence for showing the extent of the pial angioma, which appears as an area of enhancement covering the surfaces of the gyri and filling the cortical sulci. The ipsilateral choroid plexus is frequently enlarged [51]. CT frequently shows calcifications in the cerebral cortex underlying the pial angioma. The underlying white matter typically shows accentuated T2 shortening compared to the remainder of the brain, DTI show increased FA and decreased diffusivity, which likely secondary to abnormal hypermyelination. The ipsilateral cerebral hemisphere ultimately becomes atrophic in most patients.

Case1.13.3 Neurofibromatosis

Clinical Presentation

A 6-year-old girl presents with Cafe au lait spots. The genetic testing revealed an *NF1* mutation.

Imaging Findings

A. Axial T2WI showed high signal intensity in baliteral cerebellar dentate nucleus and brainstem (Fig. 1.15a).
B. Axial T2WI showed high signal intensity in brainstem (Fig. 1.15b).
C. Axial T2WI showed multiple lisions of high signal intensity in baliteral thalamus and basal ganglia (Fig. 1.15c).
D. Axial T2WI showed multiple lisions of high signal intensity in baliteral thalamus (Fig. 1.15d).

Discussion

Neurofibromatosis type 1 (NF1), formerly known as von Recklinghausen disease, is an autosomal dominant genetic disorder and is a relatively common neurocutaneous syndrome or phakomatosis, the incidence is 1/3000 live births [52].

Cafe au lait spots are the most common manifestation of NF1, other cutaneous lesions include freckling within the axilla, neurofibromas, and Lisch nodules. Other characteristic features are gliomas of the optic pathway, kyphoscoliosis, phenoid wing dysplasia, vascular dysplasias, nerve sheath tumors, and macrocephaly [53].

Except the CNS tumors, MRI has demonstrated the characteristic hyperintense T2/FLAIR lesions, located in the cer-

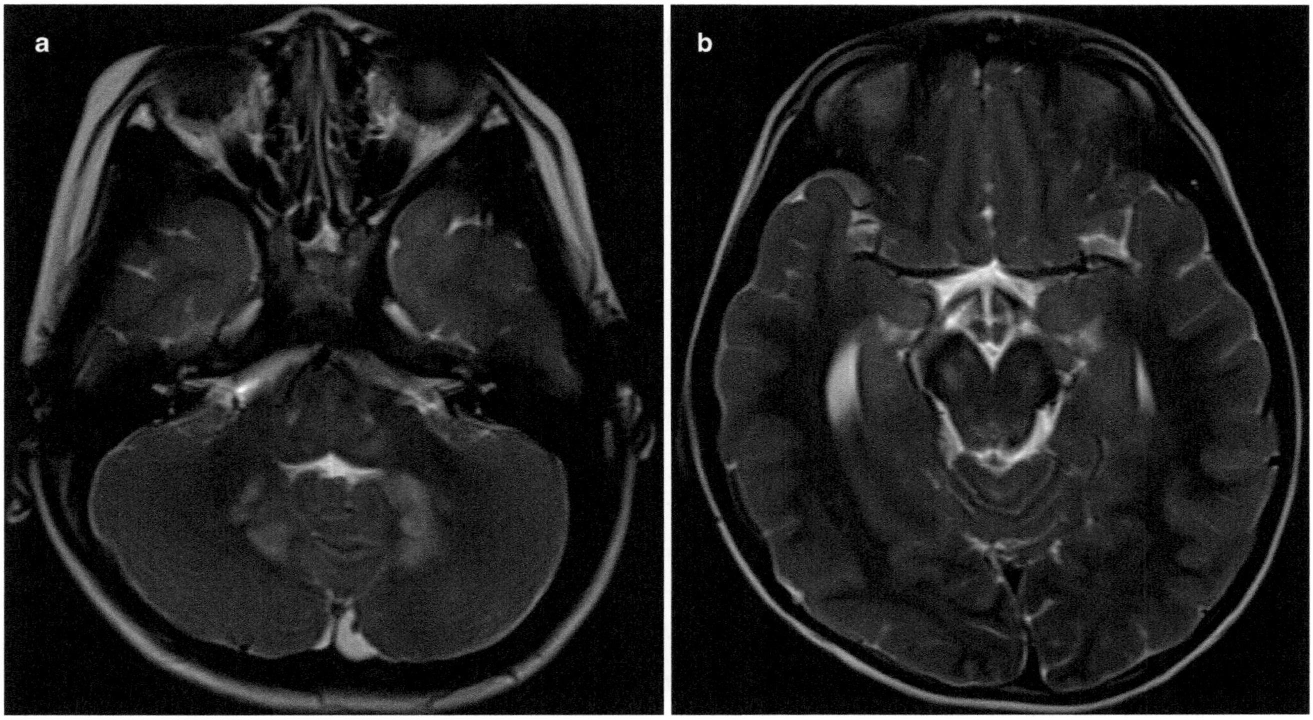

Fig. 1.15 Neurofibromatosis

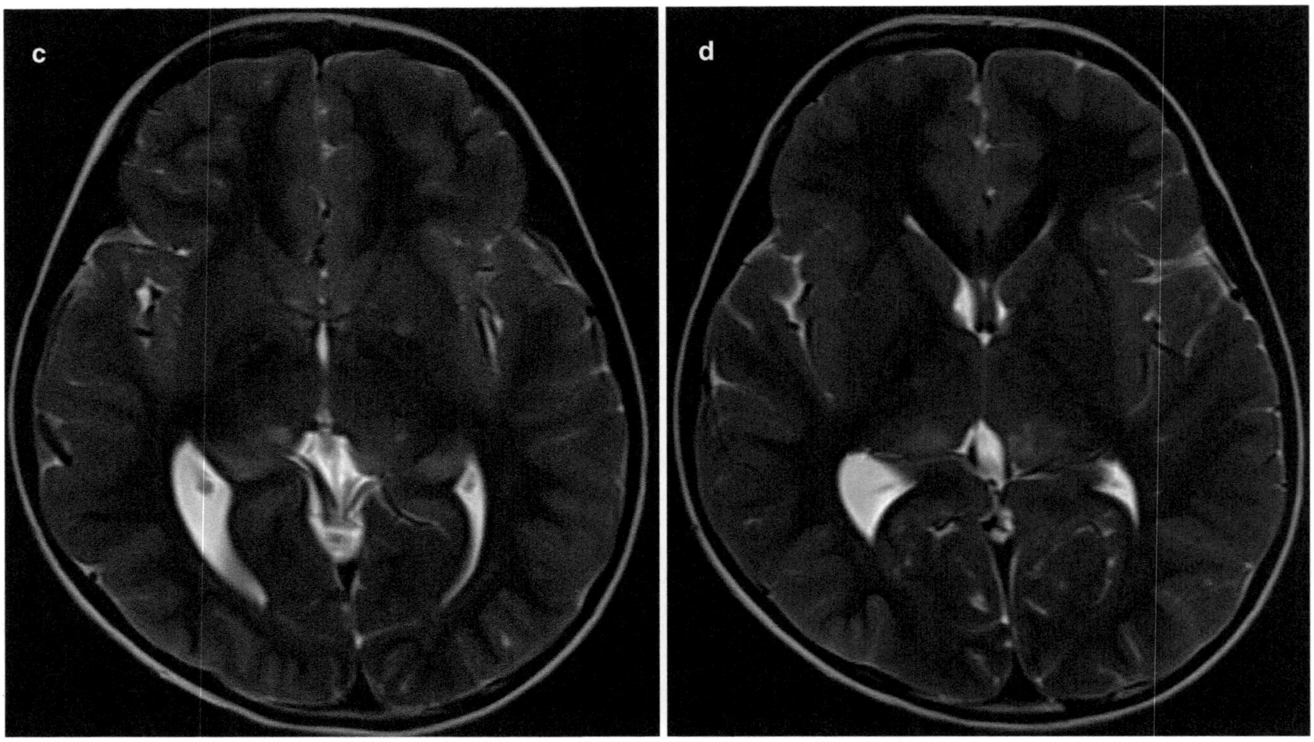

Fig. 1.15 (continued)

ebellar white matter, brainstem, thalamus, basal ganglia, internal capsule, corpus callosum. These lesions are characteristically multiple, with little or no mass effect; their signal appears normal on T1-weighted images, and do not enhance after intravenous administration. These lesions appear from late infancy to about the age of 12 years, and start to regress late in the first decade of life. A pathologic analysis has shown that these are regions of myelin vacuolation, where the layers of myelin become separated as they spiral around the axon.

References

1. Cherian EV, Shenoy KV, Bukelo MJ, et al. Racing car brings tear drops in the moose. BMJ Case Rep. 2013;2013:bcr2012008165.
2. Schell-Apacik CC, Wagner K, Bihler M, et al. Agenesis and dysgenesis of the corpus callosum: clinical, genetic and neuroimaging findings in a series of 41 patients. Am J Med Genet A. 2008;146A(19):2501–11.
3. Nagwa S, Saran S, Sharma Y, et al. Imaging features of complete agenesis of corpus callosum in a 3-year-old child. Sudan J Paediatr. 2018;18(2):69–71.
4. Brown WS, Paul LK. The neuropsychological syndrome of agenesis of the corpus callosum. J Int Neuropsychol Soc. 2019;25(3):324–30.
5. Guion-Almeida ML, Richieri-Costa A, Saavedra D, et al. Frontonasal dysplasia: analysis of 21 cases and literature review. Int J Oral Maxillofac Surg. 1996;25:91–7.
6. Kakita A, Inenaga C, Kameyama S, et al. Cerebral lipoma and the underlying cortex of the temporal lobe: pathological features associated with the malformation. ActaNeuropathol (Berl). 2005;109:339–45.
7. Yildiz H, Hakyemez B, Koroglu M, Yesildag A, Baykal B. Intracranial lipomas: importance of localization. Neuroradiology. 2006;48:1–7.
8. Nahas Z, Tatlipinar A, Limb CJ, et al. Spontaneous meningoencephalocele of the temporal bone: clinical spectrum and presentation. Arch Otolaryngol Head Neck Surg. 2008;134:509–18.
9. Fleming A, Copp AJ. A genetic risk factor for mouse neural tube defects: defining the embryonic basis. Hum Mol Genet. 2000;9:575–81.
10. Noden DM, Trainor PA. Relations and interactions between cranial mesoderm and neural crest populations. J Anat. 2005;207:575–601.
11. Lo BW, Kulkarni AV, Rutka JT, et al. Clinical predictors of developmental outcome in patients with cephaloceles. J Neurosurg Pediatr. 2008;2:254–7.
12. Kotil K, Kilinc B, Bilge T. Diagnosis and management of large occipitocervical cephaloceles: a 10-year experience. Pediatr Neurosurg. 2008;44:193–8.
13. Mei D, Lewis R, Parrini E, et al. High frequency of genomic deletions and duplication in the LIS1 gene in lissencephaly: implications for molecular diagnosis. J Med Genet. 2008;45:355–61.
14. Aicardi J. The agyria-pachygyria complex: a spectrum of cortical malformations. Brain Dev. 1991;13:1–8.
15. Barkovich AJ, Koch TK, Carrol CL. The spectrum of lissencephaly: report of ten cases analyzed by magnetic resonance imaging. Ann Neurol. 1991;30:139–46.
16. Yakovlev PI, Wadsworth RC. Schizencephalies. A study of the congenital clefts in the cerebral mantle. 1. Clefts with fused lips. J Neuropathol Exp Neurol. 1946;5:116–30.
17. Tietjen I, Erdogan FS, Currier S, et al. EMX2-independent familial schizencephaly: clinical and genetic analyses. Am J Med Genet Part A. 2005;135A(2):166–70.

18. Tietjen I, Bodell A, Apse K, et al. Comprehensive EMX2 genotyping of a large schizencephaly case series. Am J Med Genet Part A. 2007;143A(12):1313–6.
19. Simon E, Hevner R, Pinter J, et al. Assessment of deep gray nuclei in holoprosencephaly. Am J Neuroradiol. 2000;21:1955–61.
20. Roessler E, Muenke M. Holoprosencephaly: a paradigm for the complex genetics of brain development. J Inherit Metab Dis. 1998;21:481–97.
21. Olsen CL, Hughes JP, Youngblood LG, et al. Epidemiology of holoprosencephaly and phenotypic characteristics of affected children: new York State, 1984–1989. Am J Med Genet. 1997;73:217–26.
22. Fitz CR. Holoprosencephaly and related entities. Neuroradiology. 1983;25:225–38.
23. de Arruda JA, Figueiredo E, Monteiro JL, et al. Orofacial clinical features in Arnold Chiari type I malformation: a case series. J Clin Exp Dent. 2018;10(4):e378–82.
24. Bhimani AD, Esfahani DR, Denyer S, et al. Adult Chiari I malformations: an analysis of surgical risk factors and complications using an international database. World Neurosurg. 2018;115:e490–500.
25. Rogers JM, Savage G, Stoodley MA. A systematic review of cognition in Chiari I malformation. Neuropsychol Rev. 2018;28(2):176–87.
26. Jayamanne C, Fernando L, Mettananda S. Chiari malformation type 1 presenting as unilateral progressive foot drop: a case report and review of literature. BMC Pediatr. 2018;18(1):34.
27. Goel A, Gore S, Shah A, et al. Atlantoaxial fixation for Chiari 1 formation in pediatric age-group patients: report of treatment in 33 patients. World Neurosurg. 2018;111:e668–77.
28. Lin W, Duan G, Xie J, et al. Comparison of results between posterior fossa decompression with and without duraplasty for the surgical treatment of chiari malformation type I: a systematic review and meta-analysis. World Neurosurg. 2018;110:460–474.e5.
29. Hickey CL, Sherman JC, Goldenberg P, et al. Cerebellar cognitive affective syndrome: insights from Joubert syndrome. Cerebellum Ataxias. 2018;5:3–23.
30. Revenkova E, Liu Q, Gusella GL, et al. The Joubert syndrome protein ARL13B binds tubulin to maintain uniform distribution of proteins along the ciliary membrane. J Cell Sci. 2018;1319:5.
31. Suzuki T, MiyakeN TY, et al. Molecular genetic analysis of 30 families with Joubert syndrome. Clin Genet. 2016;906:526–35.
32. Reith W, Haussmann A. Dandy-Walker-malformation [Dandy-Walker malformation]. Radiologe. 2018;58(7):629–35.
33. Orrea GG, Amaral LF, Vedolin LM. Neuroimaging of Dandy-Walker malformation: new concepts. Top Magn Reson Imaging. 2011;22(6):303–12.
34. Takami H, Shin M, Kuroiwa M, Isoo A, et al. Hydrocephalus associated with cystic dilation of the foramina of Magendie and Luschka. J Neurosurg Pediatr. 2010;5(4):415–8.
35. Kau T, Marterer R, Kottke R, et al. Blake's pouch cysts and differential diagnoses in prenatal and postnatal MRI: a pictorial review. Clin Neuroradiol. 2020;30(3):435–45.
36. Wüest A, Surbek D, Wiest R, et al. Enlarged posterior fossa on prenatal imaging: differential diagnosis, associated anomalies and postnatal outcome. Acta Obstet Gynecol Scand. 2017;96(7):837–43.
37. Niesen CE. Malformations of the posterior fossa: current perspectives. Semin Pediatr Neurol. 2002;9(4):320–34.
38. Passi GR, Bhatnagar S. Rhombencephalosynapsis. Pediatr Neurol. 2015;52(6):651–2.
39. Aldinger Kimberly A, Dempsey Jennifer C, Tully Hannah M, et al. Rhombencephalosynapsis: fused cerebellum, confused geneticists. Am J Med Genet C Semin Med Genet. 2018;1784:432–9.
40. Paktinat M, Inaloo S, Serati Z, et al. Ataxia and developmental delay as the main manifestation of rhombencephalosynapsis. Iran J Neurol. 2018;171:56–7.
41. Poretti A, Boltshauser E, Doherty D. Cerebellar hypoplasia: differential diagnosis and diagnostic approach. Am J Med Genet C Semin Med Genet. 2014;166C(2):211–26.
42. Ward DJ, Connolly DJA, Griffiths PD. Review of the MRI brain findings of septo-optic dysplasia. Clin Radiol. 2021;76(2):160.e1–160.e14.
43. Alt C, Shevell MI, Poulin C, et al. Clinical and radiologic spectrum of septo-optic dysplasia: review of 17 cases. J Child Neurol. 2017;32(9):797–803.
44. Cemeroglu AP, Coulas T, Kleis L. Spectrum of clinical presentations and endocrinological findings of patients with septo-optic dysplasia: a retrospective study. J Pediatr Endocrinol Metab. 2015;28(9–10):1057–63.
45. Volpi A, Sala G, Lesma E, et al. Tuberous sclerosis complex: new insights into clinical and therapeutic approach. J Nephrol. 2019;32(3):355–63.
46. Ekure EN, Addissie YA, Sokunbi OJ, et al. Tuberous sclerosis in a patient from Nigeria. Am J Med Genet A. 2019;179(8):1423–5.
47. Chihi M, Gembruch O, Oppong MD, et al. Intracranial aneurysms in patients with tuberous sclerosis complex: a systematic review. J Neurosurg Pediatr. 2019;24(2):174–83.
48. Thomas-Sohl KA, Vaslow DF, Maria BL. Sturge-Weber syndrome: a review. Pediatr Neurol. 2004;30(5):303–10.
49. Sudarsanam A, Ardern-Holmes SL. Sturge-Weber syndrome: from the past to the present. Eur J Paediatr Neurol. 2014;18(3):257–66.
50. Slasky SE, Shinnar S, Bello JA. Sturge-Weber syndrome: deep venous occlusion and the radiologic spectrum. Pediatr Neurol. 2006;35(5):343–7.
51. Nemmi F, Cignetti F, Assaiante C, et al. Discriminating between neurofibromatosis-1 and typically developing children by means of multimodal MRI and multivariate analyses. Hum Brain Mapp. 2019;40(12):3508–21.
52. DeBella K, Poskitt K, Szudek J, et al. Use of "unidentified bright objects" on MRI for diagnosis of neurofibromatosis 1 in children. Neurology. 2018;54(8):1646–51.
53. Aydin S, Kurtcan S, Alkan A, et al. Relationship between the corpus callosum and neurocognitive disabilities in children with NF-1: diffusion tensor imaging features. Clin Imaging. 2016;40(6):1092–5.

2 Brain Tumors

Shuai Wang, Yuanting Lu, Zidong Zhou, Wangchun Dai, Bin Ai, Honglei Shang, Hongsheng Liu, Xin Zhao, and Xiaoan Zhang

The incidence of brain tumors in children is second only to lymphohematopoietic system tumors, ranking first among solid tumors in children. In recent years, with the popularization of imaging examination methods and the improvement of scanning technology, the detection rate of brain tumors in children is increasing. Children's brain tumors are significantly different from adult brain tumors in type, occurrence site, genetics, and prognosis and are not microversions of adult brain tumors. The adult brain tumors are mainly glioblastoma, pituitary tumor, meningioma, and metastatic tumor. The top five brain tumors in children are astrocytoma, craniopharyngioma, medulloblastoma, germ cell tumor, and ependymoma. The majority of brain tumors in children are malignant, but metastatic tumors are rare. Brain tumors in children can occur at any age, and different types of brain tumors have different occurrence ages, with the onset peak at 5–8 years. Computed tomography (CT) and magnetic resonance imaging (MRI) are the most commonly used imaging methods to examine brain tumors. However, due to high soft-tissue resolution and no radiation injury, MRI is the preferred method for the evaluation of brain tumors, which can provide effective information for tumor localization and characterization.

S. Wang · Y. Lu · Z. Zhou
Division of Diagnostic, Guangzhou Women and Children's Medical Center, Guanzhou, Guangdong, China

W. Dai · B. Ai
Department of Radiology, Guangzhou Women and Children's Medical Center, Guangzhou City, Guangdong, China

H. Shang
Department of Radiology, The Third Affiliated Hospital of Zhengzhou University, Zhengzhou, Henan, China

H. Liu (✉)
Guangzhou Women and Children's Medical Center, Guangzhou City, Guangdong, China

X. Zhao · X. Zhang
Department of Radiology, The Third Affiliated Hospital of Zhengzhou University, Institute of Neuroscience, Zhengzhou University, Zhengzhou, Henan, China
e-mail: zdsfyzx@zzu.edu.cn; zxa@zzu.edu.cn

2.1 Supratentorial Astrocytoma

Case 2.1.1 Pilocytic Astrocytoma

Clinical Presentation

A 2-year-old girl was admitted to neurosurgery for tremor and fatigue in the right limb for more than 10 days.

Imaging Findings

A. Axial T2-weighted image demonstrates a cystic-solid mass in the left basal ganglia and surrounded by little edema. The solid component is sligjhtly hyperintense and the cystic component is homogeneously hyperintense (Fig. 2.1a).
B. Axial T1-weighted shows the slightly hypointense solid component and the homogeneously hypointense cystic component (Fig. 2.1b).
C. Axial T2WI-FLAIR demonstrates cystic component with hypointensity (Fig. 2.1c).
D. Axial contrast-enhanced T1-weighted images show marked enhancement in the solid component and cystic wall (Fig. 2.1d).
E. Sagittal contrast-enhanced T1-weighted images show marked enhancement in the solid component and cystic wall (Fig. 2.1e).
F. Coronal contrast-enhanced T1-weighted images show marked enhancement in the solid component and cystic wall (Fig. 2.1f).

Discussion

The supratentorial location of astrocytoma is less common than infratentorial ones in pediatrics, accounting for about 30% of supratentorial brain tumors in children. It could occur in all pediatric groups. Astrocytoma can be divided into four grades according to WHO grade classification: grade I and grade II astrocytomas are well differentiated which are considered benign and usually follow a relatively indolent course with a better prognosis; grade III and grade IV astrocytomas are poorly differentiated and diffuse infiltrating with cystic degeneration, necrosis, and hemorrhage

H. Liu, X. Zhang (eds.), *Pediatric Neuroimaging*, https://doi.org/10.1007/978-981-16-7928-5_2

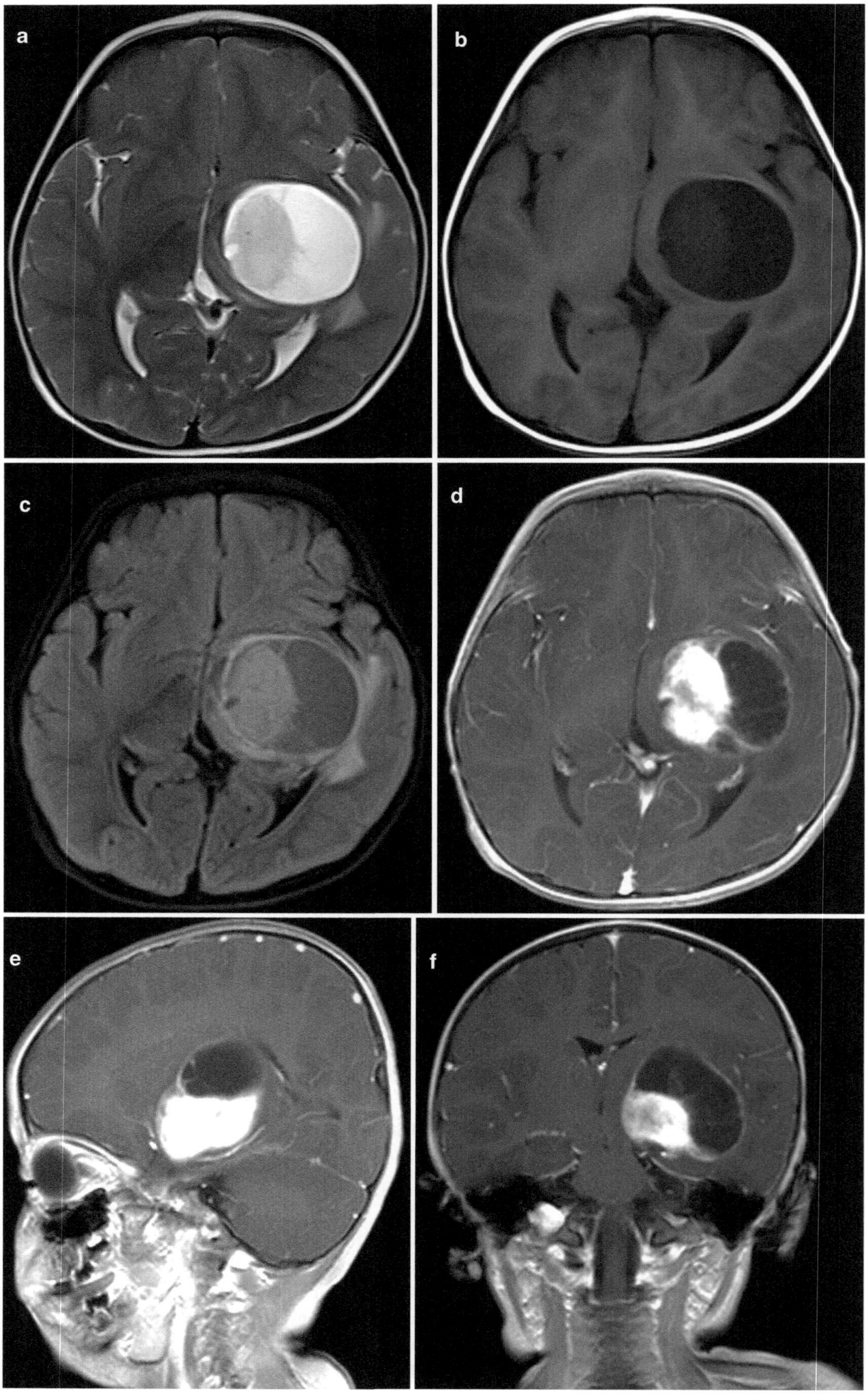

Fig. 2.1 Pilocytic astrocytoma

that are prone to relapse and malignant transformation with a poor prognosis.

Pilocytic astrocytoma (PA) was classified as WHO grade I in the 2016 WHO Classification of Tumors of the Central Nervous System. PA is the most common glioma during the first two decades of life [1]. Supratentorial PA accounts for 36% in all of PAs, including the cerebellum, brainstem, and optic pathway [2].

The symptoms depend on the age at the time of presentation and the location of the lesions. Infants present with increasing head circumference, nausea, vomiting, lethargy, and strabismus. Children usually complain of headache due to elevated intracranial pressure and may develop partial onset seizures or focal neurological deficit, such as truncal and limb ataxia, tremor, hemiparesis, and aphasia.

Histologically, PA is characterized by Rosenthal fibers, eosinophilic granular bodies, and alternating cystic regions with densely cellular regions (biphasic architecture). Transmission electron microscopic shows fenestrae and infolding vacuoles. Extracapillary space is expanded, and a common basement membrane formed by astrocytic processes is seen [3].

On CT and MR scans, the cystic portion of PA is hypoattenuated and slightly hyperintense to CSF on both T1- and T2WI, and it often does not suppress completely on FLAIR. The solid portion often appears isodense on CT, iso/hypointense on T1WI, and iso/hyperintense on T2WI/FLAIR. After contrast administration, the solid component presents with intense but heterogeneous enhancement in many cases. The cyst wall enhances from none to moderate. Besides, diffusion-weighted imaging shows no restriction of diffusion.

The diagnosis of PA should be differentiated from other tumors, such as pleomorphic xanthoastrocytoma (PXA) and germinoma. The common site of PXA in children is mainly in the temporal lobe, followed by the frontal and parietal lobe, often close to the meningeal side. The involvement of the adjacent leptomeninges (dural tail sign) has been reported to be a characteristic feature of PXA. Germinoma is iso-hypointense on T2WI, while slightly high density on CT. Germinoma is predominantly solid mass, with multiple small cysts or calcification.

Case 2.1.2 Pleomorphic Xanthoastrocytoma

Clinical Presentation

A 7-year-old boy presented to the department of neurological rehabilitation with dizziness for 4 months and unstable holding for half a month. His past medical, surgical, and family histories were negative.

Imaging Findings

A. Axial T2-weighted image demonstrates a cystic-solid mass with mural nodule close to the meningeal side in the left frontal lobe and surrounded by little edema. The mural nodule is iso-hyperintense and the cystic component is homogeneously hyperintense (Fig. 2.2a).
B. Axial T2WI-FLAIR demonstrates cystic component with iso- or hyperintensity (Fig. 2.2b).
C. Axial T1-weighted shows the iso-hypointense mural nodule and the homogeneously hypointense cystic component (Fig. 2.2c).
D. Axial contrast-enhanced T1-weighted images show marked enhancement in the mural nodule and cystic wall (Fig. 2.2d).
E. Coronal contrast-enhanced T1-weighted images show marked enhancement in the mural nodule and cystic wall (Fig. 2.2e).
F. Sagittal contrast-enhanced T1-weighted images show marked enhancement in the mural nodule and cystic wall (Fig. 2.2f).

Discussion

Pleomorphic xanthoastrocytomas (PXAs) are WHO grade II tumors that are believed to arise from the astrocyte in the pia mater. PXAs are rare neoplasms comprising less than 1% of all astrocytic tumors. They are more frequently encountered in childhood and young adulthood. They usually occur in the peripheral part of the lobe, mainly in the temporal lobe, followed by fontal and parietal lobe. PXAs are benign tumors but are accompanied by aggressive behaviors. Symptoms of 71% patients include a long history (median 3 years) of epilepsy [4].

The term "pleomorphic" refers to the variegated histologic appearance of the tumor with mono- or multi-nuclear giant cells, the nuclei of which display great variation in size and staining. The second term "xanthoastrocytoma" refers to the fact that many tumor cells in this neoplasm show intracellular accumulation of lipids, usually in the form of droplets and quite often occupy much of the cell's body.

Typically, PXAs appear cystic, mixed cystic-solid, or solid lesions. Cystic components of tumors are hypointense on T1WI and hyperintense on T2WI, whereas the solid components of tumors are hypointense or isointense on T1WI and mildly hyperintense on T2WI. CE-T1WI typically shows marked enhancement of the solid component, with little or no mass effect or peritumoral edema. The involvement of the adjacent leptomeninges (dural tail sign) has been reported to be a characteristic feature of PXA.

PXAs should be differentiated from tumors which are superficial part of the lobe, including pilocytic astrocytoma (PA), ganglioglioma, and meningioma. When located in supratentorial, the imaging presentation of PA can be a solid mass, or a cystic mass with mural nodule. The involvement of the adjacent leptomeninges (dural tail sign) is a characteristic feature of PXA, which may be useful in differentiating PXA from supratentorial PA. Ganglioglioma is also characterized by a large cyst with mural nodule; however, ganglioglioma shows signs of calcification, not involvement of leptomeninges. Middle age onset, rare incidence of necrosis, and cystic degeneration are features of meningioma, which are different from that of PXA.

Case 2.1.3 Diffuse Astrocytoma

Clinical Presentation

A 1-year-old boy was sent to neurosurgery for 2 months of continuous weakness in the right limb. His clinical manifestations are weakness in the right limb and swinging while walking. His past medical, surgical, and family histories were negative.

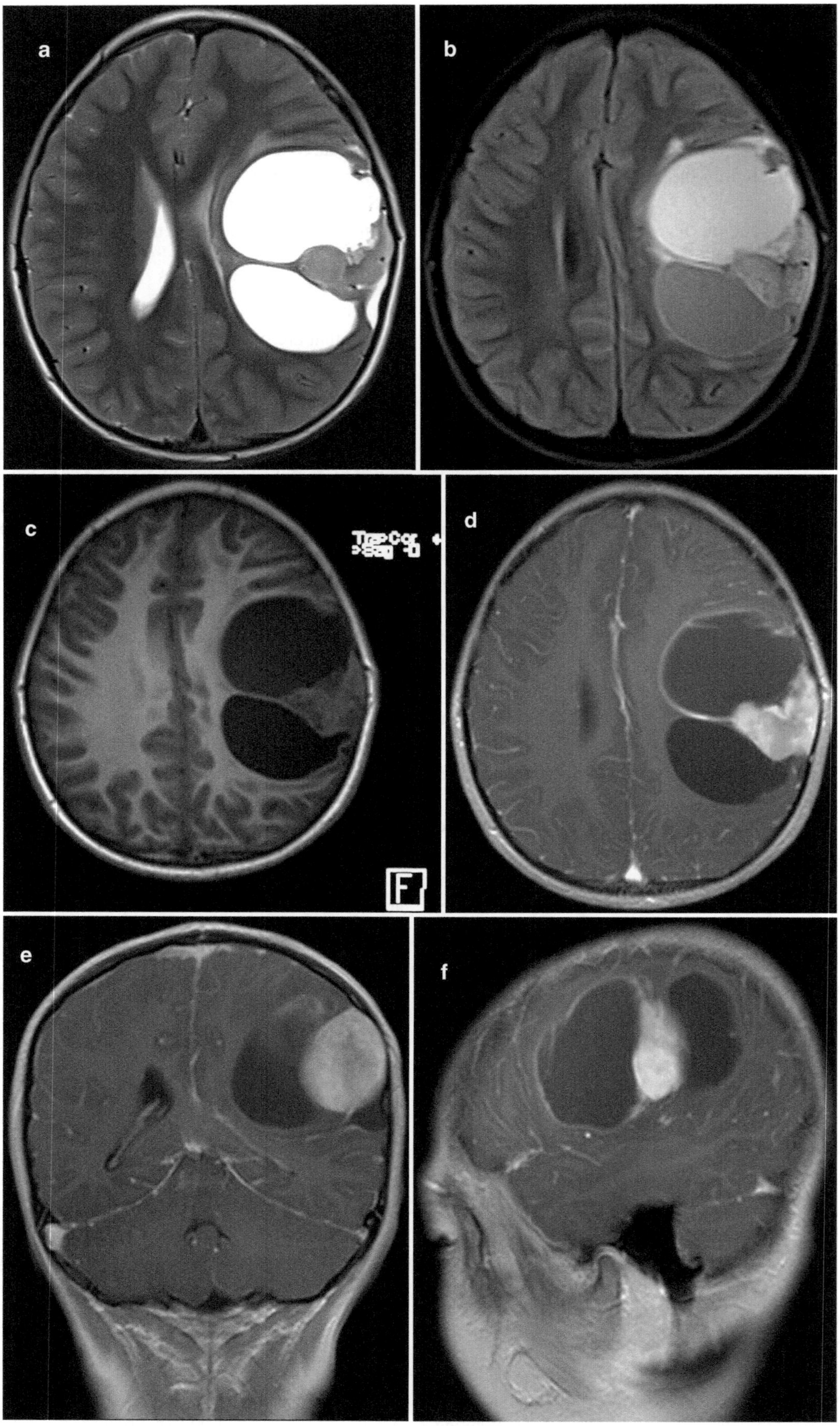

Fig. 2.2 Pleomorphic xanthoastrocytoma

Imaging Findings

A. Axial T1WI image showed a large round-like hypointense mass located in the left frontal lobe (Fig. 2.3a).
B. Axial T2WI image showed that the tumor was hyperintense (Fig. 2.3b).
C. Axial T1WI enhanced scan showed patchy enhancement in the center of the mass (Fig. 2.3c).
D. Coronal T1WI enhanced scan showed a huge tumor spanning the midline and invading the right cerebral hemisphere, and the left basal ganglia was obviously compressed (Fig. 2.3d).

Discussion

Diffuse astrocytoma, also known as low-grade diffuse astrocytoma, is the most common low-grade astrocytic tumor, WHO class II. It is more common in adults; the peak age of onset is 30–40 years, slightly more in men. Pathologically, it is characterized by tumors without capsules, local brain tissue swelling, occasional cystic changes, calcification, and

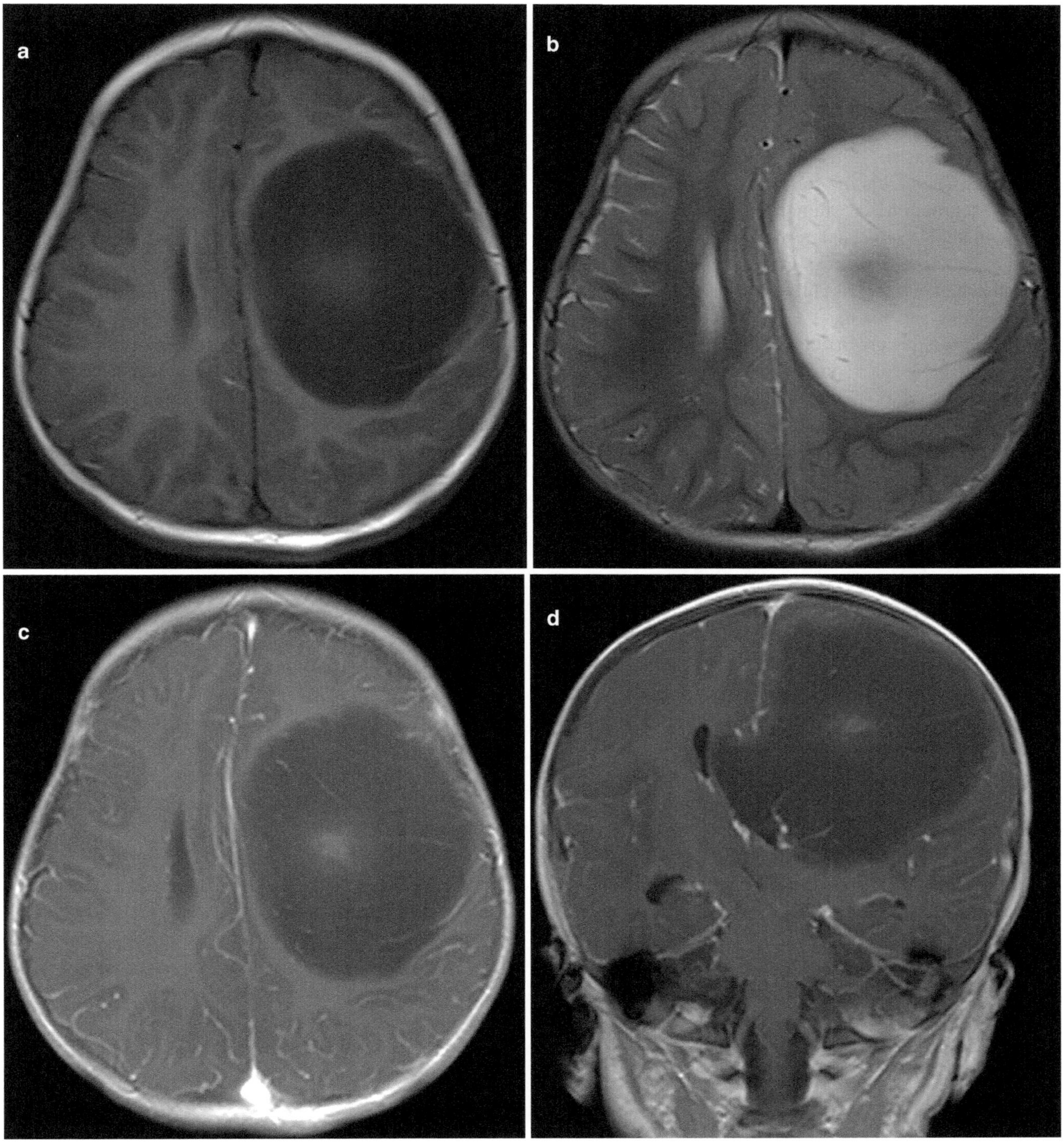

Fig. 2.3 Diffuse astrocytoma

hemorrhage [5]. The clinical manifestations are related to the location of the tumor, and convulsions are the most common symptom. The disease has a good prognosis and slow progress, but easy to relapse [6].

Diffuse astrocytoma occurs in the cerebral hemisphere, with the most common site being the frontal lobes (about 2/3). Diffuse astrocytoma in the cerebral cortex often forms cystic masses in the cortex, which grows slowly and expands. The tumor has multiple boundaries, the occupancy effect is light, and edema and hemorrhage are rare. About 1/5 of the lesions showed calcification, and the enhanced scan showed no enhancement or slight enhancement. MRI mainly showed low signal on T1WI, high signal on T2WI and FLAIR, and DWI showed no diffusion limitation or mild diffusion limitation with ADC value decreased. Enhanced scan showed 40% light boost. MRS showed no specificity.

The diffuse astrocytoma of the cerebral cortex needs to be differentiated from the following diseases: dysembryoplastic neuroepithelial tumor (WHOI grade): occurs mostly in adolescents, and cystic lesions such as "triangular sign" and "small vesicle sign" can be seen on the image: no enhancement or slightly nodular, small ring-like enhancement and no mass effect. Ganglion cell glioma (WHO I grade) occurs in children and adults under the age of 30, can be located on the surface of the brain, and can be expressed as cystic predominant; enhanced posterior wall nodules showed a uniform enhancement. Oligodendroglioma (WHO class II) is well involved in the cerebral cortex, cerebral edema is more obvious, and the cystic change is relatively light, because it is often accompanied by cord-like calcification and uneven signal; after the enhancement, it is mostly mild enhancement.

Case 2.1.4 Glioblastoma Multiforme

Clinical Presentation

A 1-year-old girl was sent to neurosurgery for 10 days of continuous weakness in the right limb. Her clinical manifestations are that she cannot grasp and cannot stand. Her past medical, surgical, and family histories were negative.

Imaging Findings

A. Axial T1WI showed a huge and irregular mass in the left frontal lobe, and the solid component is slightly hypointense (Fig. 2.4a).
B. Axial T2WI showed that the solid part of the tumor was slightly hyperintense, and small patchy hyperintensities were seen inside. The cystic part was hyperintense. Large areas of hyperintense edema were seen in the brain parenchyma surrounding the tumor (Fig. 2.4b).
C. Axial T2WI-FLAIR showed that the solid part of the tumor was isointense (Fig. 2.4c).
D. Axial DWI sequence showed that the ADC value of the solid part of the tumor decreased (Fig. 2.4d).
E, F. Axial T1WI-enhanced scan showed that the solid part of the tumor was significantly enhancement, but the cystic part was not. The mass effect of the lesion was obvious, and the midline structure, the third ventricle, and the frontal angle of the left ventricle were obviously compressed (Fig. 2.4e, f).

Discussion

Glioblastoma multiforme (GBM) is a rare tumor of the central nervous system. It originates from neuroepithelial tissue and accounts for 22.3% of neuroepithelial tumors. It occurs in adults and is rare in children. It is mostly located in the cerebral hemisphere within the white matter. GBM is a malignant transformation of astrocytoma and is the most malignant type of astrocytoma. GBM is generally considered to be the result of progressive variability in astrocytoma, mixed astrocytoma, and oligodendroglioma [7].

The clinical manifestations of GBM are mostly symptoms of increased intracranial pressure and signs of neuronal damage such as headache, vomiting, convulsions, and decreased vision. GBM tumors grow rapidly and are highly malignant, and the disease progresses generally faster, with an average survival of about 12 months.

GBM tumor cells are pleomorphic with obvious nuclear abnormalities; mitotic figures are common, accompanied by microvascular proliferation and necrosis. The necrosis of the tumor is located in the center of the lesion, and dense fusiform glial cells are arranged around the pseudo-fence. GBM is mainly located in the white matter of the cerebral hemisphere. It often invades the frontal, temporal, and parietal lobes. The occipital lobe is less common. The basal ganglia and the corpus callosum are often involved. The tumor tissue can invade the contralateral cerebral hemisphere by S-shaped growth or the corpus callosum. In the deep part of the cerebral hemisphere, butterfly growth is common, and the GBM of the thalamus is not uncommon. GBM in children and young people is very rare. Due to the high degree of variability and immature tumor cells, poor vascular structure, thrombosis, etc., there is often extensive degenerative hemorrhage and necrosis, so the tumor is characterized by pleomorphism [8].

When the lesions were mainly necrotic components or all necrotic, long T1 and long T2 signal was present, and the solid lesions T1WI, T2WI, and FLAIR showed equal signals, and DWI diffusion first showed high signal. The tumor showed infiltration and growth, and the edge was blurred. Because of the high degree of malignancy, the volume was generally large and had obvious occupying effect. The affected ventricle was reduced or even disappeared, and the midline was shifted to the contralateral side. Because the enhanced pathological basis is related to the different types of peritumoral cells, small blood vessels proliferate around the necrotic foci, and the hyperplastic small blood vessel wall is irregular, so the solid part of the tumor is irregular, clump-like, or garland-like. GBM needs to be differentiated from primitive neuroectodermal tumor (PNET) and lymphoma [9].

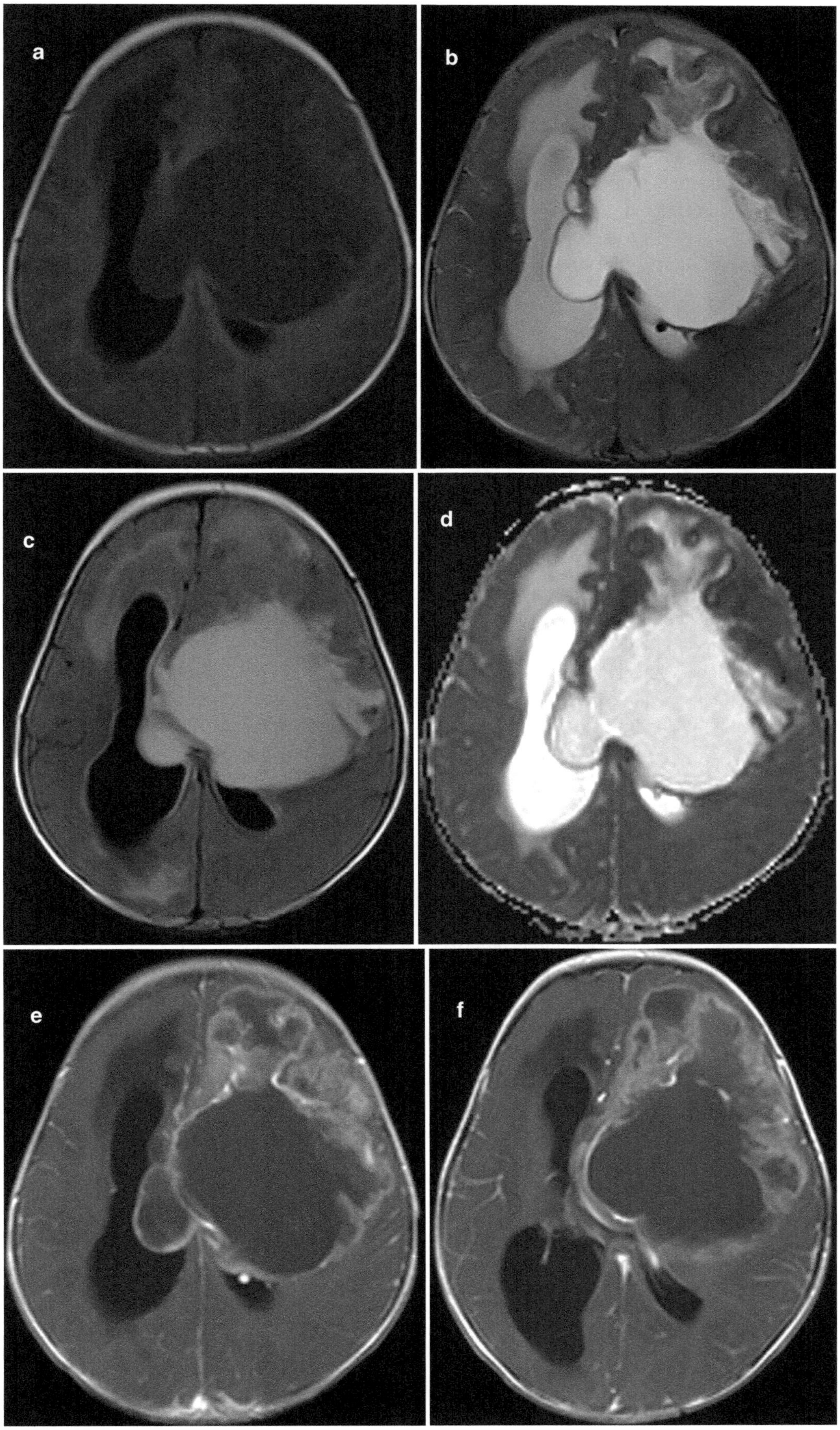

Fig. 2.4 Glioblastoma multiforme

PNET occurs in children over 5 years. The peritumoral edema is light or even absent. It is prone to dissemination and metastasis. GBM is less likely to spread and metastasize, and peritumoral edema is heavier. Lymphoma mostly occurs around the cerebral ventricle, with less edema around it, enhanced uniform nodular enhancement, and less cystic necrosis; GBM is unevenly enhanced, is easy to hemorrhage, and has necrosis and hemorrhage; peripheral edema is very obvious.

Case 2.1.5 Subependymal Giant Cell Astrocytoma

Clinical Presentation

A 6-old-year girl visited our hospital due to paroxysmal weakness in both lower extremities for 2 years.

Imaging Findings

A. Axial T2-weighted image demonstrates an isointense solid mass located in the left lateral ventricles, close to the foramen of Monro (Fig. 2.5a).
B. On axial T1-weighted image the mass is also isointense (Fig. 2.5b).
C. Axial contrast-enhanced T1-weighted image show slightly heterogeneous enhancement in the mass (Fig. 2.5c).
D. Coronal contrast-enhanced T1-weighted image show slightly heterogeneous enhancement in the mass (Fig. 2.5d).
E. Axial T2-weighted image demonstrates multiple iso-hypointense subependymal nodules in the wall of the lateral ventricles (Fig. 2.5e).
F. Axial T1-weighted image demonstrates multiple iso-hyperintense subependymal nodules in the wall of the lateral ventricles (Fig. 2.5f).

Discussion

Subependymal giant cell astrocytoma (SEGA) is a rare benign tumor, WHO grade I. SEGAs constitute approximately 1–2% of all intracranial pediatric tumors. SEGAs are originated from mixed glioneuronal cells including giant cells. SEGAs seem to develop only in tuberous sclerosis (TSC) patients and their prevalence ranges from 2.2 to 5% to up to 20% of TSC patients within the first two decades of life. However, SEGAs without TSC have been spotted by the bookwriter rarely. SEGAs are often located in the lateral ventricles, near the foramen of Monro. The clinical presentations are varied, such as obstructive hydrocephalus, neurologic deficits, and seizures.

On CT, SEGA tumors appear heterogeneous with calcification, while they are heterogeneous masses with uniform enhancement on T1-weighted images on MRI. On FLAIR images, they show heterogeneous hyperintense signal. The apparent diffusion coefficient (ADC) values for these tumors are within the range of ADC values for normal brain parenchyma [10]. MRS shows a nonspecific pattern with high choline-to-creatine ratios and low NAA-to-creatine ratios.

The radiological aspects of the two types of intraventricular lesions, subependymal nodules (SEN) and SEGAs, are not specific for one or another. Both might contain calcifications, appear slightly more intense than gray matter on T1 images usually, and might be either hyperintense or hypointense (calcifications) on T2-weighted images. There might be some gadolinium enhancement in both entities; however, there is predominant contrast uptake in SEGAs. Whereas SEGAs have only been described near the foramen of Monro, SENs might be located anywhere around the ventricular wall [11–13]. SEGAs will progressively enlarge, whereas SENs will remain stable. According to the literature, lesions, which are bigger than 5–12 mm with incomplete calcification and contrast enhancement, tend to be SEGAs rather than SENs.

Case 2.1.6 Dysembryoplastic Neuroepithelial Tumors

Clinical Presentation

A 7-year-old boy presented to the department of neurological rehabilitation with unstable walked for 1 week, head discomfort for half a month, and vomiting many times. His past medical, surgical, and family histories were negative.

Imaging Findings

A. Axial T2-weighted image shows a hyperintense lesion in the right temporal lobe (Fig. 2.6a).
B. Axial T1-weighted image shows a hypointense lesion in the right temporal lobe (Fig. 2.6b).
C. Axial T2WI-FLAIR imaging showed hypointensity in the central region and hyperintensity in the peripheral region (Fig. 2.6c).
D. Axial contrast-enhanced T1-weighted image show no enhancement (Fig. 2.6d).
E. Coronal contrast-enhanced T1-weighted image show no enhancement (Fig. 2.6e).
F. Sagittal contrast-enhanced T1-weighted image show no enhancement (Fig. 2.6f).

Discussion

Dysembryoplastic neuroepithelial tumors (DNTs) are benign tumors with WHO grade I. They arise from mixed neural-glial cells [14]. They usually occur in the supratentorial cortex of temporal and frontal lobes. The symptom often presents with epilepsy. Incidence peaks are 10–30 years at presentation.

Typically, DNTs show a wedge-shaped configuration, presenting hypointense on T1-weighted images and hyperintense on T2-weighted images. Minimal or no enhancement is seen. T2-FLAIR imaging shows a bright rim without mass effect and perilesional edema. DNTs are usually found intracortical; however, they can be seen as enlarged gyrus with septalike structures which cause cystic appearance. This cystic appearance may be explained by glioneuronal element within the tumor. Highest ADC values are shown in DNTs among benign tumors according to the research [15]. MRS is nonspecific and possibly shows a lactate peak.

MRI features are classified as follows: type 1 (cystic/polycystic-like, well-delineated, strongly hypointense on

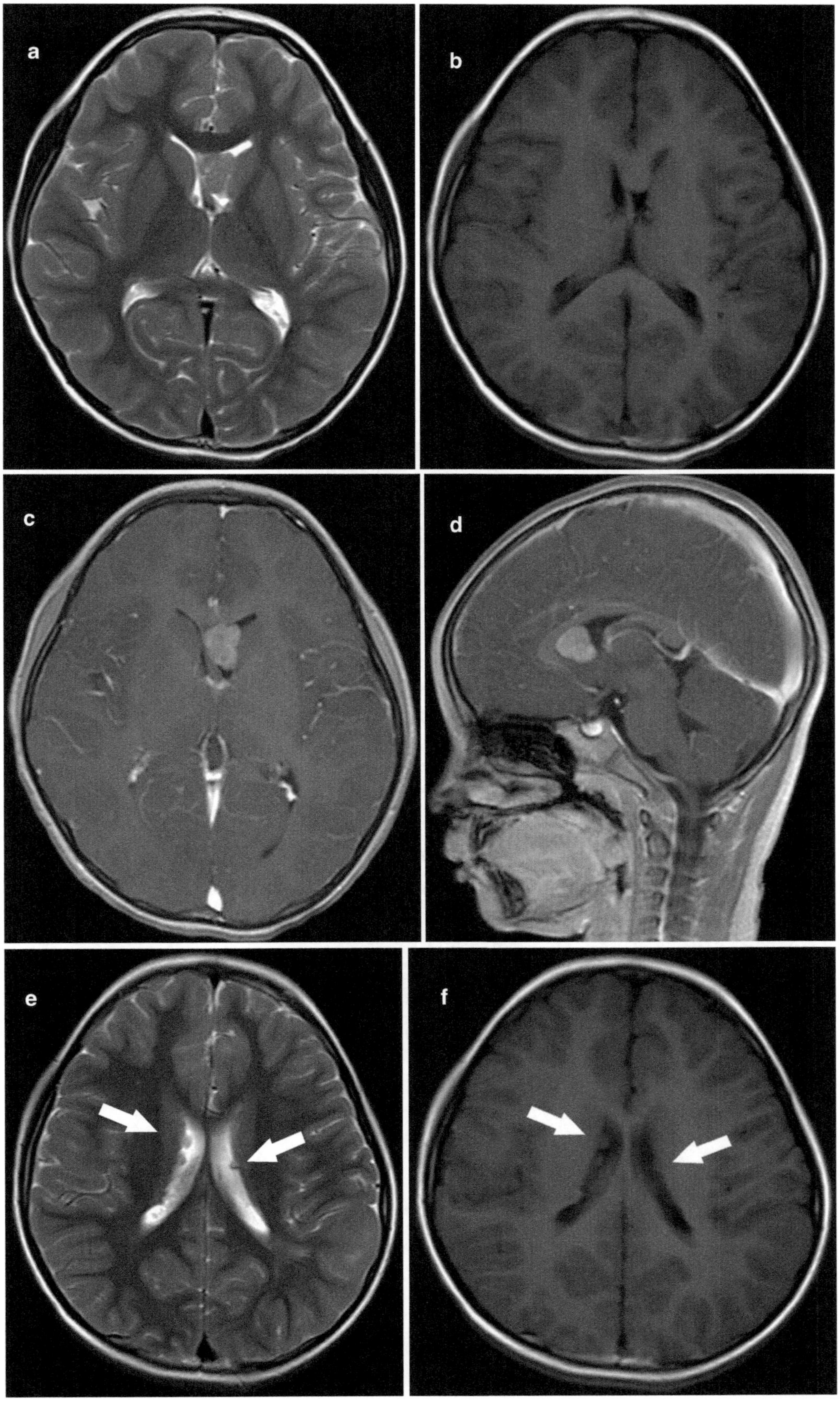

Fig. 2.5 Subependymal giant cell astrocytoma

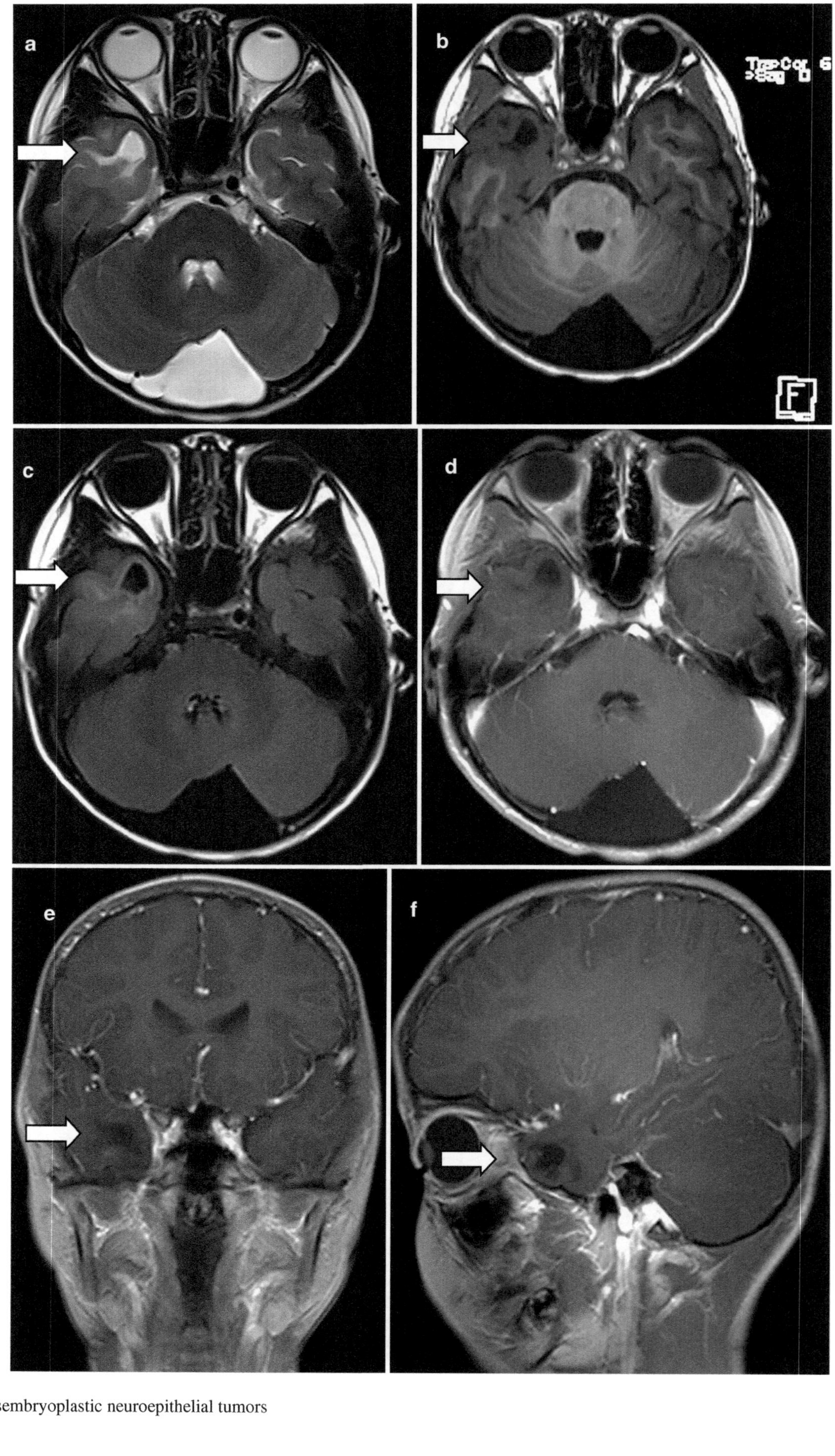

Fig. 2.6 Dysembryoplastic neuroepithelial tumors

T1), type 2 (nodular-like, heterogeneous signal), or type 3 (dysplastic-like: iso/hyposignal T1, poor delineation, gray-white matter blurring). Different MRI types show correlation to different histologic DNT subtypes [16]. Hippocampal sclerosis or malformations (15% of DNTs involving the temporal lobe) and FCD are mainly associated with type 3 MRI. There are usually calcifications in type 2 MRI and bone deformation in types 1 and 2. Contrast enhancement is relatively rare (12%) and found equally in all MRI subtypes. True cysts are also rare and are found only in types 2 and 3.

The main differential diagnosis remains gangliogliomas in which malignant evolution is not rare. When a true cyst and associated nodular contrast enhancement are seen, imaging features may suggest a ganglioglioma; this is much more frequently seen than in DNTs. Secondly, gangliogliomas, typically exhibiting granular bodies and perivascular lymphocytic cuffing, often extend within arachnoid spaces, and they contain an intercellular reticulinic frame, and these latter features are absent in DNTs.

The second differential diagnosis that merits discussion is low-grade diffuse glioma, when the glial component is exclusively made up of isolated tumoral cells. In these "diffuse" variants (corresponding to the nonspecific "dysplastic-like" DNT), the cortex–white matter interface is usually blurred, thus rendering the diagnosis particularly difficult. However, on T1-weighted MRI sequences, the diffuse variants of DNT are isointense to normal cortex, whereas diffuse gliomas are hypointense.

The third diagnosis that may be discussed is FCD when MRI shows a poorly limited lesion in the temporal lobe with blurring of the gray and white matter junction, also corresponding to nonspecific dysplastic-like DNT. However, FCD type 2 lesions are mainly located in extratemporal areas, while FCD type 1 lesions are usually associated with normal MRI. Moreover, histologic examination allows identification of tumor cells mixed with the FCD when present [17].

Case 2.1.7 Central Neurocytoma

Clinical Presentation

An 18-year-old male presented with headache for 2 months. The laboratory test was negative.

Imaging Findings

A. The axial T2WI image demonstrates a cystic-solid mass in the bilateral ventricles, showing heterogeneous high signal, lobulated, and clear boundaries (Fig. 2.7a).
B. The axial enhanced-T1WI image demonstrates that the mass was heterogeneous and obviously enhanced (Fig. 2.7b).

Discussion

Central neurocytoma (CN),is a rare neuronal tumor, WHO grade II, with a biological behavior of low-grade malignancy [18]. The tumor usually occurs in the lateral ventricle and the third ventricle. The foramen of Monro is a typical site of the disease, and occasionally occurs in the fourth ventricle [19]. CNs are more common in young and middle-aged people, with an average age of about 30 years, and there is no obvious gender difference. The clinical symptoms are not obvious at the beginning of the onset, but when the tumor is large and obstructs the foramen of Monro, the third ventricle, or the midbrain aqueduct, it can cause hydrocephalus, headache, nausea, vomiting, and other symptoms of increased intracranial pressure. Complete surgical resection is the preferred treatment for CNs. The histological and biological behaviors of most central neurocytomas are benign, and the prognosis is good.

The typical CN imaging manifestations are round or lobulated masses in the body of the lateral ventricle, the third ventricle, or the midline. T1WI showed equal or low signal; T2 WI showed high signal. Because tumors are often accompanied by cysts of varying sizes, the tumors are mostly cystic or solid masses. A solid cystic mass has a soap bubble-like appearance on T2WI. On enhanced scan, the mass showed heterogeneous enhancement [20]. On DWI, CNs showed a heterogeneous high signal, while ADC showed a slightly low signal [21]. The tumor usually has a clear demarcation from the surrounding tissues. In a few cases, the lesion invades the paraventricular brain parenchyma, resulting in unclear demarcation, indicating a poor prognosis. CNs showed equal or high density on CT, and cystic low-density foci and high-density calcification were seen in the tumor.

CNs need to be differentiated from other intraventricular tumors. (1) Ependymoma: Tumors in children are mostly located in the fourth ventricle and in adults are mostly located in the triangle of the lateral ventricle. There is often hemorrhage in the tumor. (2) Subependymal giant cell tumor: It is common in children, located in the Monro hole. Tumors are generally solid, cystic transformation is rare, and it manifests as a homogeneous mass with a clear boundary. In patients it is mostly accompanied by tuberous sclerosis, which is conducive to diagnosis. (3) Choroidal papilloma: Occurs in children, usually in the triangle of the lateral ventricle, often involving the subependymal white matter, relatively homogeneous lesions, and marked enhancement, often causing communicating hydrocephalus.

Case 2.1.8 Ependymoma

Clinical Presentation

A 1-year-old boy was diagnosed with neurosurgery for half a month of repeated convulsions of his right hand. He was consciously awake during the attack, and both sleep and wakefulness could occur. He was diagnosed for language and motor development retardation in a foreign hospital 3 months ago.

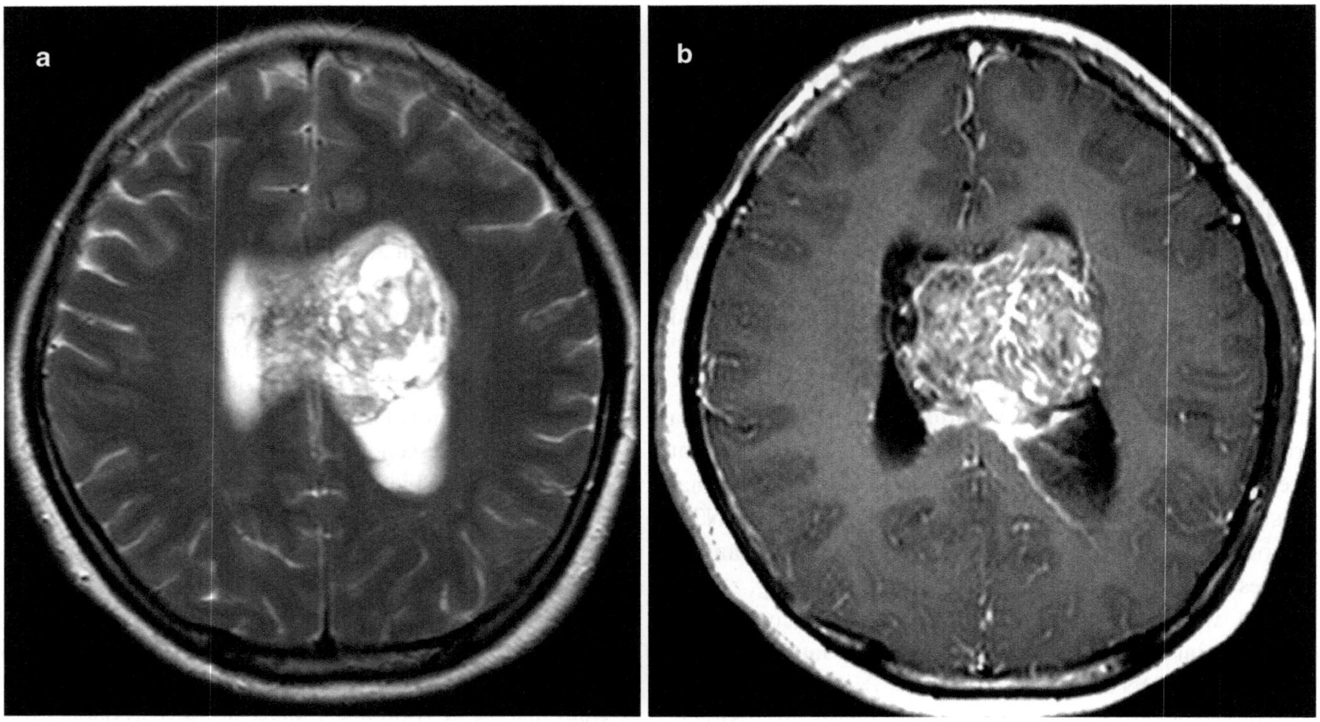

Fig. 2.7 Central neurocytoma

Imaging Findings

A. Axial T1WI showed that a round-like cystic-solid mixed tumor located in the left parietal lobe, and the solid part was slightly hypointense (Fig. 2.8a).
B. Axial T2WI showed that slightly high signal in the solid part of the tumor and high signal in the cystic part (Fig. 2.8b).
C. Axial T2WI-FLAIR showed high signal in the solid part of the tumor (Fig. 2.8c).
D. Axial T1 enhanced scan showed that the solid part of the tumor and the intracapsular septum were significantly enhanced, but the cystic part was not enhanced (Fig. 2.8d).

Discussion

Ependymoma is a common tumor in the central nervous system of children, accounting for 10% of primary neurological tumors, mostly located in the posterior fossa, second only to medulloblastoma, cerebellar astrocytoma, and brainstem glioma; it is the fourth tumor of the posterior fossa; the supratentorial ependymoma is rare. Ependymoma is a slow-growing glioma with varying degrees of tumor differentiation [22]. Among them, 70% of childhood ependymoma is located subtentorially, and the fourth ventricle is the most common site; 30% occurs in the lateral ventricle, third ventricle, midbrain, white matter, and spinal cord [23].

The general morphology of ependymoma can be nodular or lobulated, and the shape of the tumor often varies according to its position. There is tumor swelling and growth—the boundaries are clear; there is also infiltration growth—the boundaries are not clear. Ependymoma can occur with glassy changes, hemorrhage, necrosis, and cystic changes, and occasionally a large sac can be formed. Histological features of ependymoma can be divided into cell type, epithelial type, papillary type, and clear cell type.

On the MRI, the solid part of the tumor showed low or equal signal on T1WI and equal or high signal on T2WI; the cystic part showed low signal on T1WI and high signal on T2WI. After enhancement, the substantial part of the tumor often appears to be enhanced, and the cystic part is not enhanced. The solid components of the tumor are strengthened in a variety of forms, from obvious enhancement to no enhancement. Mild edema can be seen around the tumor [24].

The ependymoma of the supratentorial brain parenchyma needs to be differentiated from supratentorial pilocytic astrocytoma and atypical teratoid/rhabdoid tumor (AT/RT). The supratentorial pilocytic astrocytoma is mostly found in adults. It is characterized by a typical cystic mass with well-defined borders and wall nodules. On MRI, the cystic part of the mass shows long T1 and long T2 signal, and the tumor has no calcification. If calcification occurs, it often shows spotted calcification. AT/RT is also rare, often accompanied by compressive degeneration, hemorrhage, necrosis and calcification, increased DWI signal of solid components, and delay enhancement.

Case 2.1.9 Anaplastic Ependymoma

Clinical Presentation

A 2-year-old girl was sent to neurosurgery due to vomiting. Symptoms were repeated. The symptoms of vomiting suddenly aggravated 1 h ago, accompanied by convulsions, and resolved after a few minutes. The past medical history of the child and family history were negative; there was no history of trauma.

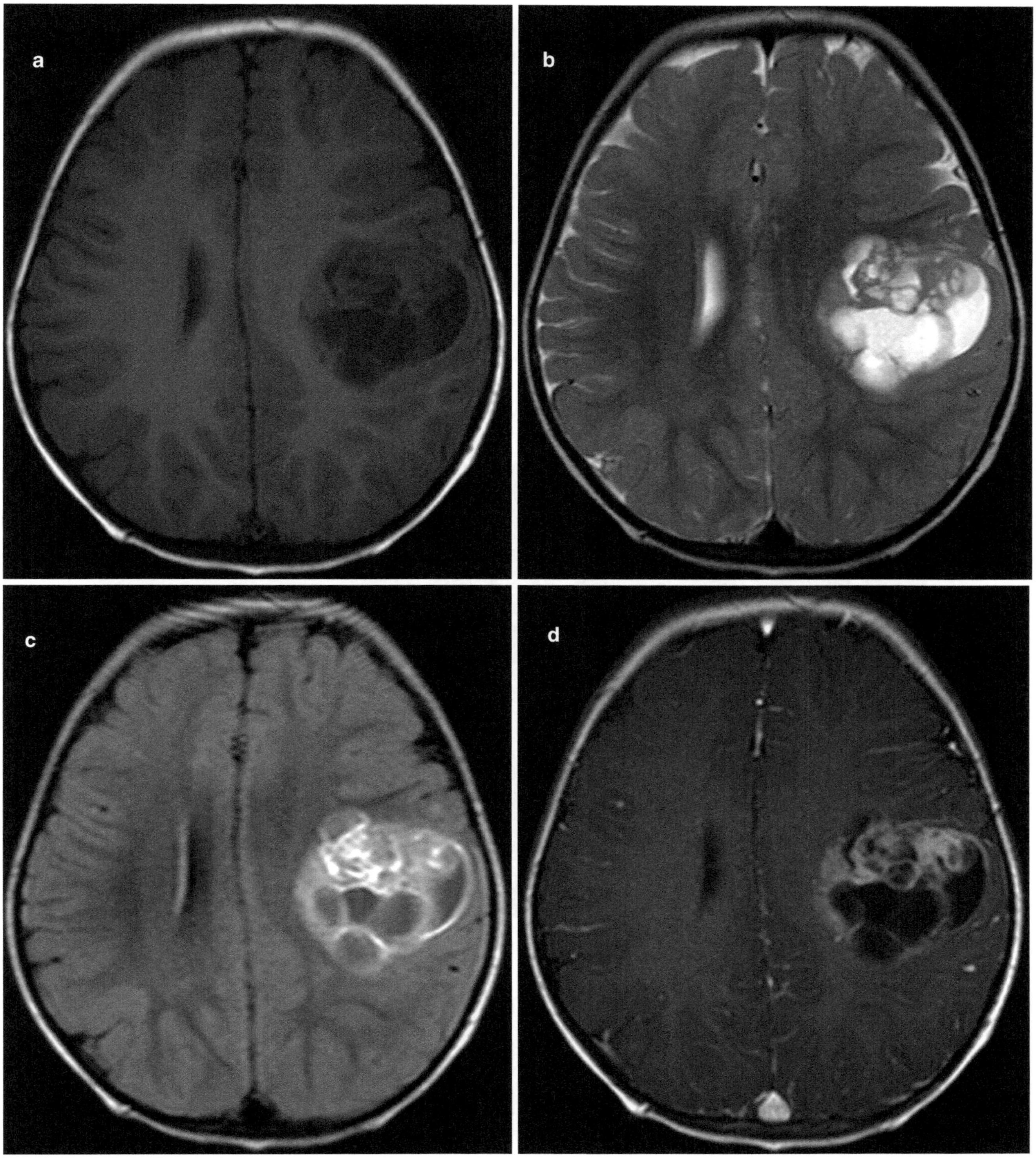

Fig. 2.8 Ependymoma

Imaging Findings

A. Axial T1WI showed a huge cystic-solid tumor in the left parieto-occipital region, and the solid part was slightly hypointense (Fig. 2.9a).
B. Axial T2WI showed slightly high signal in the solid part of the tumor and high signal in the cystic part (Fig. 2.9b).
C. Axial T2WI-FLAIR showed slightly high signal in the solid part of the tumor (Fig. 2.9c).
D. Axial DWI sequence showed that the ADC value of the solid part of the tumor decreased (Fig. 2.9d).
E. Axial T1WI-enhanced scan showed marked enhancement of the solid component of the tumor (Fig. 2.9e).
F. Axial T1 contrast-enhanced scan showed that the cyst wall was significantly enhanced in a ring shape (Fig. 2.9f).

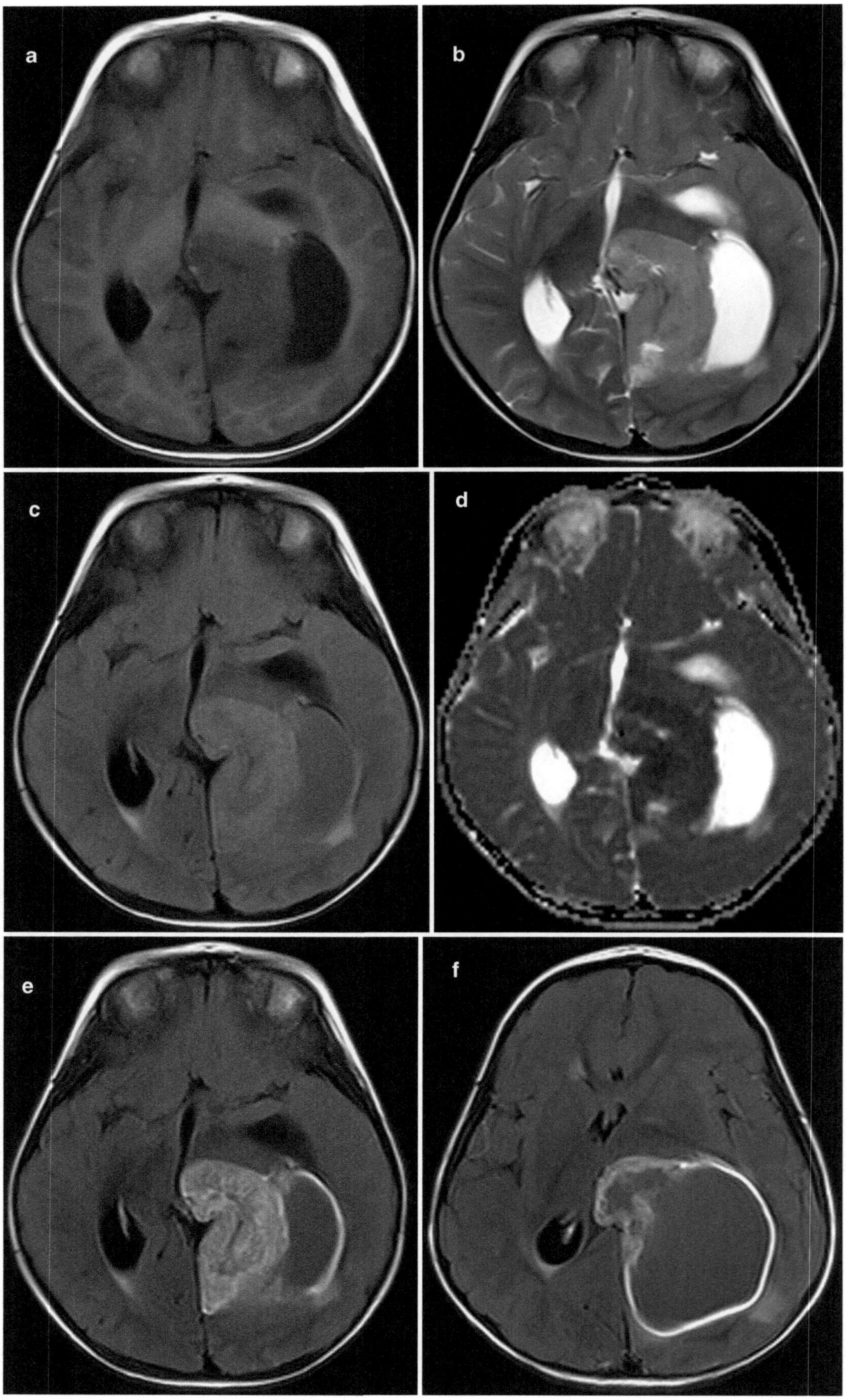

Fig. 2.9 Anaplastic ependymoma

Discussion

Anaplastic ependymoma originates from the ventricular surface ependymal epithelial cells, 90% occur in the brain, can occur in any part of the ventricular system, most are located in the posterior fossa, the fourth ventricle is the most common site, and the peak age of onset is 1–5 years. The supratentorial anaplastic ependymoma is often located in the brain parenchyma, accounting for about 30%. It can be divided into complete parenchymal and cystic mixture. The complete substance mainly occurs in adults. The cystic mixture mainly occurs in children and adolescents. Most of the symptoms depend on the location of tumor growth and are nonspecific: often headache, nausea, vomiting, ataxia, nystagmus, etc. Epilepsy and elevated intracranial pressure are common causes of treatment [25].

The gross morphology of the tumor may be nodular or lobulated, depending on the morphology of the space in which the tumor is located; anaplastic ependymoma is mostly expansively growing, with clear boundaries and infiltration growth; varicose chambers occur in the cerebral hemisphere. The imaging performance of the membranous tumor is related to the age of the patient. In the pediatric and adolescent population, the tumor is mostly located at the frontal lobe and the junction of the temporal lobe and occipital lobe, and the larger part of the tumor can be seen [26]. MRI showed that the tumor was low signal or equal signal on T1WI, and T2WI was high signal. Enhanced scan showed that the tumor parenchyma was mostly enhanced, and there was edema around the lesion, and the degree of edema was light.

The anaplastic ependymoma of the supratentorial brain parenchyma is prone to misdiagnosis due to the atypicality of the site and the lack of characteristic imaging signals of the tumor itself. It needs to be differentiated from supratentorial pilocytic astrocytoma and atypical teratoid/rhabdoid tumor (AT/RT) [27]. The supratentorial pilocytic astrocytoma is common in adults and is rare in children. It is characterized by a typical cystic mass with well-defined borders and wall nodules. MRI has a long T1 and long T2 signal, and the tumor is almost spotted calcification. AT/RT is also rare, often accompanied by compressive degeneration, hemorrhage, necrosis and calcification, increased DWI signal of solid components, and enhanced scan display delay enhancement.

Case 2.1.10 Germinoma

Clinical Presentation

An 11-year-old boy presented with uncoordinated left limbs, headache, vomiting, abnormal muscle tone, and progressively worsening symptoms. There is no special medical history or family history of the child.

Imaging Findings

A. Axial T1WI showed that the tumor was located in the third ventricle and the right basal ganglia, with ill-defined borders, uneven signal, and isointense in the solid part (Fig. 2.10a).
B. Axial T2WI showed isointense in the solid part of the tumor and hyperintensity in the cystic part (Fig. 2.10b).
C. Axial T2WI-FLAIR sequence showed isointense in the solid part of the tumor (Fig. 2.10c).
D. Axial T1WI-enhanced scan showed marked enhancement in the solid part of the tumor (Fig. 2.10d).

Discussion

Germinoma is the most common tumors of the pineal gland, accounting for 50–75% of tumors in the pineal region. Germinoma is derived from primitive germ cells. In intracranial germ cell tumors, 55–60% occur in the pineal region, 30% in the sella region, and 15% in the basal ganglia or hypothalamus. Germinoma can be single or multiple, with approximately 15% of the pineal and sella region [28]. Germinoma is a malignant tumor that can spread along the ependymal and cerebrospinal fluid. Because germ cell tumors are very sensitive to radiotherapy, experimental radiotherapy is powerful evidence for the diagnosis of germ cell tumors.

Germinoma usually occurs in adolescents aged 10–15 years. Clinical symptoms may include increased intracranial pressure, nausea, vomiting, central diabetes insipidus, and endocrine disorders depending on the tumor site. Microscopically, the tumor is composed of two types of cells: one is a round or polygonal cell, the size is basically the same, the nucleus is large, and the cytoplasm is rich. The other is a small cell with little cytoplasm and deep staining, which may be lymphocytes. Tumor cells secrete embryonic alkaline phosphate. Germinoma is sensitive to radiotherapy and is significantly different from non-germ cell tumors.

The morphology of germ cell tumor is not regular, the edge is clear, the density on the CT image is slightly higher, the tumor on the MRI image is T1WI slightly low signal and T2WI high signal, the peripheral edema is not obvious, and the tumor often causes obstruction in the posterior part of the third ventricle and hydrocephalus. Enhanced scans showed lesions with clear boundaries and enhanced enhancement, banding, or nodular enhancement of the ventricular wall [29]. MRI-enhanced scans help detect tumors that have been implanted through the cerebrospinal fluid. Calcification is a characteristic change in germ cell tumors in the pineal region, but other parts of the germinoma may be calcified.

The pineal and sella region germinomas are easily diagnosed due to the specific site of the disease and the age of proneness. The germinoma that occurs in the ventricle needs to be differentiated from meningioma; the germinoma located in the anterior third ventricle needs to be differentiated from tumors in the sellar region. Area tumor identification. Experimental radiotherapy is strong evidence for the diagnosis of germ cell tumors.

Case 2.1.11 Teratoma

Clinical Presentation

A 1-year-old girl was sent to neurosurgery for 5 days of continuous weakness in the left limb. Her clinical manifestations

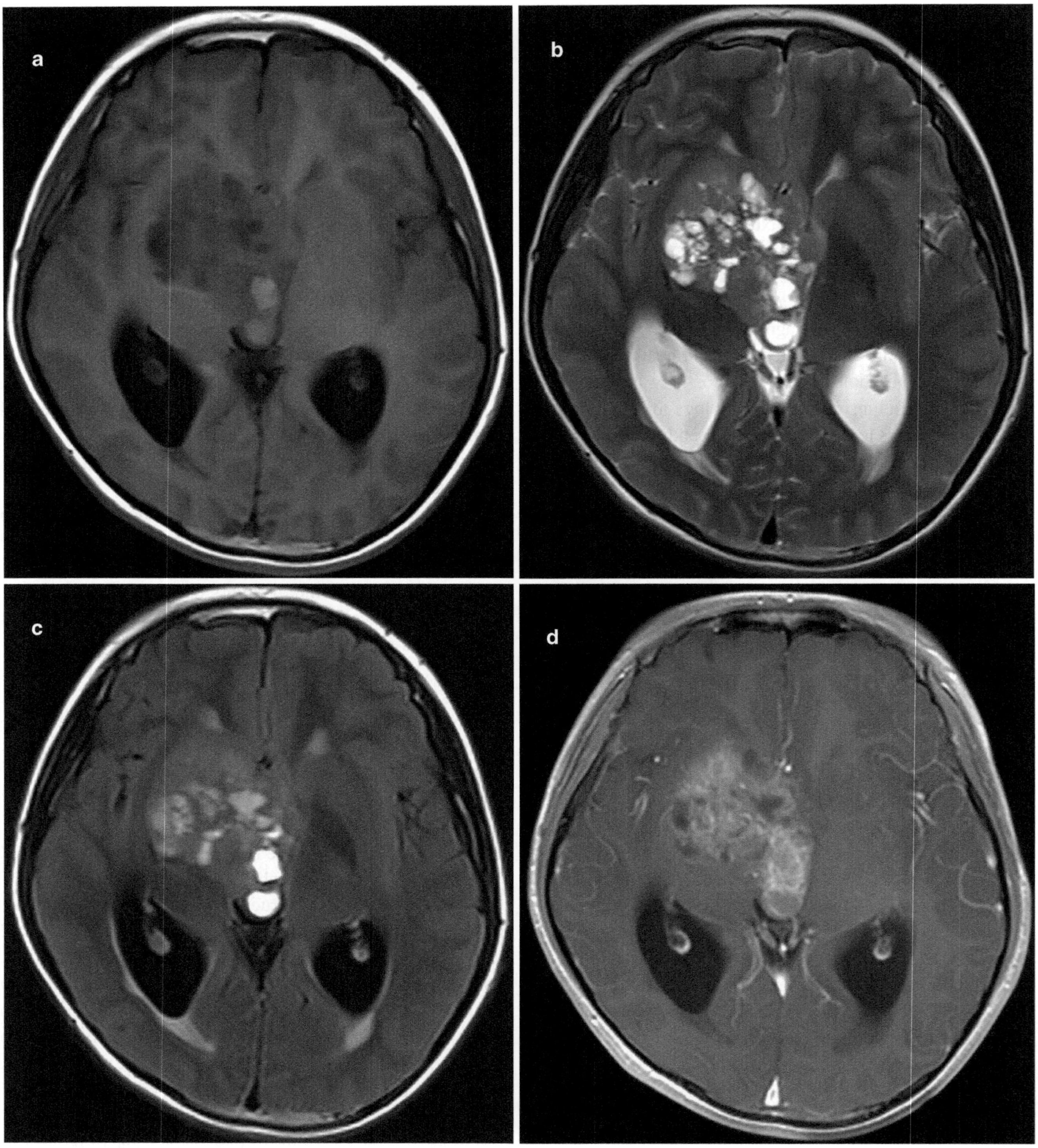

Fig. 2.10 Germinoma

continued to worsen. Her past medical, surgical, and family histories were negative.

Imaging Findings

A. Axial T1WI showed a huge round cystic-solid mass in the right cerebral hemisphere, the solid part was located in the center of the tumor, and a small cystic structure was seen inside. The solid part was isointense (Fig. 2.11a).
B. Axial T2WI showed that the cystic part of the tumor was mainly located around the tumor and showed high signal. Signs of hyperintense edema were seen around the tumor. The tumor invaded the right basal ganglia and right thalamus. The right ventricle was significantly compressed, and the midline structure was shifted to the left (Fig. 2.11b).
C. Axial T2WI-FLAIR sequence showed slightly higher signal in the solid part of the tumor (Fig. 2.11c).

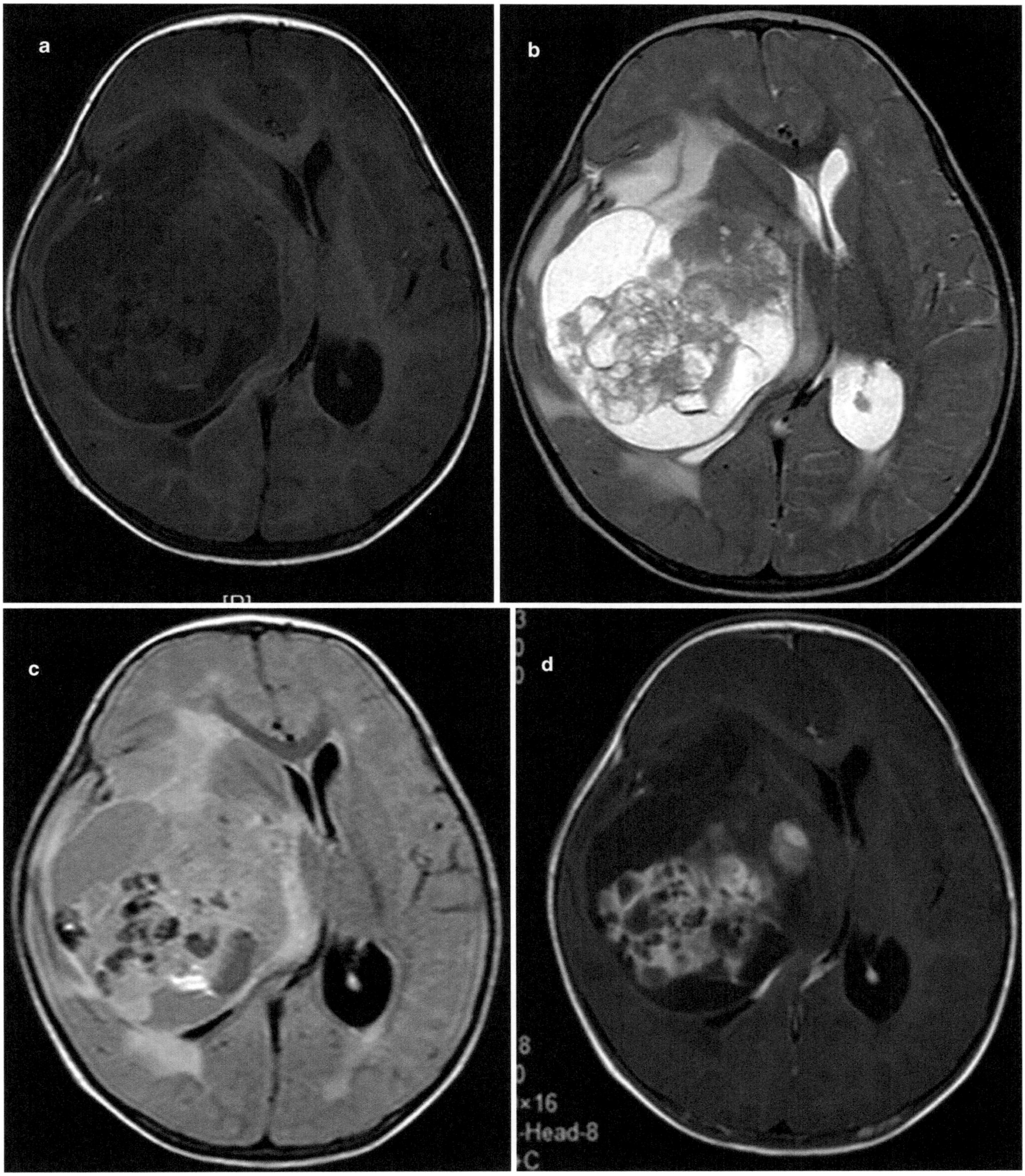

Fig. 2.11 Teratoma

D. Axial T1WI-enhanced scan showed obvious enhancement in the solid part of the tumor, but no enhancement in the cystic part (Fig. 2.11d).

Discussion

Teratomas are divided into fully differentiated mature teratomas and immature teratoma with incomplete differentiation. The incidence of intracranial immature teratoma accounts for 6.28% of intracranial germ cell tumors. The most common sites are the pineal region, sella region, and basal ganglia. The incidence of basal ganglia is relatively low. The immature teratoma is a malignant germ cell tumor [30].

Immature teratoma is mainly composed of three germ layer components that are undifferentiated or poorly differentiated [31]. The endodermal structures in the tumor contain digestive and respiratory tissues and various glands that secrete mucus. Mesodermal structures include tissues such as bone, cartilage, and muscle. The postganglionic ectoderm typically contains squamous and neuroepithelium, glial cells, neurons, neural tube, and choroid plexus [32]. The clinical manifestations will have different neurological symptoms depending on the location of the tumor. The early stage of the tumor in the sellar region mainly manifests as polydipsia and polyuria, followed by visual field change and hydrocephalus. Some children may have hypopituitarism and the symptoms such as sexual developmental delay; patients in the basal ganglia have early hemiparesis of the contralateral limbs, accompanied by awkward movements, hydrocephalus, and visual field loss with tumor enlargement; Tumors originating in the pineal region, the main clinical features are hydrocephalus, Parinaud syndrome, abducens palsy, ataxia, and other symptoms; the main body located in the third ventricle is mainly characterized by hydrocephalus.

The immature teratoma has complex MRI signals, mostly irregular long T1 and long T2 mixed signals. Most of the borders are clear, and there may be multiple chamber capsule changes. The enhanced scan shows heterogeneous enhancement, still observed after fat suppression and obvious peritumoral edema in some patients. Intracranial immature teratoma needs to be differentiated from choroid plexus papilloma, ependymoma, and central neurocytoma. Choroid plexus papilloma is more common in children and adolescents, the lateral ventricle is the majority, and the tumor signal is mixed and generally without peritumoral edema. Significant enhancement can be seen in the tumor and the normal choroid plexus, which is not the manifestation of immature teratoma. Ependymoma occurs in the fourth ventricle, which is more common in the age of 10–20. Intratumoral hemorrhage is rare. Most of lesions show significant heterogeneous enhancement. The capsule is not obvious in immature teratoma. Most of the central neurocytomas are located near the foramen of Monro in the lateral ventricle. Cystic degeneration is common, which may be associated with hemorrhage and calcification. The immature teratoma is rarely located in the foramen of Monro.

Case 2.1.12 Atypical Teratoid/Rhabdoid Tumor

Clinical Presentation

An 8-month-old boy was sent to neurosurgery due to a week of weakness in the right side of his limbs. He was admitted to the hospital with hemiplegia. His past medical, surgical, and family histories were negative. He had no recent trauma.

Imaging Findings

A. Axial T1WI showed a large cystic-solid mass in the left cerebral hemisphere with isointense in the solid part. The tumor involved the left frontal, temporal, and parietal lobes, as well as the left basal ganglia and thalamus (Fig. 2.12a).
B. Axial T2WI showed isointense in the solid part of the tumor and hyperintensity in the cystic part. There was no obvious edema around the tumor (Fig. 2.12b).
C. Axial T2WI-FLAIR sequence showed that the solid part of the tumor was isointense. Left ventricle was compressed (Fig. 2.12c).
D. Axial DWI sequence showed that the ADC value of the local solid part of the tumor decreased (Fig. 2.12d).
E. Axial T1WI-enhanced scan showed that the tumor was garland-like and significantly enhanced. There is no enhancement in the cystic part (Fig. 2.12e).
F. Cranial MRA showed abnormal tumor-supplying vessels in the horizontal segment of the left middle cerebral artery (Fig. 2.12f).

Discussion

Atypical teratoid rhabdoid tumor (AT/RT) is a rare, invasive, childhood embryonic tumor that can occur anywhere in the central nervous system [33]. The most common site of tumors is in the lower part of the brain, and the on-screen people account for about 39%; the ones that occur on the screen are more common in older children. Adults are located in the cerebral hemisphere.

The clinical manifestations of AT/RT depend on the location of the lesion and the age of onset. Children younger than 3 years of age usually present with nonspecific signs and symptoms such as vomiting, lethargy, irritation, weight loss, increased head circumference, and limited growth. Older children often present with increased intracranial pressure or local signs, cranial nerve palsy, headache, and hemiplegia.

The exact diagnosis of AT/RT depends on pathology, which consists of a mixture of various tumor cell components. Rhabdomyoid cells are typically seen in the lesion, which may be eccentric round nuclei with prominent nucleoli and expanded eosinophils, small spindle cells with oval nuclei, or large cells with marginal shrunken nuclei. The tumor components are diverse, so the immunohistochemical results are complex. The expression of EMA, VIM, and SMA is more significant, and the negative expression of INI-1 is specific [33].

AT/RT images lack specificity and lesions are usually large. CT showed mixed lesion density, cystic changes, hemorrhage, calcification, and peritumoral low-density edema. The plain tumor has a high density of parenchymal components. On the MRI images, T1WI and T2WI were mainly based on equal signals, and there were cystic changes and hemorrhages. The signals were mixed, and the enhancement of the substantial part of the scan showed moderate to significant enhancement [34].

On-screen AT/RT mainly needs to be differentiated from PENT, oligodendroglioma, glioblastoma, and ependymoma. There is a significant overlap in histology between PENT and AT/RT, so the imaging findings of the two tumors are similar and difficult to identify. When the patient is younger than 5 years, especially less than 2 years, the diagnosis of AT/RT

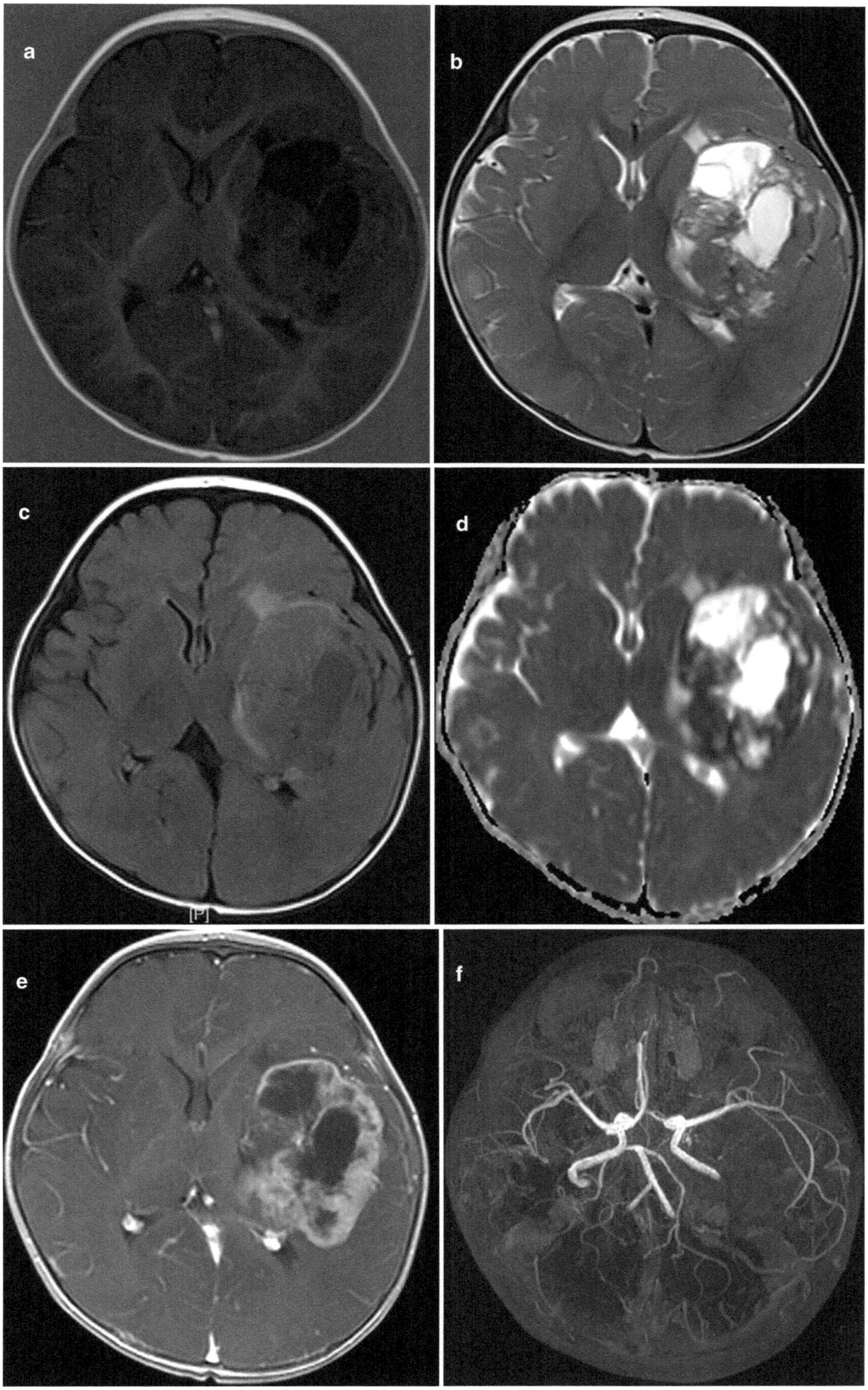

Fig. 2.12 Atypical teratoid rhabdoid tumor

should be considered first. The clinical manifestations of oligodendroglioma are epilepsy, the most common in the frontal lobe, generally involving the cortex, mixed with MR signals, no or mild enhancement after CT and MRI enhancement, mass effect and peritumoral edema, and no midline structure. The DWI (shift or slight shift) is mostly a slightly higher signal. Glioblastoma is more common in the elderly. The solid part of the CT has low-density, long T1 and long T2 signals. The tumor boundary is unclear, and the peritumoral edema and mass effect are obvious. About half of the supratentorial ependymoma is located in the brain parenchyma, which is closely related to the lateral ventricle. The solid part of the CT has a low-density, long T1 and long T2 signal, and the peritumoral edema and mass effect are more obvious.

2.2 Tumors of Pineal Gland Region

Case 2.2.1 Germinoma

Clinical Presentation

A 5-year-old boy was admitted to the Guangzhou Women and Children Medical Center. A pineal tumor was accidentally found in MRI with 1 month history of premature puberty.

Imaging Findings

A. Axial T1-weighted image shows an iso-hypointense solid mass in the pineal region (Fig. 2.13a).
B. Axial T2-weighted image shows an iso-hyperintense solid mass in the pineal region (Fig. 2.13b).
C. Axial contrast-enhanced T1WI shows markedly heterogeneous enhancement (Fig. 2.13c).
D. Sagittal contrast-enhanced T1WI shows markedly heterogeneous enhancement (Fig. 2.13d).
E. Axial DWI image (b = 800 s/mm^2) shows hyperintensity (Fig. 2.13e).
F. Axial ADC map shows hypointensity (Fig. 2.13f).

Discussion

Germinomas account for approximately 50–70% of germ cell tumors (GCTs). The peak incidence is during the second decade of life. The sites are commonly located in the pineal gland (50–60%) and the suprasellar region (30–40%) [35]. Less common sites include the basal ganglia and other regions of the brain. Approximately 5–10% of patients have both suprasellar and pineal gland involvement at the same time, which is referred to as bifocal germinoma.

The origin of extragonadal GCTs remains unknown. Recent studies mainly focus on the molecular pathology of central nervous system germ cell tumors. The frequent chromosome variations are the amplification of 12p [36]. Alterations of the p14 and c-kit gene have been reported in germinomas [37]. However, there is no link between these variations and clinical data, such as diagnosis and prognosis [36].

The clinical presentation varies by location and size, which frequently includes endocrine abnormalities, visual changes, and signs of increased intracranial pressure. Laboratory studies show that the levels of β-hCG and AFP are not typically elevated in germinomas. However, the β-hCG level is increased in a small number of germinomas due to its syncytiotrophoblast element, whereas the vast majority of β-hCG levels will not exceed the threshold of 50 IU/L [37, 38].

Germinomas are composed of sheets or lobules of large and uniform cells surrounded by varying amounts of vascularized connective tissue stroma. The tumor cells are round or oval with abundant clear or slightly eosinophilic cytoplasm. The centrally located vesicular nucleus is large, usually containing one prominent nucleolus, and sometimes a few smaller nucleoli. Mitotic activity is always detectable. Lymphocytes are found. In some instances, a few plasma cells, and occasionally neutrophils and eosinophils, are also found. Granulomatous reactions with aggregates of epithelioid histiocytes, some psammoma bodies, or gross cystic change are also present in some instances [39].

Imaging features of pineal germinoma demonstrate a mass with iso-hypointensity on T1WI and iso-hyperintensity on T2WI. Contrast enhancement shows markedly homogenous enhancement. Multiple small cysts or calcification are often seen in the tumor.

Differential diagnosis should include pineocytoma, pineoblastoma, and teratoma. A large and relatively homogeneous mass in the pineal region is shown in pineocytoma: CT scan, with peripheral displacement of pineal calcification. Contrast-enhanced CT scan shows homogeneous enhancement in the mass. MR image shows hyperintense lesions in T2WI with homogeneous enhancement without associated restricted diffusion or increased perfusion.

As the second most common pineal region tumor, pineal teratoma accounts for approximately 15% of all masses. In imaging studies, teratomas tend to be heterogeneous, multilocular, ring, or ring-enhanced lesions. They may have areas of mixed CSF, lipid, and soft-tissue characteristics, as well as calcification. Some of teratomas are circumscribed masses with fatty areas, a feature notably absent from all the other tumor types.

Low to intermediate signal on T1-weighted images and intermediate to high signal on T2-weighted images are shown on MRI for pineoblastomas, demonstrating contrast enhancement. Given their highly malignant nature, it is not uncommon to see hemorrhage and necrosis within the lesion, with infiltration into adjacent structures with cerebral spinal fluid seeding and dissemination within the subarachnoid space. Pineoblastomas usually have low minimum ADC and restricted diffusion on DWI.

Case 2.2.2 Teratoma

Clinical Presentation

An 8-year-old boy was referred to our hospital with progressive weakness in his left extremities. He had no vomiting,

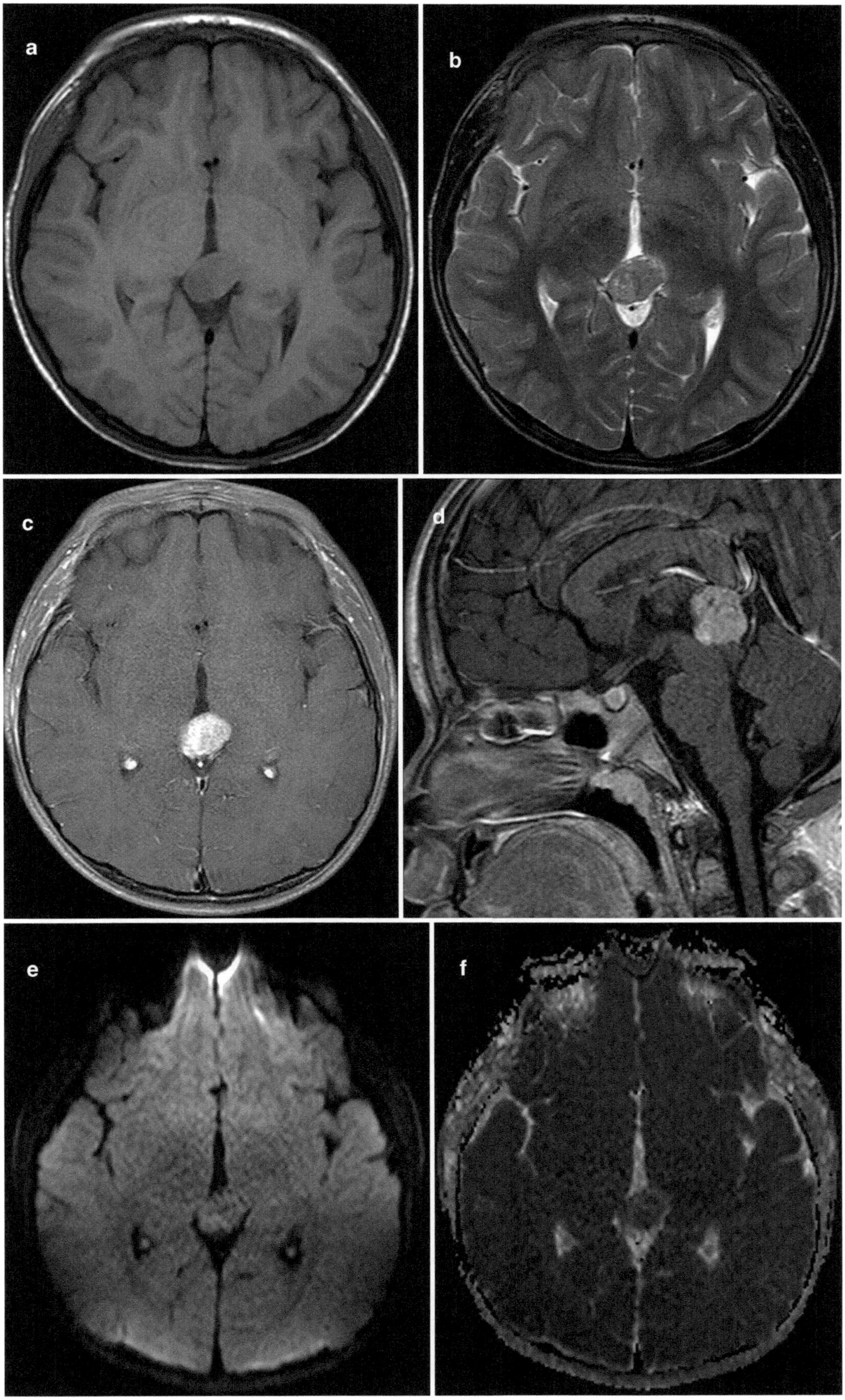

Fig. 2.13 Germinoma

convulsion, or fever. CT in other hospital showed a mass lesion in the midline region.

Imaging Findings

A. Axial T1-weighted shows a hypo-hyperintense mass in the pineal region (Fig. 2.14a).
B. Axial T2-weighted image shows a hypo-hyperintense mass in the pineal region (Fig. 2.14b).
C. FLAIR T2-weighted images show no obvious edema (Fig. 2.14c).
D. Sagittal contrast-enhanced T1-weighted image shows no enhancement (Fig. 2.14d).
E. Axial DWI image ($b = 800\ s/mm^2$) shows iso-hypointense (Fig. 2.14e).
F. Axial ADC image shows iso-hyperintense (Fig. 2.14f).

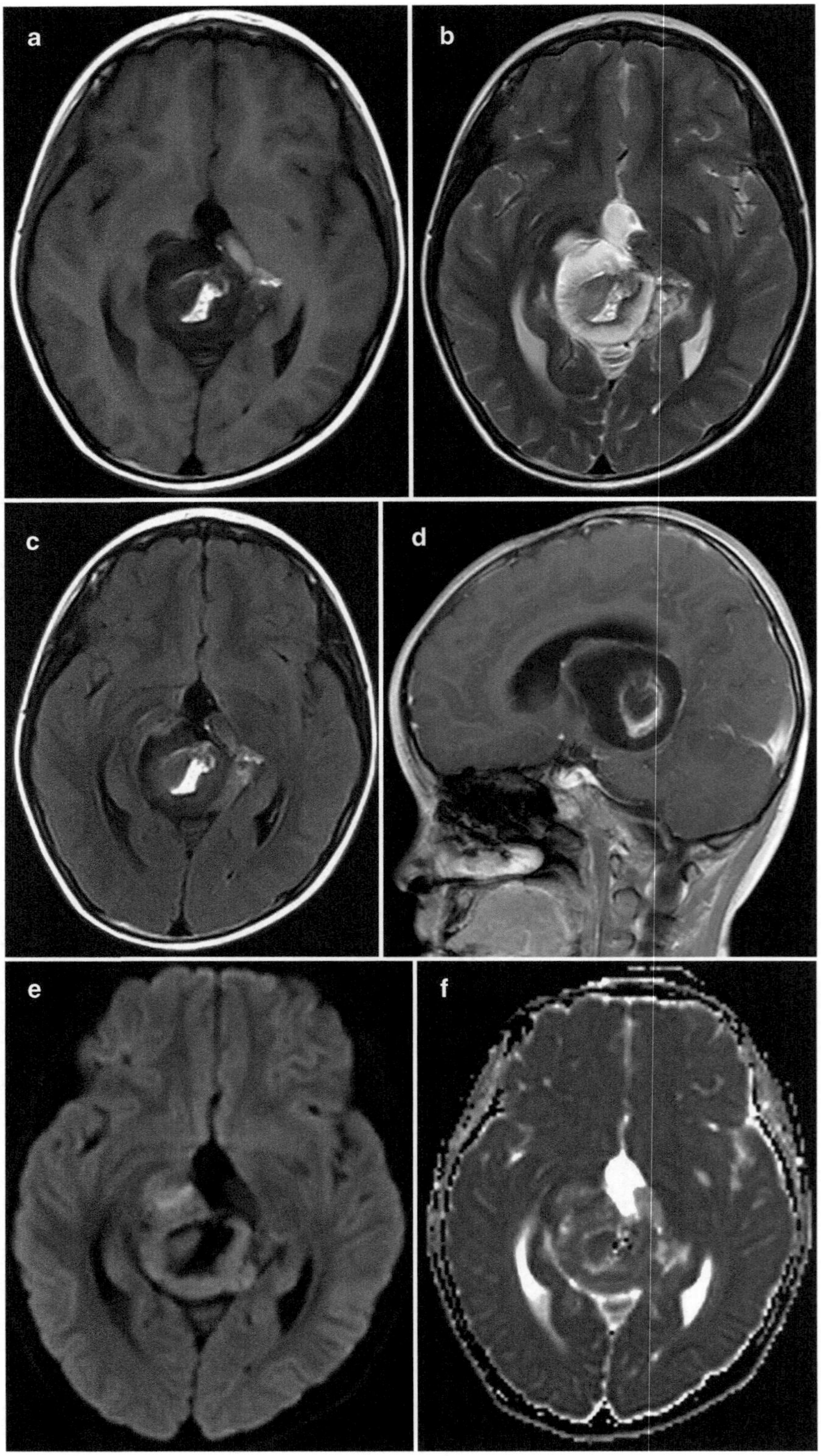

Fig. 2.14 Teratoma

Discussion

Germ cell tumors are composed of teratomas and germinoma. The incidence rate of pineal teratoma is relatively low. Teratomas are usually located either in the pineal region or in the sellar region. Its clinical manifestations depend on the location and size of the tumor. Pineal teratomas manifest as an increase in intracranial pressure, which are caused by a blockade of the upper orifice of the aqueduct of midbrain. Sellar teratomas commonly manifest as polydipsia, polyuria, and oftentimes, vision disorders.

The radiological appearance of teratoma varies with the contents. Mature teratomas are often large. The masses are irregular in shape and well-demarcated and show mixed density on plain CT scan. In all cases, multiple calcified regions and multiple cystic components are identified. Immature or malignant teratomas show isodense, low-density, mixed density masses. The shape is irregular, and the margin is partly or totally obscure. Small calcified areas and cystic components are also observed. Contrast enhancement shows marked but heterogenous enhancement [40]. However, it is not possible to make the diagnosis of teratoma on the basis of radiology alone in most instances. Therefore, in order to make a diagnosis of teratoma in such cases, a high index of suspicion and thorough histopathological examination of the encephalocele sac and contents are warranted.

Differential diagnosis: Several imaging features have been analyzed including calcifications, presence of cysts, and pattern of contrast enhancement as possible findings to differentiate pure germinomas from non-germinomatous germ cell tumors. However, there are no specific radiological appearances, which would enable such a distinction with certainty.

Differentiation from pineal parenchymal tumors (pineocytoma, pineal parenchymal tumor with intermediate differentiation, pineoblastoma) is not easy, because of the overlapping imaging findings on conventional techniques, including T1WI, T2WI, and pattern of enhancement. However, germinomas show higher ADC values than the pineal cell tumors.

Case 2.2.3 Pineocytoma

Clinical Presentation

A 1-year-old girl was admitted due to a sudden onset for 4 days of apathy, narcolepsy, and vomiting.

Image Findings

A. Axial T1-weighted image shows a hypointense mass in the pineal region (Fig. 2.15a).
B. Axial T2-weighted image shows a hypointense mass in the pineal region (Fig. 2.15b).
C. Axial contrast-enhanced T1-weighted image shows heterogeneous enhancement (Fig. 2.15c).
D. Sagittal contrast-enhanced T1-weighted image shows heterogeneous enhancement (Fig. 2.15d).

Discussion

Pineocytomas are rare benign tumors classified as WHO grade I, which arise from pineal parenchymal cells. Pineocytomas constitute about 14–30% of tumors in the pineal region within all ages, but mostly present in adults from age 30 to 60 [41]. Signs and symptoms are hydrocephalus, increased intracranial pressure with consequent headaches, nausea, visual changes, and ataxia.

Histologically, pineocytomas are composed of medium-sized neoplastic cells resembling mature pineocytes. These tumor cells are uniform and show a diffuse to loosely nested-growth pattern. Round to oval nuclei are seen with a delicate or "salt-and-pepper" chromatin. Pineocytomatous rosettes are a characteristic feature of pineocytomas, but are not present in all cases. Endothelial hyperplasia is not a distinctive feature, although it has been reported in some cases; necrosis is typically absent [42]. Ganglionic and glial differentiation can sometimes be observed [43, 44].

On CT, pineocytomas are well-demarcated, usually less than 3 cm, and iso- to hyperattenuating. On MR imaging, they can appear as hyperintense lesions on T2WI with homogeneous enhancement without associated restricted diffusion or increased perfusion. Furthermore, cysts and hemorrhage can be found within these lesions. The lesion may be entirely cystic, with a fluid–fluid level.

Differential diagnosis: compared with gray matter on both T1- and T2-weighted images, germinomas can appear as a solid pineal mass with intermediate to slightly high signal. In 20–52% of cases, cystic components are commonly identified, and post-contrast enhancement is usually present on MRI.

Demonstrating a multi-loculated and lobulated lesion with mixed signal, teratomas include areas of high signal intensity on T1-weighted images due to the presence of fat or lipid components, and areas of low signal due to calcification. There is usually a low to intermediate signal of soft-tissue components on T2-weighted images. Enhancement of the soft-tissue components can be shown in post-contrast images. There is a more homogeneous imaging appearance with fewer cysts and calcifications for teratomas with malignant transformation.

A low to intermediate signal on T1-weighted images and intermediate to high signal on T2-weighted images are shown on MRI for pineoblastomas, demonstrating contrast enhancement. Given their highly malignant nature, it is not uncommon to see hemorrhage and necrosis within the lesion, with infiltration into adjacent structures with cerebral spinal fluid seeding and dissemination within the subarachnoid space. Pineoblastomas usually have low minimum ADC and restricted diffusion on DWI.

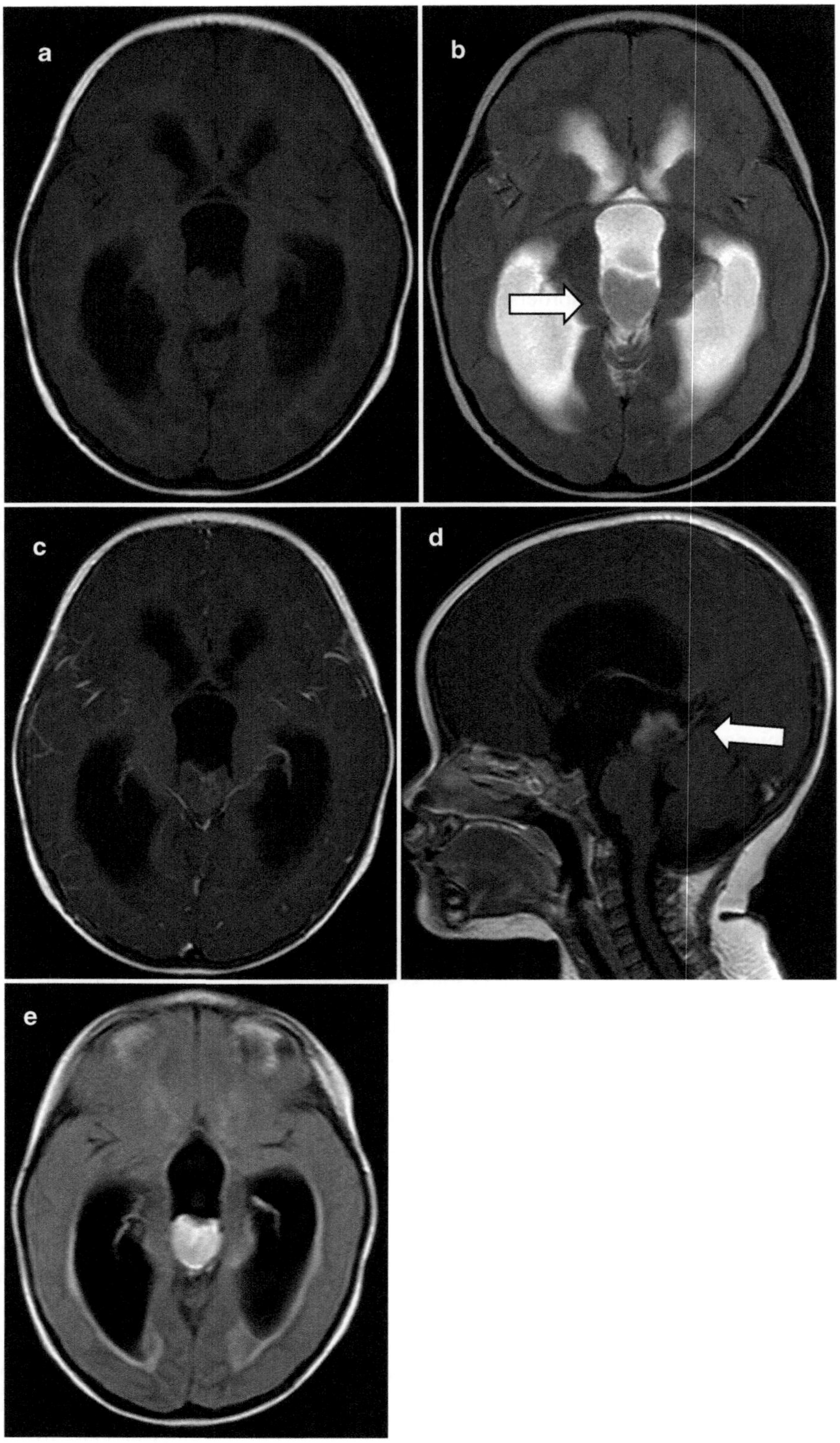

Fig. 2.15 Pineocytoma

2.3 Choroid Plexus Tumors

Case 2.3.1 Choroid Plexus Papilloma

Clinical Presentation

A 9-month-old girl had vomiting with reaction difference for 2 days.

Imaging Findings

A. Axial T1WI showed an irregular vegetative mass in the posterior part of the left ventricle, with a clear boundary and a size of about 2.0 cm × 3.1 cm × 3.3 cm. It was an equal signal on T1WI (Fig. 2.16a).
B. Axial T2WI showed the signal intensity of the mass is equal (Fig. 2.16b).

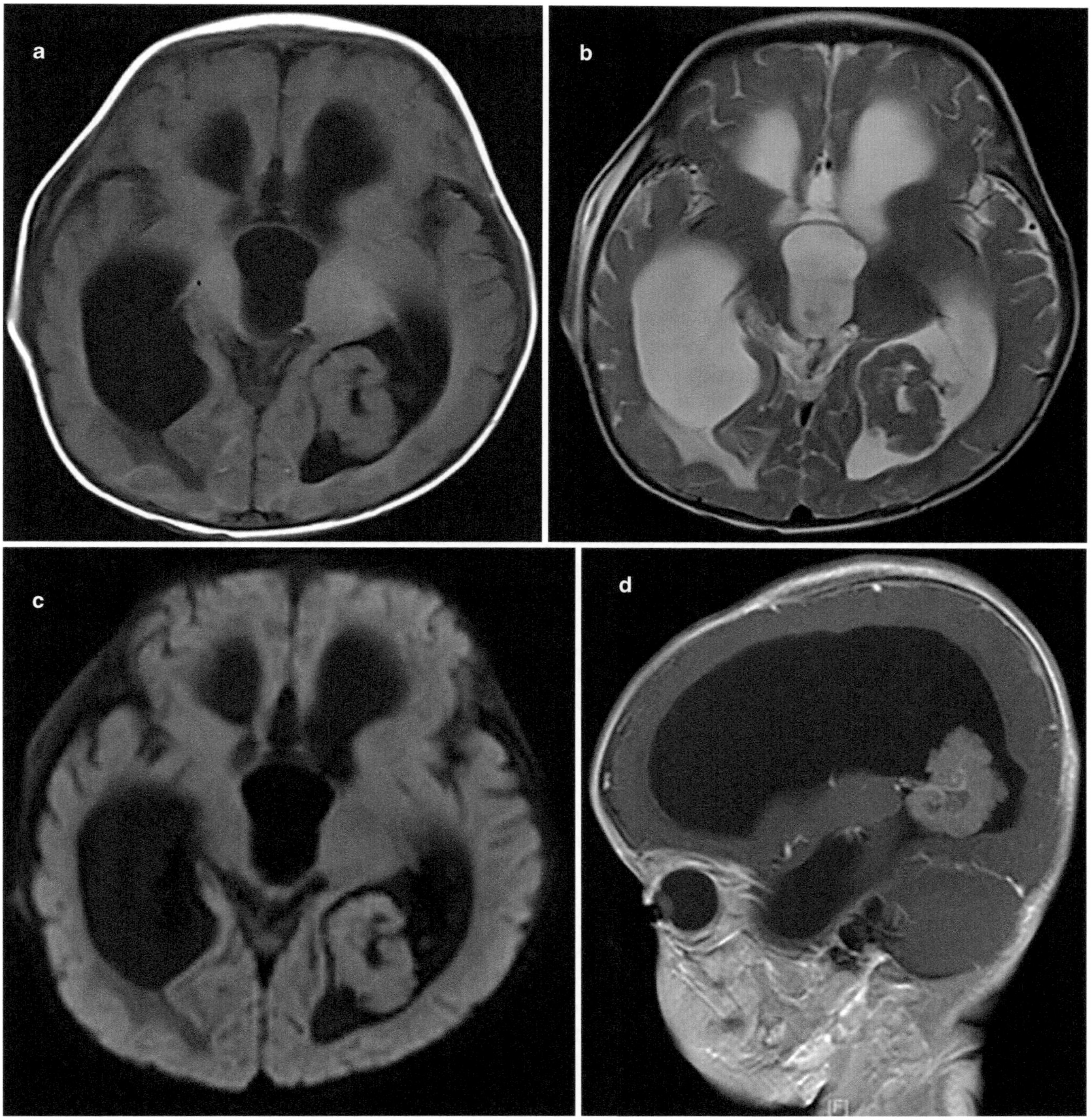

Fig. 2.16 Choroid plexus papilloma

C. DWI showed the mass with equal signal (Fig. 2.16c).
D. Sagittal T1WI-enhanced showed mild uniform enhancement after enhancement. The ventricular system was dilated, and stromal edema was seen beside the ventricles on both sides (Fig. 2.16d).

Discussion

Choroid plexus tumor originates from the choroid plexus papillomatous epithelial cells of the ventricle. The most common sites are the fourth ventricle and the lateral ventricle; only a very small fraction arises from the outside of the ventricle. Its incidence is relatively low, accounting for 0. 3 ~ 0. 6%. In 2016, according to the WHO Classification of Tumors of the Central Nervous System, choroid plexus tumor is divided into benign choroid plexus papilloma (WHO grade I), atypical choroid plexus papilloma (WHO grade II), and choroid plexus papilloma carcinoma (WHO grade III). The overall sex difference of choroid plexus papilloma is not obvious, and the incidence in the lateral ventricle is mostly in children, especially children under

2 years, while the incidence in the subtentorium is mostly in adults. The most common complication of tumor is hydrocephalus, which is considered to be an important diagnostic indicator. Its reasons are mainly as follows: The tumor directly leads to cerebrospinal fluid circulation obstruction (obstructive hydrocephalus) and the generation of cerebrospinal fluid and absorb disorder (traffic sex hydrocephalus); its most main expression is the size of tumor and hydrocephalus degree is out of proportion; smaller tumor often causes heavier hydrocephalus. The supratentorial tumor is mostly traffic hydrocephalus, and subtentorial tumor is mostly obstructive hydrocephalus. Immunohistochemical staining showed almost all of the choroid plexus papillomas express cytokeratin and vimentin; about 90% of the cases express S-100 and at the same time express negative EMA.

Under the microscope, the tumor cells are well differentiated and have the appearance of normal choroid plexus tissue, presenting as single rectangular or columnar epithelial cells neatly arranged in the basal interstitium. Under electron microscope, the tumor cells present a single columnar appearance, arranged into a mastoid shape, and the surface of the tumor cells is rich in the microvilli of tumor flourishing growth. The tumor cells could be shed and planted and disseminated along the cerebrospinal fluid circulation. The transthyretin thought to be associated with choroid plexus papilloma has relative specificity.

The tumor grows slowly, rarely produces malignant change, and grows more along cerebral interior; the form is cauliflower-shaped or nodular; the surface shows irregular papillary process appearance protuberant, with clear circumferential brain organization delimit, rarely cystic change, hemorrhage necrotic, and visible fine calcification grain. On CT plain scan, it is shown to have slightly uniform density or slightly dense or mixed density shadow, with a few cystic changes or calcification. T1-weighted MR shows slightly lower signal; t2-weighted MR shows high signal, clear boundary with CSF, and irregular tumor profile. CT and MRI have obvious enhancement. It is the most important imaging feature of the tumor that the small granular signal can be distinguished by MRI.

Usually, the fourth brain choroid plexus papilloma needs to be distinguished from the following [45] Medulloblastoma: It occurs in the midline, with common cysts, little calcification, and moderate uneven enhancement after enhanced scan. (2) Ependymoma: Mixed signal/density, clear but not smooth tumor margin, common bleeding, calcification, cystic degeneration and necrosis, and other secondary manifestations of tumors; enhanced scan shows obvious uniform enhancement. Usually, it is difficult to distinguish between the tumors originated in the choroid plexus papillary epithelial cells and those originated in ependymal epithelium. But maybe immunohistochemical staining will help the differential diagnosis.

Case 2.3.2 Atypical Choroid Plexus Papilloma

Clinical Presentation

A 2-month-old boy vomited with reaction difference for 2 days. After delivery, MR suggested the consideration of subendymal cyst due to "mass in the head."

Imaging Findings

A. Axial T1WI showed a large cystic solid space-occupying lesion was seen in the left ventricle, mainly cystic lesions, which presented CSF signals. The solid part had a slightly lower signal on T1WI (Fig. 2.17a).
B. Axial T2WI showed the signal intensity of the mass solid is slightly higher (Fig. 2.17b).
C. DWI showed the mass with equal signal (Fig. 2.17c).
D. Coronal T1WI-enhanced showed obvious enhancement, while the cystic part did not show enhancement.The parenchyma around the tumor was compressed, and the midline was significantly compressed. Bilateral ventricles dilate and deform (Fig. 2.17d).

Discussion

Atypical choroid plexus papilloma is between choroid plexus papilloma and choroid plexus carcinoma. Compared to choroid plexus papilloma, the atypical choroid plexus papilloma will have higher density, multi-line nucleus, necrosis, and substantial growth, but the main difference between them is increased nuclear fission, and the only diagnostic criteria is fission ≥ 2/10 HPE [46], but cannot reach the standard in the diagnosis of cancer. But it does not meet the criteria for cancer diagnosis. It tends to strike young people in their 20 s. The boundary of the atypical choroid plexus papilloma is not clear. Edema around the choroid plexus is seen. It is lobulated or granular. Because the incidence of atypical choroid plexus papilloma is low and the tumor is new, few scholars research at home and abroad. Because of only a few case reports in imaging, no characteristic analysis, and clinical lack of awareness, it is difficult for preoperative diagnosis. Surgical excision may lead to recovery. Compared to choroid plexus papilloma, it is more prone to recurrence and can occur in CSF disseminated implantation. In imaging, it is similar to choroid plexus papilloma. However, it is more likely to invade the periphery of the ventricle [47], without obvious midline structural shift, and it is more likely to have small cystic degeneration.

Case 2.3.3 Choroid Plexus Carcinoma

Clinical Presentation

A 1-month-old boy presented with vomiting for 6 days, and the examination in the other hospital revealed a ventricular tumor for half a day.

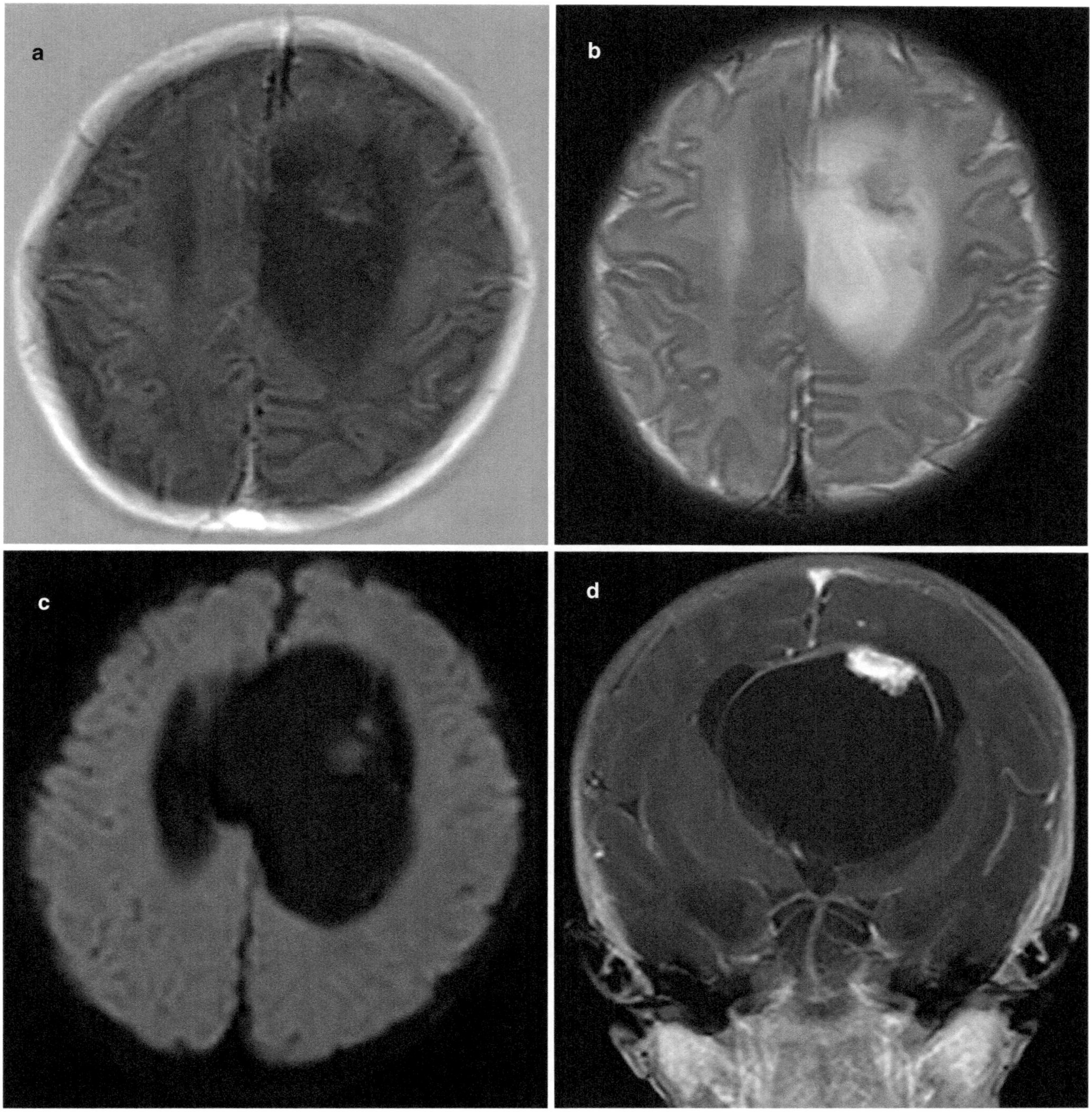

Fig. 2.17 Atypical choroid plexus papilloma

Imaging Findings

A. Axial T1WI showed a cystic solid mass spreading to the interventricular pore in the left lateral ventricle, and the boundary between the left basal ganglia and the pineal gland was not clear. The solid components of the tumor showed slightly lower signal on T1WI (Fig. 2.18a).

B. Axial T2WI showed the solid component of the tumor slightly higher signal (Fig. 2.18b).

C. DWI showed the mass with slightly higher signal (Fig. 2.18c).

D. Coronal T1WI-enhanced showed obvious enhancement in the solid component and the capsule wall of the tumor. The third ventricle was narrowed and the left basal ganglia is not clear with the compression (Fig. 2.18d).

Discussion

The etiology of choroid plexus carcinoma is not completely clear; some scholars think it may be related to choroid plexus papilloma. It mainly occurs in the lateral

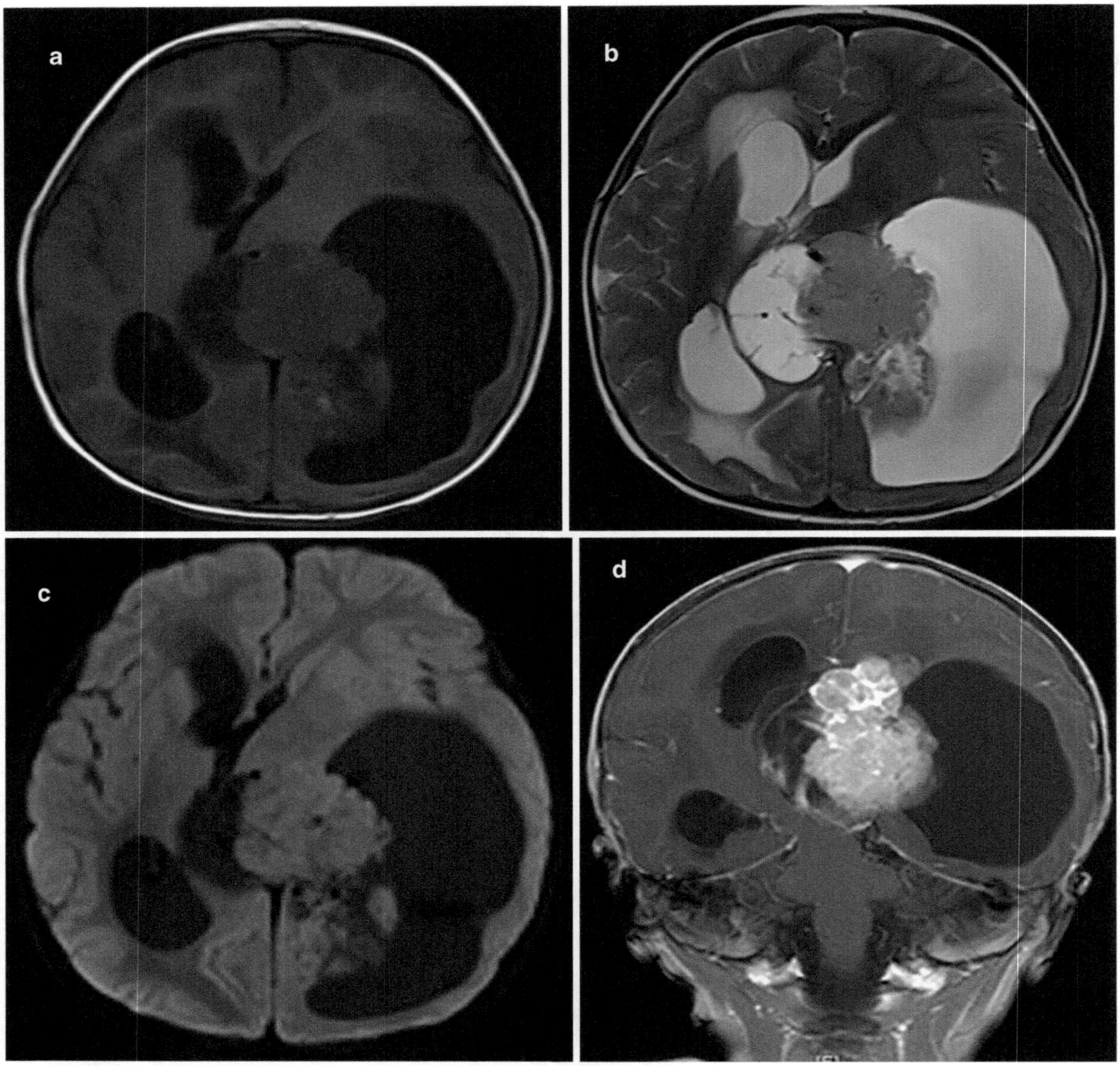

Fig. 2.18 Choroid plexus carcinoma

ventricle and the fourth ventricle. Its pathological manifestations are higher cell density, obvious nuclear atypia, and more frequent nuclear division. In imaging, the tumor is lobulated or cauliflower-shaped, often located in the ventricle or close to the wall of the ventricle, and beyond the edge of the ventricle to the brain parenchyma growth; boundary is not clear, some with calcification, bleeding, and necrosis. CT showed uneven density, and showed uneven enhancement after enhancement, with multiple invasions of the lateral ventricle wall and expansion to the brain tissue, causing vasogenic edema, and the tumor was often accompanied by hemorrhage and cystic changes. On MR, T1WI showed slightly lower signal and T2WI higher signal, which could invade adjacent tissues. The tumor can spread through CSF, grow rapidly, and have a poor prognosis [48].

2.4 Posterior Fossa Tumors

Case 2.4.1 Medulloblastoma

Clinical Presentation

A 5-year-boy presented with unsteady walk for 2 months. Previously, he had intermittent headache, persistent more intense dull pain, vomiting, and blurred vision.

Imaging Findings

A. Axial T1WI showed a round mass in vermis with hypointense signal (Fig. 2.19a).
B. Axial T2WI showed the tumor with slightly hyperintense (Fig. 2.19b).
C. T2WI-FLAIR showed the mass with slightly higher signal (Fig. 2.19c).

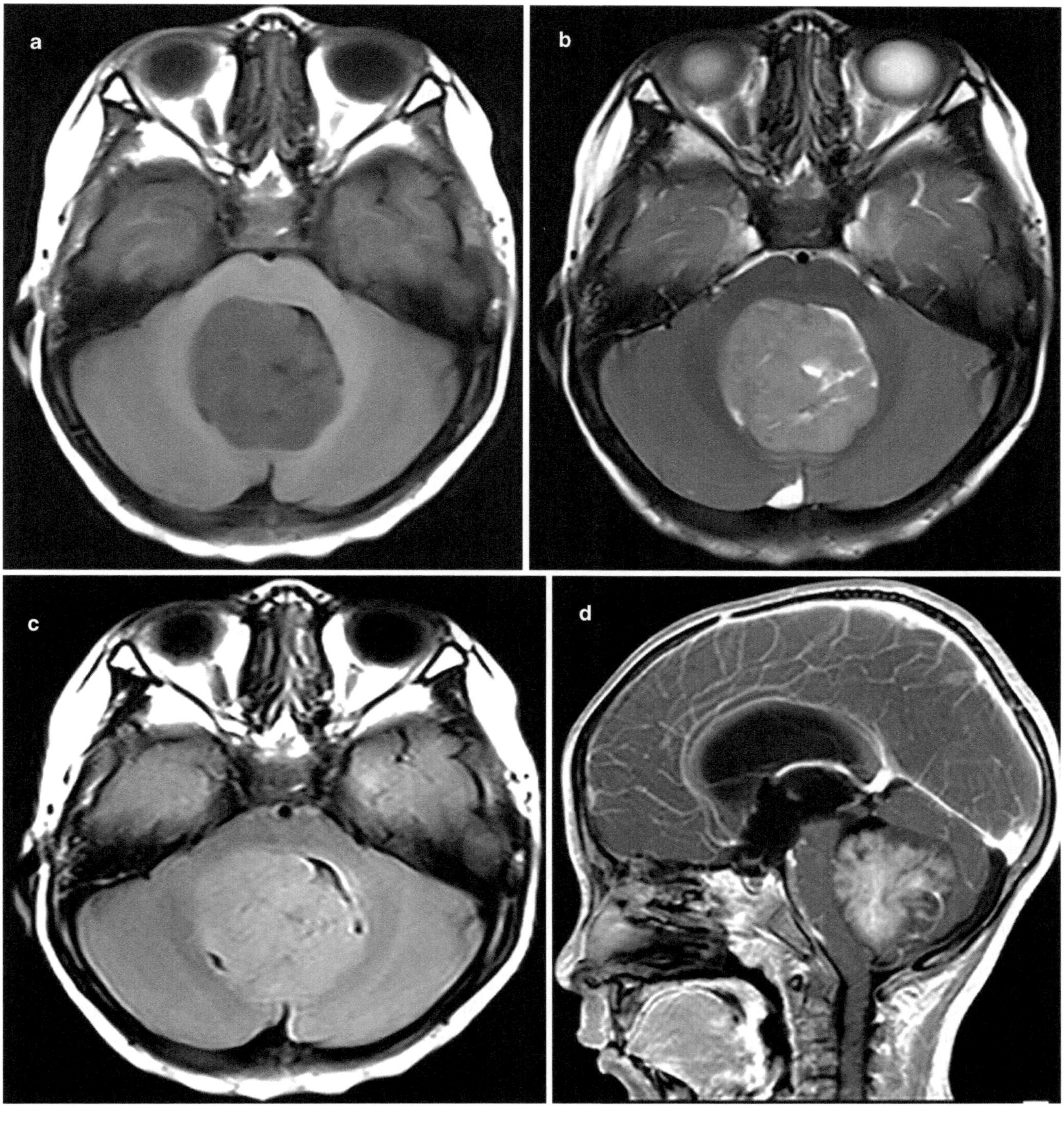

Fig. 2.19 Medulloblastoma

D. Coronal T1WI-enhanced showed the tumor with obvious uneven enhancement after enhancement scanning. The cerebellum and brainstem were compressed and displaced obviously (Fig. 2.19d).

Discussion

Medulloblastoma is the most common embryonal malignant tumor of the central nervous system during childhood, especially 5–10 years, accounting for 25% of all childhood intracranial tumor. Medulloblastoma is the most common malignant tumor in the posterior fossa. Usually, the first symptom is headache, vomiting, and gait instability; then diplopia, ataxia, and decreased visual acuity appear. Severe cases can have subarachnoid hemorrhage and the cerebellum crisis.

According to WHO 2016 classification definition, pathology can be divided into the following different subtypes: (1) classic, (2) desmoplastic/nodular (DN), (3) medulloblastoma with extensive nodularity (MBEN), and (4) large cell/anaplastic (LC/A). In recent years, MB genotyping gradually reached a consensus in the world. It is divided into the following four kinds of molecular subtypes: WNT, SHH, Group3, and Group4 type. In 2016, the WHO classified SNH into TP53 mutations type and wild type. Each performance is as follows:

1. MB WNT-activation type: the rarest. It accounts for only 11% of MB, with the median age of 10 ~ 12 years. Pathology is more typical. The overall survival is more than 90%.
2. MB SHH activation and TP53 mutations, MB SHH activation, and TP53 wild: about 28% of MB. The incidence is bidirectional, under the age of 4 and more than 16 years. Almost all of the connective tissue hyperplasia MB belong to the SHH group, but SHH can also be seen in typical and large cell/mesenchymal MB. Its prognosis was second to WNT group, but SHH with TP53 mutation had a poor prognosis.
3. Group3 type: It accounts for about 28%, with worst prognosis and very distant metastases. Pathological type is more typical and large cell/between variant. The pathologic types are typical and large cell /intercellular variant.
4. Group4 type: It is the most common and accounts for about 34%, about two-thirds of patients have abnormal chromosome 17 q (i17q). The peak age of onset is 10 years, and it is rare under 3 years. Compared with Group3, the prognosis was relatively good.

CT manifestations: MB usually occurs near the midline of the superior vermis of the cerebellum and can penetrate into the fourth ventricle. A few occur in the cerebellar hemisphere and cerebellopontine angle. CT findings are usually round, nodular, or slightly dense; bleeding and calcification are rare. The mass with more necrotic sac and less parenchyma presents low-density shadow, and the internal density is more uneven. Most of the tumor parenchyma show uniform moderate or obvious enhancement on enhanced scanning. MB can also spread along CSF to the supratentorial meninges and brain parenchyma. Vertebral body and distant bone tissue metastasis can also occur [49].

MRI manifestations: The tumor morphology is mostly circular, and a small part is deeply lobulated, with low signal on T1WI and iso- or slightly high signal on T2WI; multiple dotted or circular cystic areas were mostly visible inside. Edema signals are often present around the tumor. More importantly, the diffuse diffusion-weighted image of medulloblastoma is diffusion limited.

Differential diagnosis: (1) The ependymomas of the fourth ventricle: Ependymomas tend to grow along the lateral foramen of the fourth ventricle to the orifice of cerebellopontine angle on both sides, and calcification is common. MB is, however, rarely located in the fourth ventricle for growth, and calcification is rare. When the above two points to identify difficult, according to the origin of differential between, namely MB originated in the cerebellar vermis top four ventricle wall, sagittal position or axis of MRI is the front line of cerebrospinal fluid signal tumor is separated from the brain stem, which originated in the bottom of the fourth ventricle ependymoma, sagittal position or axis of an MRI is the rear line samples of cerebrospinal fluid shadow parts tumors with cerebellar vermis. (2) Astrocytoma: Most of them were cystic masses with mural nodules, and the lesions on CT are mostly low-density shadows, which are more likely to occur in the vermis of the cerebellum. MB is dominated by solid masses, which can have cystic changes. The density of plain CT scan and enhanced CT scan is higher than that of astrocytomas. The differential diagnosis is not difficult to be familiar with the typical imaging manifestations of the two.

Case 2.4.2 Pilocytic Astrocytoma

Clinical Presentation

A 12-year-old girl was admitted to the hospital with intermittent headache for a year, with dyskinesia and personality changes for more than 10 days.

Imaging Findings

A. Axial T1WI showed a cystic solid mass in the cerebellar vermis—left cerebellar hemisphere with clear boundary (Fig. 2.20a).
B. Axial T2WI showed the solid part of the tumor with high signal,and cystic component with higher signal (Fig. 2.20b).
C. Sagittal T1WI-enhanced showed the tumor with obvious after enhanced scanningin. The cerebellum and brainstem were compressed and displaced obviously. The cystic part showed fluid signal and no enhanced. The fourth ventricle was raised by push press (Fig. 2.20c).

Discussion

Childhood pilocytic astrocytoma is more common in the cerebellum and brainstem, WHO grade I. Pilocytic astrocytoma of the cerebellar hemisphere is one of the most common brain tumors in children with the highest incidence of gliomas, most of which occur at the age of 5–19 years, with the peak age of 5–9 years, and most of them are astrocytomas [50]. Tumors can compress the fourth ventricle, resulting in cerebrospinal fluid circulation disturbance, intracranial hypertension, ataxia, headache, vomiting, gait instability, and other clinical manifestations.

According to the types of cysts, there are three types of pilocytic astrocytomas: (1) cyst type, presenting as non-walled nodules or solid masses, (2) cyst nodule type, cystic lesion with wall nodule, and (3) solid mass type, mainly solid or not accompanied by cystic changes. Pilocytic astrocytoma in the posterior fossa is rare.

Imaging findings: CT shows that pilocytic astrocytoma is usually low-density lesions with clear boundary and no obvi-

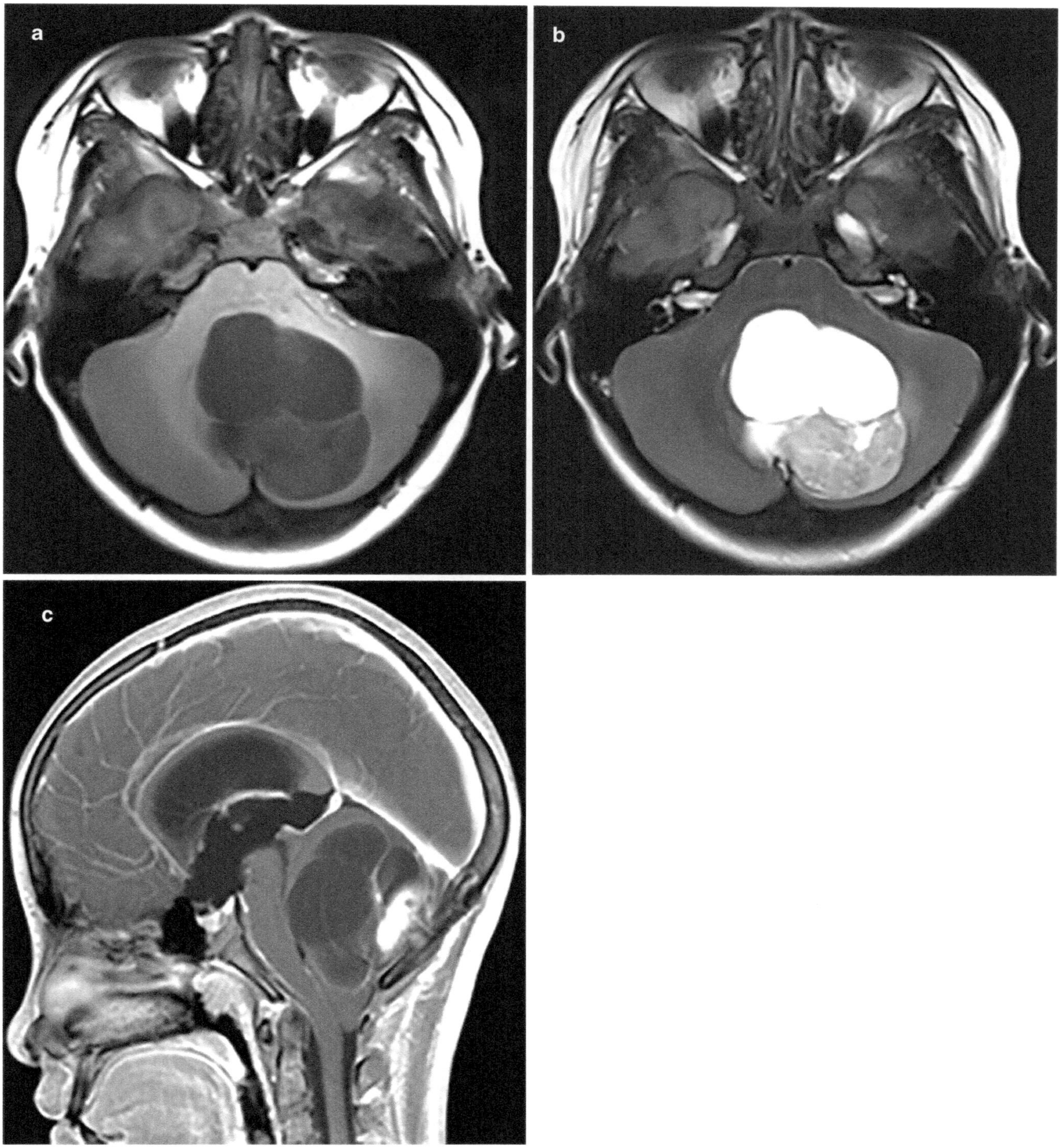

Fig. 2.20 Pilocytic astrocytoma

ous edema around. On MRI, tumor signals often show low signal on T1WI and high signal on T2WI, and uneven signal when calcification occurs. The diffusion-weighted image shows that the dispersion is not restricted. It may be significantly unevenly enhanced after enhancement.

Usually, pilocytic astrocytomas in the posterior fossa need to be distinguished from the following: (1) Medulloblastoma: It occurs in the midline, with common cysts, little calcification, and moderate uneven enhancement after enhanced scan. It is diffusion-constrained in diffusion-weighted images. This is an important basis for identification of pilocytic astrocytomas. (2) Ependymoma: Mixed signal/density, clear but not smooth tumor margin, common bleeding, calcification, cystic degeneration and necrosis, and other secondary manifestations of tumors; enhanced scan show obvious uniform enhancement.

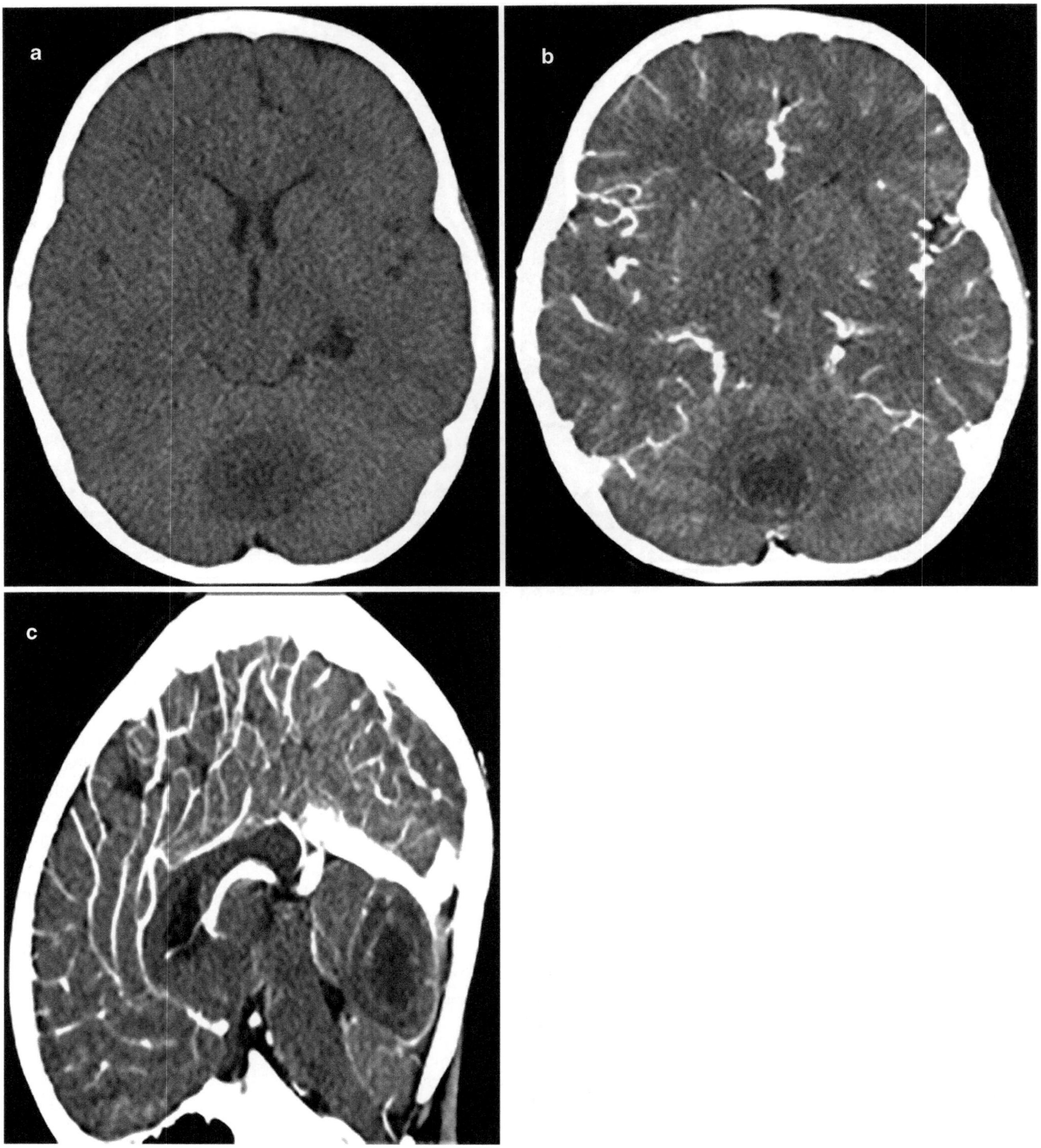

Fig. 2.21 Pilomyxoid astrocytoma (PMA)

Case 2.4.3 Pilomyxoid Astrocytoma (PMA)

Clinical Presentation

A 6-year-old girl was not able to walk steadily for a month.

Imaging Findings

A. Axial CT shows a solid mass in the cerebellum vermis with uneven and slightly lower density (Fig. 2.21a).

B. Axial enhanced CT scan showed mild uneven enhancement (Fig. 2.21b).
C. Sagittal T1WI-enhanced shows the fourth ventricle was slightly compressed. There was no peripheral edema (Fig. 2.21c).

Discussion

Pilomyxoid astrocytoma, a subtype of pilocytic astrocytoma, is a new classification defined by the WHO in 2016 for central nervous system tumors. It is an invasive pilocytic astrocytoma with a myxoid matrix, multipolar cells surrounding blood vessels, and no Rosenthal fibers or eosinophilic granule bodies. Recent studies have shown that PMA has a unique age and location of onset and has different histological and clinical characteristics from pilocytic astrocytoma. It is more invasive, prone to local recurrence, and prone to implant metastasis through cerebrospinal fluid, with a poor prognosis. It is more common in children under the age of 4; there is no significant gender difference. Most of the tumors were located near the midline, mainly involving the hypothalamus, optic chiasm, sella region and thalamus, and rarely the posterior fossa.

Its histological diagnosis can be summarized as follows [51]: (1) The tumor cells are monophasic and composed of bipolar spindle cells. (2) The tumor has a large mucinous background and is free of the dense and loose structure of the two-phase pilocytic astrocytoma. (3) The blood vessels were obviously proliferated. Some tumor cells were distributed around the blood vessels and arranged radially around the blood vessels. (4) There are free Rosenthal free fibers and eosinophilic granule bodies.

Immunohistochemical staining showed diffuse strong positive expression of glial fibrillary acidic protein, S-100 protein, and vimentin. It needs to be distinguished from mucus papillary ependymoma, spinal cord glioma, and hemangioblastoma of the cerebellum [52].

Most of the tumors were solid, while a few were mainly solid and partly cystic, with rare hemorrhage and calcification. On CT, the tumor mostly showed low density, followed by high and low mixed density, and high density was related to intratumoral hemorrhage. PMA on MRI plain scan is more complex, most of which is low signal on T1WI, part of which is equal signal, followed by low, high, or low mixed signal. Hydrocephalus is more common; tumor edema is rare. Compared with the pilocytic astrocytoma, the pilomyxoid astrocytoma is more prone to bleeding.

Case 2.4.4 Yolk Sac Tumor

Clinical Presentation

A 1-year-old boy presents with repeated vomiting for 10 days. Laboratory showed AFP greater than 1000.0 ng/mL.

Imaging Findings

A. Axial T2WI shows a solid neoplasm in the midline of the cerebellum with high signal intensity (Fig. 2.22a).
B. Axial T1WI showed the neoplasm with low signal intensity (Fig. 2.22b).
C. The tumor showed high signal on ADC, (Fig. 2.22c).
D. Sagittal image of the tumor was significantly enhanced by gadolinium contra-enhancement scan, accompanied by dilated hydrocephalus of superior mu ventricle (Fig. 2.22d).

Discussion

Yolk sac tumor as well as endodermal sinus tumor is a rare and highly malignant tumor derived from pluripotent primitive germ cells. It often occurs in the gonads of infants and children. The primary tumor is rare in intracranial and even rarer in the cerebellum. Intracranial yolk sac tumor is more common in men.

The clinical manifestations of intracranial yolk sac tumor are related to tumor size and location. The main manifestations of vitellocystic tumor in the cerebellum are recurrent vomiting of intracranial hypertension, vestibular dysfunction, and convulsion [53]. In addition, AFP was significantly elevated in cerebellar yolk sac tumor.

In cerebellar yolk cystic tumor, MR is well bounded, low signal intensity on T2WI, and high signal intensity on T2WI. When the tumor is larger, it may be accompanied by cystic degeneration and necrosis, with mixed signals and varying degrees of obstructive hydrocephalus. There was obvious enhancement after enhancement scan. It should be noted that the ADC of cerebellar yolk sac tumor showed high signal intensity, suggesting unrestricted diffusion, which may be related to the loose network structure of tumor tissue. Cerebellar yolk cyst tumor is mainly differentiated from astrocytoma, medulloblastoma, and atypical teratoma/rhabdomyoid tumor (AT/RT).

The diagnosis of cerebellar yolk sac tumor can be difficult. If combined with MR, ADC, and clinical AFP elevation, the diagnosis can be improved.

Case 2.4.5 Atypical Teratoid/Rhabdoid Tumor (AT/RT)

Clinical Presentation

A 2-year-old boy presented to the department of neurological rehabilitation with unstable walk for 2 month, head discomfort for half a month, and vomiting many times. His past medical, surgical, and family histories were negative. He had no recent trauma.

Imaging Findings

A. Axial T1WI showed a irregular mixed cystic mass and abnormal signal can be seen in the vermis cerebelli.

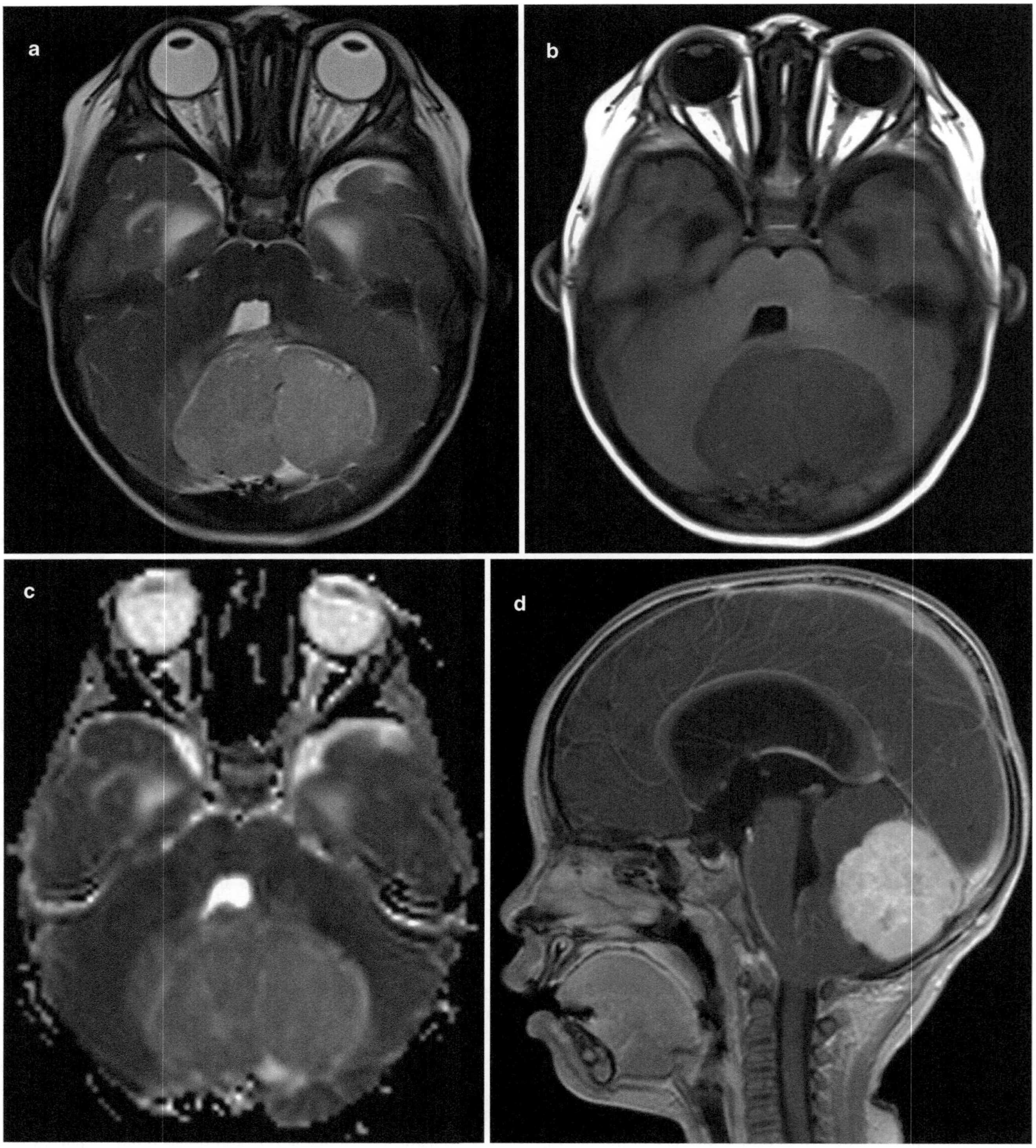

Fig. 2.22 Yolk sac tumor

T1WI showed low to intermediate signal intensity (Fig. 2.23a).

B. Axial T2WI showed showed high signal (Fig. 2.23b).

C. The solid component was uneven high signal on DWI (Fig. 2.23c).

D. Sagittal CE-T1WI sequence showed slight heterogeneous enhancement (Fig. 2.23d).

Discussion

Atypical teratoid/rhabdoid tumor (AT/RT) is a rare childhood malignant tumor of the central nervous system, with

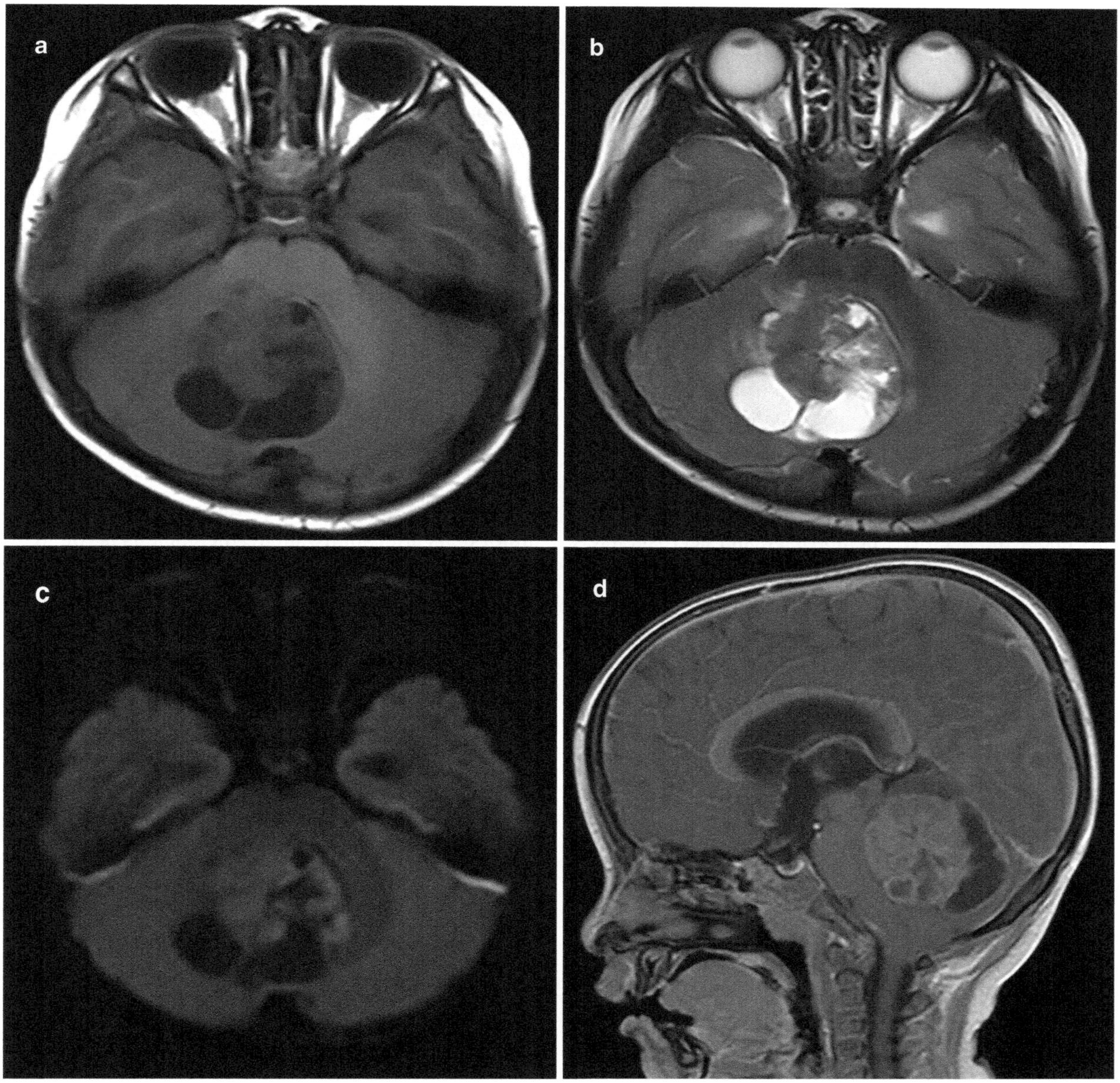

Fig. 2.23 Atypical teratoid/rhabdoid tumor (AT/RT)

invasion. AT/RT often occurs in children, especially under the age of 2 years. The tumor accounted for 1–2% of children of the central nervous system tumors, accounting for 10% of the infants. The male to female ratio is about 1.4:1. In recent years, the reports about the AT/RT are increasing by 1–2 cases, with poor prognosis, and most of the patients die in less than1 year [54].

AT/RT takes place in different parts of the body and has different manifestations. The tumors locate intracranial usually show the lesions caused by damage to the parts of the mental symptoms or neurologic. Such as side limb weakness or hemiplegia, gait instability ,sleepiness, and so on, combined with intracranial pressure, headache, and vomiting. It occurs in the spinal cord that is characterized by pain in both legs, developing into paralysis of lower limbs.

The pathogenesis of AT/RT is unclear. Maybe it relates to INI 1 mutation or missing. It is observed under light microscope. The sample contains striated muscle cells of the tumor, the original neural ectoderm and leaf which is between epithelial tissue and tumor tissues, but some cases do not have the typical sample striated muscle cells. Focal necrosis is one of its characteristics. Immunohistochemical staining often shows the tumor expresses EMA and vimentin and also expresses SMA, GFAP, NFP, and CK, and other germ cell tumor markers are negative. INI1 lack of expression is the most sensitive and specific indicator of tumor diagnosis. AT/RT and neuroectodermal tumor/medulloblastoma are very similar; differentiations rely on immunohistochemical staining.

Most tumors in children with AT/RT occur in the brain parenchyma, slightly more in the supratentorial region than infratentorial; part of tumor is grown across the cerebellum awning and rare within the brain and spinal cord. Usually, the tumor has larger size and rapid growth. The tumor size in supratentorial region is larger than infratentorial. Usually, the signal or density on MRI or CT was mixed, accompanied by cystic degeneration, hemorrhage, necrosis, and calcification. Solid composition is high signal on DWI; accordingly the ADC is characterized by low signal. Most of the tumors are moderate or obvious reinforcement, and individual cases can be mild. Dynamic enhancement was delayed reinforcement on CT.

The tumor needs to be differentiated from pilocytic astrocytoma and germ cell tumors, especially MB3 [55]. AT/RT is similar to MB in radiology and pathological histology. MB peak age is 5–7 years, and has rare cystic change, necrosis, and hemorrhage. Usually, AT/RT more often occurs in patients under the age of 2, hemorrhage and necrosis likely appear, and the prognosis is worse. Pilocytic astrocytoma occurs in the midline, and which is the act to pouch or solid, solid on screen to see more, few bleeding, calcification. As AT/RT is a highly malignant tumor, is aggressive, has tumor cell density, and is diffusion limited.

Case 2.4.6 Ependymoma

Clinical Presentation

A 3-year-old boy presented with intermittent vomiting for more than a month, accompanied by abdominal pain.

Imaging Findings

A. Axial T1WI showed the fourth ventricle was enlarged and there was a large lobu lated mass shadow with equal and low signal (Fig. 2.24a).
B. Axial T2WI showed slightly high and high signal (Fig. 2.24b).
C. DWI showed equal signal (Fig. 2.24c).
D. Sagittal CE-T1WI sequence showed mild enhancement. The tumor extended downward into the foramen occipital region, and the outlet of the fourth ventricle was compressed and narrowed (Fig. 2.24d).

Discussion

Ependymoma is a central nervous system tumor of spinal cord central canal; ependymal cells nests in the white matter between ventricle and ventricle or ependymal cells. It is also more common in children. In 2016, the ependymoma is divided into I–III level by the WHO Classification of Tumors of the Central Nervous System (2). WHO I ependymoma is a benign tumor, WHO II is between benign and malignant, and WHO III type according to variant ependymoma is a malignant ependymoma, spread easily with cerebrospinal fluid. It is aggressive, has a poorer prognosis, and is easy to relapse. Ependymomas are slow growing and tend to be distended rather than aggressive. Its clinical manifestations are closely related to the site of growth, size, age, and presence of pia mater metastasis.

Ependymomas are mostly located in the fourth ventricle and can be classified into three relatively fixed positions: (1) The most common occurrence is at the bottom of the fourth ventricle. In the process of tumor growth, the lower part of the fourth ventricle was first filled and through the posterior median hole extended to the back of the cervical spinal cord. Therefore, the patients showed torticula and ataxia in addition to increased intracranial pressure. (2) A small portion of it occurs in the lateral recess, where the tumor may wrap around and/or compress the pons as it grows into the quadrennial ventricle, and grows down the surface of the medulla oblongata. Patients at this site often have posterior cranial nerve symptoms, including hearing impairment, dysarthria, dysphagia, and poor pitch discrimination. (3) It occurs less frequently in the four-chambered roof. Ataxia can occur when the vermis is stressed.

Histopathological manifestations: (1) Microscopically, tumor cells are usually small; the nucleus is round or oval, with moderate cytoplasm. Tumor cells may appear as characteristic chrysanthemum or pseudochrysanthemum clusters. (2) Under electron microscope, the tumor cells were embedded and arranged, and two or more adjacent cells formed microchrysanthemum clusters. There are a lot of microvilli and cilia on the surface of the inner lumen of microchrysanthemum group. The cilium is surrounded by cell membrane and cytoplasm and contains microtubules.

The tumors on CT plain scan were equally dense, with scattered calcification and cystic degeneration in a small number of cases. Ependymoma shows equal or slightly lower signal on TIW1 and higher signal on T2W1. Ependymoma is usually located in the fourth ventricle. It can extend to the periphery through the lateral foramen and median foramen, and the tumor is often surrounded by cerebrospinal fluid.

Ependymoma should be differentiated from the following diseases: (1) Medulloblastoma: It originated from the original embryonic residual cells of the posterior medulla of the fourth ventricle. It can occupy the whole fourth ventricle rapidly and implant metastasis is easy to occur. It has higher CT density, less bleeding, necrosis, and cystic degeneration. (2) Pilocytic astrocytoma: It often happens in the cerebellum hemisphere; more expression is seen in the cystic mass that accompanies tumor nodule. The enhancement of nodules was obvious after enhanced scanning.

2.5 Tumors and Tumor-Like Lesions of the Sellar Region

Case 2.5.1 Craniopharyngioma

Clinical Presentation

A 7-year-old boy had suffered with symptoms of vomiting and dizziness for half a year. His past medical and family histories and physical examination were negative.

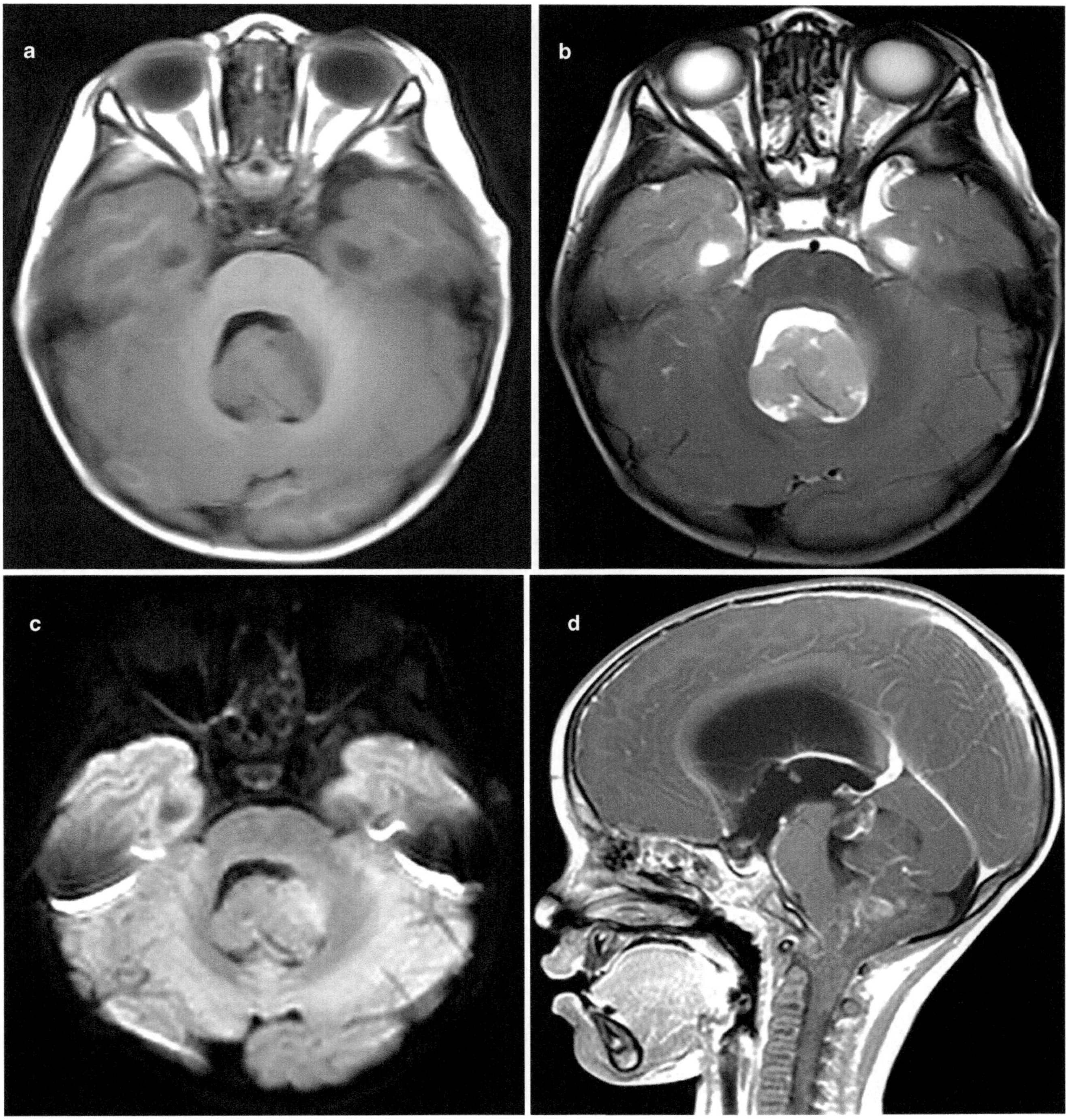

Fig. 2.24 Ependymoma

Imaging Findings

A-C. Axial MR images show a cystic-solid space-occupying heterogeneous mass in the sellar and parasellar region, high signal was shown in the right front part of the mass (Fig. 2.25a–c).

D. Sagittal T1-weighted image demonstrates the mass with remarkable hyperintense (Fig. 2.25d).

E-F. Sagittal contrast-enhanced T1-weighted images demonstrates the slightly enhancing cystic wall (Fig. 2.25e–f).

G-H. CT images show calcifications with popcorn and eggshell forms of the mass (Fig. 2.25g–h).

Discussion

Craniopharyngiomas are the most common tumors of the sellar/parasellar region in childhood, with a similar incidence in both sexes, and a bimodal age distribution has been shown: 5–10 years and 60–70 years [56].

Craniopharyngiomas can be solid, cystic, or mixed. They have two pathology subtypes: adamantinomatous and papillary. Craniopharyngiomas typically sit in the midline with low histological grade (WHO I°). The majority located above sella and other rare locations include nasopharynx, paranasal area, sphenoid bone, ethmoid sinus, and others. The Pathogenesis of craniopharyngioma is explained by two the-

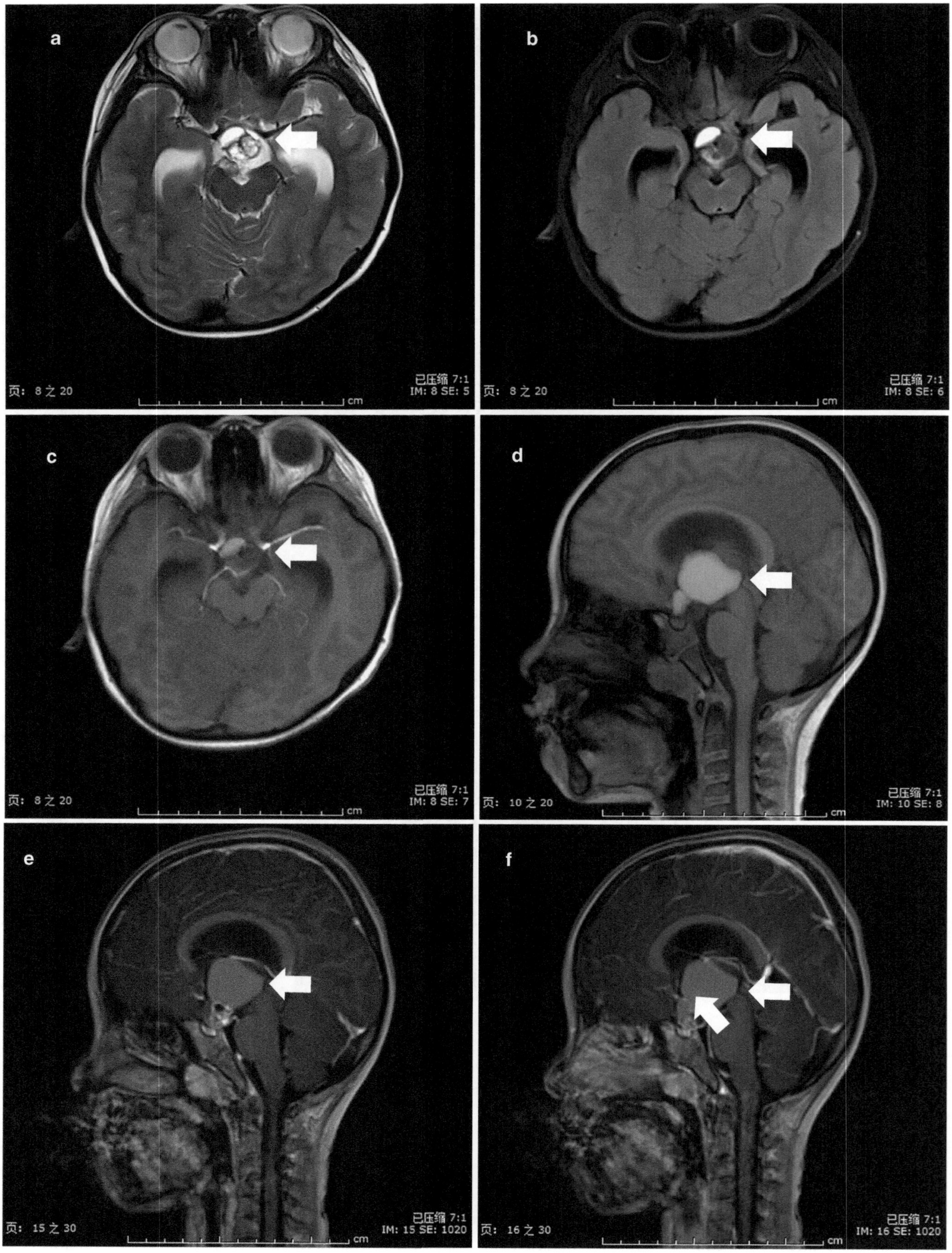

Fig. 2.25 Craniopharyngioma

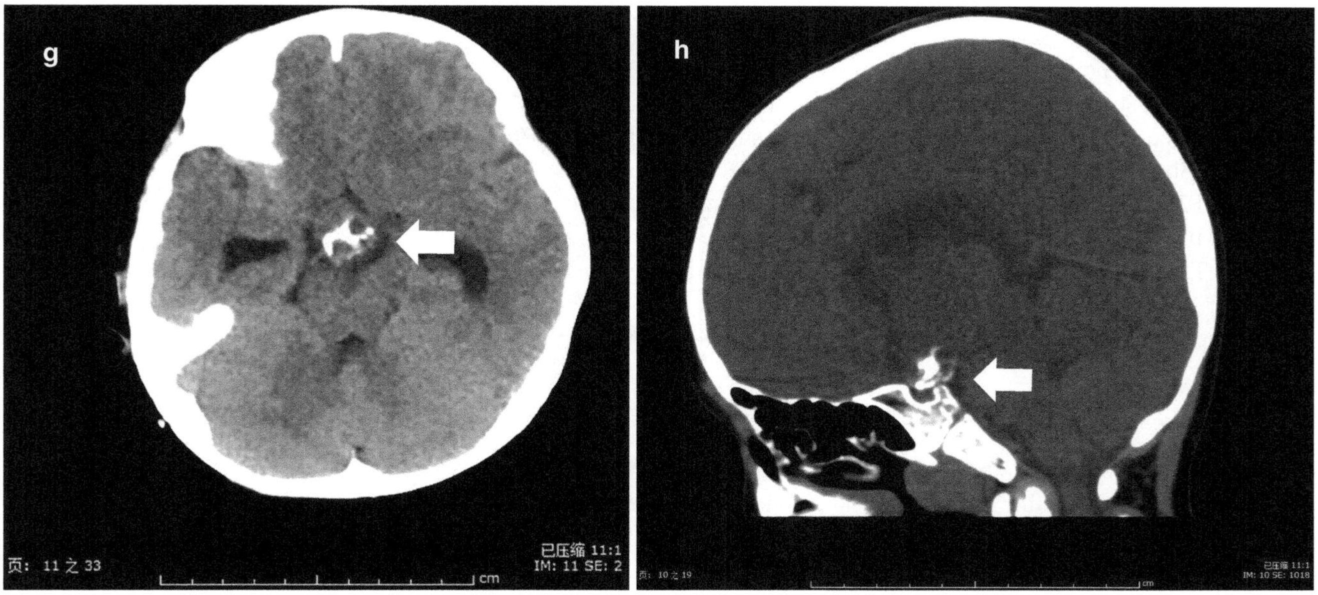

Fig. 2.25 (continued)

ories: embryonic and metaplastic, although it is not completely understood [57].

Patients with craniopharyngioma may present with neurological, endocrinological, and visual symptoms. Vision impairment and endocrine deficits are the most common symptoms [56].

Calcifications are found in up to 90% of these tumors which might be definitively detected on computerized tomography (CT). Calcifications can be ring-shaped, thick or thin, and eggshell and might have popcorn forms. The signal of the cystic component varies in magnetic resonance imaging (MRI) T1WI and T2WI according to the contents, describing different signal patterns: protein, blood, fat, and fluid. After enhancement, the solid component and the wall of the cystic component are enhanced, usually suprasellar. The differential diagnosis of sellar/parasellar masses includes Rathke's cleft cyst, pituitary adenoma, epidermoid cyst, arachnoid cysts, colloid cyst of the third ventricle, and hypothalamic glioma [58].

Treatment strategies include neurosurgery and irradiation. For cystic recurrent craniopharyngiomas, intracystic instillation of sclerosing substances has been used. Craniopharyngiomas should require constant monitoring as a chronic disease.

Case 2.5.2 Glioma of Optic Chiasm and Hypothalamus

Clinical Presentation

A 12-year-old boy presented with vison loss and temporal visual field defect of left eye for 2 years. He had a history of head trauma 7 years ago and recovered after conservative treatment. Other past medical histories were negative. Laboratory tests showed a slight decrease in cortisol and increase in prolactin.

Imaging Findings

A-B. Coronal T1-weighted and T2-weighted images demonstrate a mass with irregular shape in suprasellar and intrasellar region, isointense to slightly hypointense relative to brain on T1WI and hyperintense on T2WI (Fig. 2.26a–b).

C-D. Coronal and Sagittal contrast-enhanced T1-weighted images show obvious inhomogeneous enhancement (Fig. 2.26c–d).

Discussion

Glioma of optic chiasm and hypothalamic is a subtype of optic pathway glioma (OPG), also known as optic chiasm-hypothalamic glioma (OCHG). OCHGs are rare astrocytic tumors that appear more commonly among young children and often are unresectable [59].

OCHGs account for approximately 2% of all central nervous system (CNS) tumors, 3–5% of pediatric CNS tumors, and 10–15% of supratentorial tumors in children. The median age of diagnosis is 7 years and 90% of the patients are diagnosed before 19 years. Males and females are equally affected. The main pathologic type of OCHGs is low-grade astrocytoma, especially pilocytic astrocytoma. OCHG is closely associated with neurofibromatosis type I (NFI) when it occurs in adults. The tumors are located in the sellar region and often involve optic nerve, optic chiasm, and hypothalamus, with poor prognosis. Vision loss is the most common symptom observed in patients with OCHGs. Other visual abnormalities, such as narrowing of the visual field and pendular movement nystagmus,

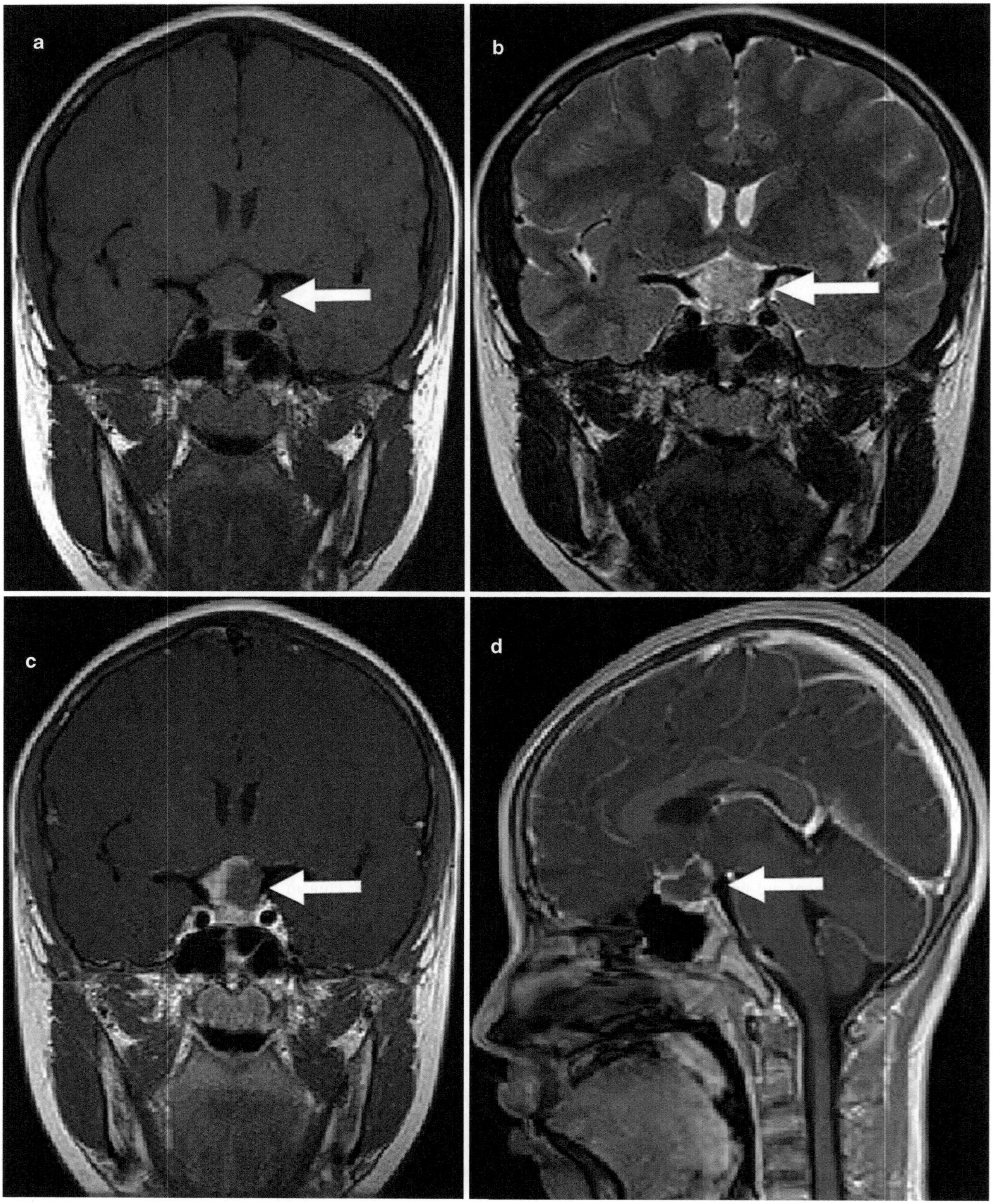

Fig. 2.26 Glioma of optic chiasm and hypothalamus

are also common. Obstruction of the third ventricle by tumors can lead to obstructive hydrocephalus. Patients often have headache, nausea, or vomiting. If this occurs in a child before 1 year of age, the head circumference will be expanded [60]. Tumors involving the hypothalamus may also present with endocrine abnormalities. The main clinical manifestations include polyuria, polydipsia, physical retardation, precocious puberty, menstrual disorders, and hypopituitarism.

Typical OCHGs are lobular masses with irregular shape. They are isointense to slightly hypointense relative to brain on T1WI and hyperintense on T2WI. The tumors are always large, but peritumoral edema is rare. Cystic elements, either microcysts or macrocysts, are common [61]. Because of the abundant vascularity of OCHGs, the solid part of the tumors often has obvious enhancement after enhanced scanning.

Although OCHGs are rare, it is necessary to differentiate them from sellar tumors. Craniopharyngiomas are the most common tumor in saddle area, accounting for about 4% of intracranial tumors. It is difficult to differentiate craniopharyngioma from OCHG on plain MRI. However, craniopharyngiomas are enhanced less than OCHGs, and the incidence of calcification is much higher than OCHGs. Suprasellar germinomas are also common in adolescents and children and may involve the optic chiasm. It can also be enhanced obviously which is similar to OCHGs. However, 75% of suprasellar germinomas are characterized by polyuria and polydipsia, while most of the first symptoms of OCHGs are visual impairment. In addition, suprasellar germinomas can be disseminated via cerebrospinal fluid. Discovery of lesions in other locations is often helpful in the diagnosis of suprasellar germinomas.

Case 2.5.3 Hypothalamic Hamartoma or Hamartoma of Tuber Cinereum

Clinical Presentation

A girl, 8 years old, presented with sexual precocity, breast development, vaginal bleeding, vulva maturation, and mental retardation. Bone age is 10 years. The uterus and ovaries had peripubertal morphology in abdominal ultrasonography The patient had generalized tonic-clonic seizures. Seizure frequency was four per year. EEG findings consisted of epileptiform spike discharges primarily in the temporal areas.

Imaging Findings

A. Sagittal T1-weighted image shows circular iso-intensity nodule in the interpodal cistern of the hypothalamus. The narrow basement is pedicled with the tuber cinereum and mammillary body (Fig. 2.27a).
B. Sagittal contrast-enhanced T1-weighted images shows no enhancement of the mass (Fig. 2.27b).
C-D. A kind of circular iso-T1 and iso T2 signal shadow could be seen in the hypothalamus coronal view MR images (Fig. 2.27c–d).
E. Coronal T1-weighted image shows iso-intensity nodule in the interpodal cistern of the hypothalamus. (Fig. 2.27e).
F. Coronal contrast-enhanced T1-weighted image shows that the non-enhancing mass is located to the left (Fig. 2.27f).

Discussion

Hypothalamic hamartoma is also called hypothalamic neuronal hamartoma, or gray nodule hamartoma, a rare developmental malformation. They are not true tumors [62]. Hypothalamic hamartomas are classified as cysts and tumor-like lesions in the revised edition [63] in WHO Classification of Tumors of the Central Nervous System 2016. Its clinical manifestations are quite special, mainly manifested as central precocious puberty and giggle-like epilepsy [63].

The components of the hypothalamus are located in the third ventricular wall between the posterior fornix of the hypothalamus, the mammillothalamic tract posteriorly, and the mammillary body inferiorly, suggesting that these structures play an important role in the transmission and occurrence of epilepsy. The symptoms of special clinical manifestation are precocious puberty (PP), giggle-like epilepsy, and abnormalities of cognition and behavior [64].

Some authors believed that the pedicle of tumors is related to clinical manifestations. The most common clinical manifestations of pedicled tumors are precocious puberty, and the manifestations of non-pedicled nodule lesions were mostly comic epilepsy.

Some hypothalamic hamartomas have no clinical symptoms, only in autopsy, but most of them have obvious clinical manifestations, and the clinical manifestations are quite special. The lesions of their shape and size decided the clinical symptoms of the patient [65]. Clinical groups could be divided into two somewhat arbitrary groups. In the first group, male patients, the main manifestation is change of voice; the genitals near puberty are close to adults, while females are superficial. It is now breast development (induration), and the external genitals are approaching puberty and maturation. Some of them have menstruation and ovary enlargement, which are manifested as acne, early growth, and advanced bone age, but epiphyseal line closes earlier; early cessation of development results in short stature by adulthood in both male and female patients.

The elevated level of serum LH, FSH, androgen in male patients, and estrogen in female patients was close to that of adolescence. In the second group, characteristic clinical manifestation is giggle-like epilepsy. The patients can present with a paroxysmal giggle that lasts for several seconds, or sudden stop in tens of seconds; loss of consciousness during seizures can occur every day dozens of times, without any inducement; with the development of the disease, other types

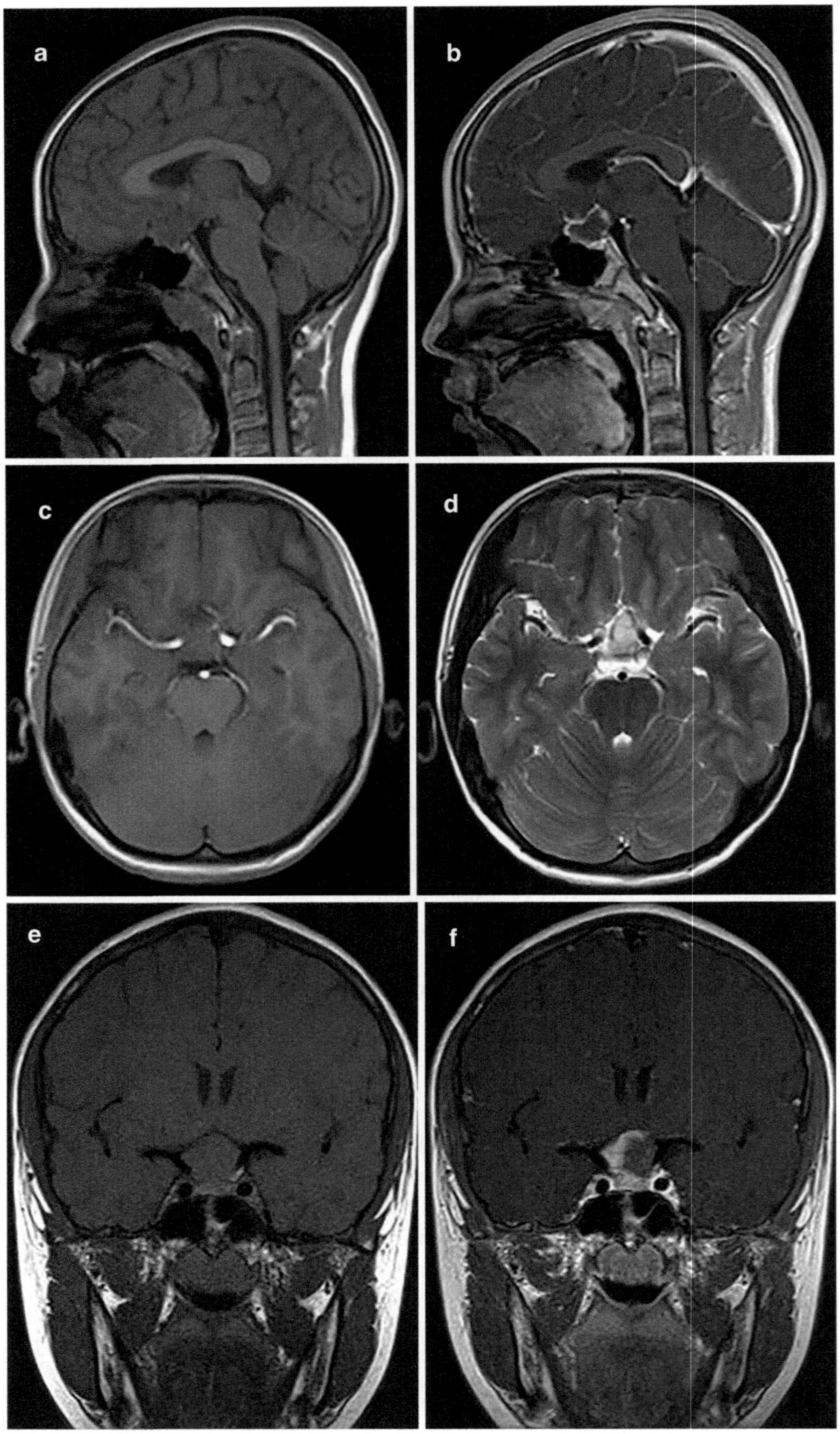

Fig. 2.27 Hypothalamic hamartoma or hamartoma of tuber cinereum

of epilepsy, cognitive impairment, and behavioral abnormalities can gradually emerge. And the main manifestations of behavioral abnormalities are irritability and hyperactivity.

With the advancement of MR imaging, we can find more and more patients of HH; the numbers are on the rise. Magnetic resonance imaging (MRI) is considered to be a definite diagnosis of this disease. The MRI findings of hypothalamic hamartoma are characteristic.

The hypothalamic margin of the suprasellar cistern is clearly smaller oval nodule closely related to the tuber cinereum and corpus callosum, diameter 5–50 mm, but most of them are 10–30 mm in diameter. Sagittal shape of T1WI and coronal scan can accurately provide the shape of the tumors and the pituitary stalk, its surroundings, and structural relationships. Lesions showed iso-signal on T1WI and iso-signal or slightly high signal intensity on T2WI; no enhancement was found in the enhanced scanning lesions.

Clinical manifestations of most hypothalamic hamartomas and MRI findings are characteristic. If the patient has precocious puberty, or giggle-like epilepsy, iso-T1 or slightly high T2 signal in the suprasellar region without enhancement, a definite diagnosis can be made.

This disease should be associated with germinoma, sellar meningioma and hypothalamic glia tumor, craniopharyngioma, tuberculoma of sellar region, and Langerhans cell histiocytosis. Clinically, the above lesions generally do not have the clinical manifestations of hypothalamic hamartoma (precocious puberty, comic epilepsy) and the volume of tumor body may increase, while the hypothalamic hamartoma is not a real tumor, so its volume usually does not change obviously.

Treatment of hypothalamic hamartoma is directed at delaying secondary sexual maturation and preventing premature epiphyseal closure. The diagnosis of HH is based on the typical MR findings [66]. Accurate diagnosis and classification is important for the selection of treatment modality.

Case 2.5.4 Germinoma

Clinical Presentation

A 13-year-old girl was admitted with polydipsia and amenorrhea as chief complaint. Laboratory examination suggested a slight increase in β-HCG, while AFP and CEA were mostly normal.

Imaging Findings

A-B. Axial T1-weighted and T2-weighted images demonstrate a well delineated iso-intensity mass in the suprasellar region (Fig. 2.28a–b).

C-D. Coronal and Sagittal MR images show the mass invaded the suprasellar cistern, resulting the pituitary structure could not be displayed (Fig. 2.28c–d).

E-F. Coronal and Sagittal contrast-enhanced T1-weighted images show obvious inhomogeneous enhancement of the mass (Fig. 2.28e–f).

Discussion

Intracranial germinoma accounts for about 1–2% of all intracranial tumors. Intracranial germ cell tumors are most commonly found in the midline region, most commonly in the pineal region, followed by suprasellar region, but it also occurs in the basal ganglia, thalamus, third ventricle, brainstem, cerebellar vermis, and cerebral hemisphere.

Suprasellar germinoma accounts for about 20–30% of intracranial germinoma [67], most commonly in children and adolescents. There are slightly more in women than men. Diabetes insipidus is the most common clinical symptom associated with hypothalamic–neurohypophysis axis involvement. Because it has no capsule and is located in the subarachnoid space, cerebrospinal fluid is prone to implantation. The pituitary gland is vulnerable to invasion, which is mainly manifested as thickening of the pituitary stalk and disappearance of high T1 signal in the posterior lobe of the pituitary gland. Laboratory examination is often accompanied by the increase of tumor indicators such as β-HCG, AFP, CEA, and placental alkaline phosphatase, and the commonly used clinical indicators are β-HCG and AFP [68].

Imaging shows clear boundary, light effect, uniform signal, obvious enhancement, and large lesions with cystic degeneration. The imaging findings of suprasellar germinoma are mainly solid with some cystic changes, calcification, and hemorrhage. In terms of MRI examination, suprasellar germinoma shows equal or slightly higher signal on T1 and T2WI. The enhancement scan shows obvious uniform enhancement.

Suprasellar germinoma needs to be differentiated from craniopharyngioma [69], pituitary tumor, meningioma, and pilocytic astrocytoma. Craniopharyngioma is common in patients under 15 years of age and over 50 years of age, often accompanied by cystic degeneration and calcification; solid part and cystic wall enhancement showed moderate—obvious enhancement. The pituitary tumor mostly grows upright toward the saddle, while the germinoma mostly grows backward and upward and can spread to the third ventricle, accompanied by thickening of the pituitary stalk and disappearance of T1 high signal in the posterior pituitary lobe. Meningioma enhancement is characterized by dural enhancement and is easily distinguished from germinoma. Pilocytic astrocytoma in suprasellar region tends to occur in adolescents, with no symptoms of pituitary or hypothalamic endocrine abnormalities. Cystic and solid masses are its characteristics, which are mostly manifested as hypo-iso on T1WI and hyper on T2WI, with obvious enhancement.

Case 2.5.5 Pituitary Adenomas

Clinical Presentation

A 7-year-old girl came to the hospital for a headache, vision loss, and short stature. Her past medical, surgical, and family histories were negative. She had no recent trauma or traveling in the epidemic area.

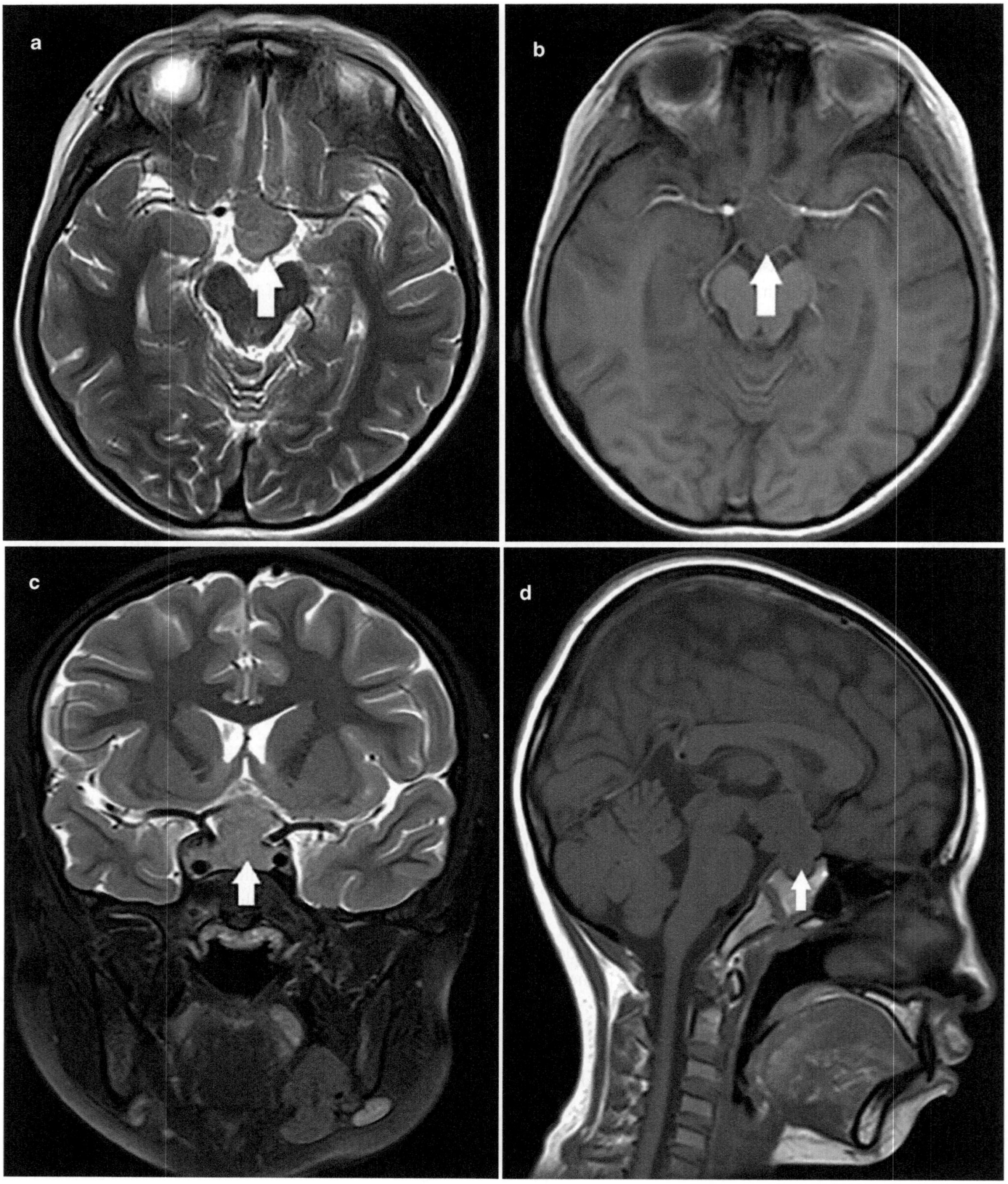

Fig. 2.28 Germinoma

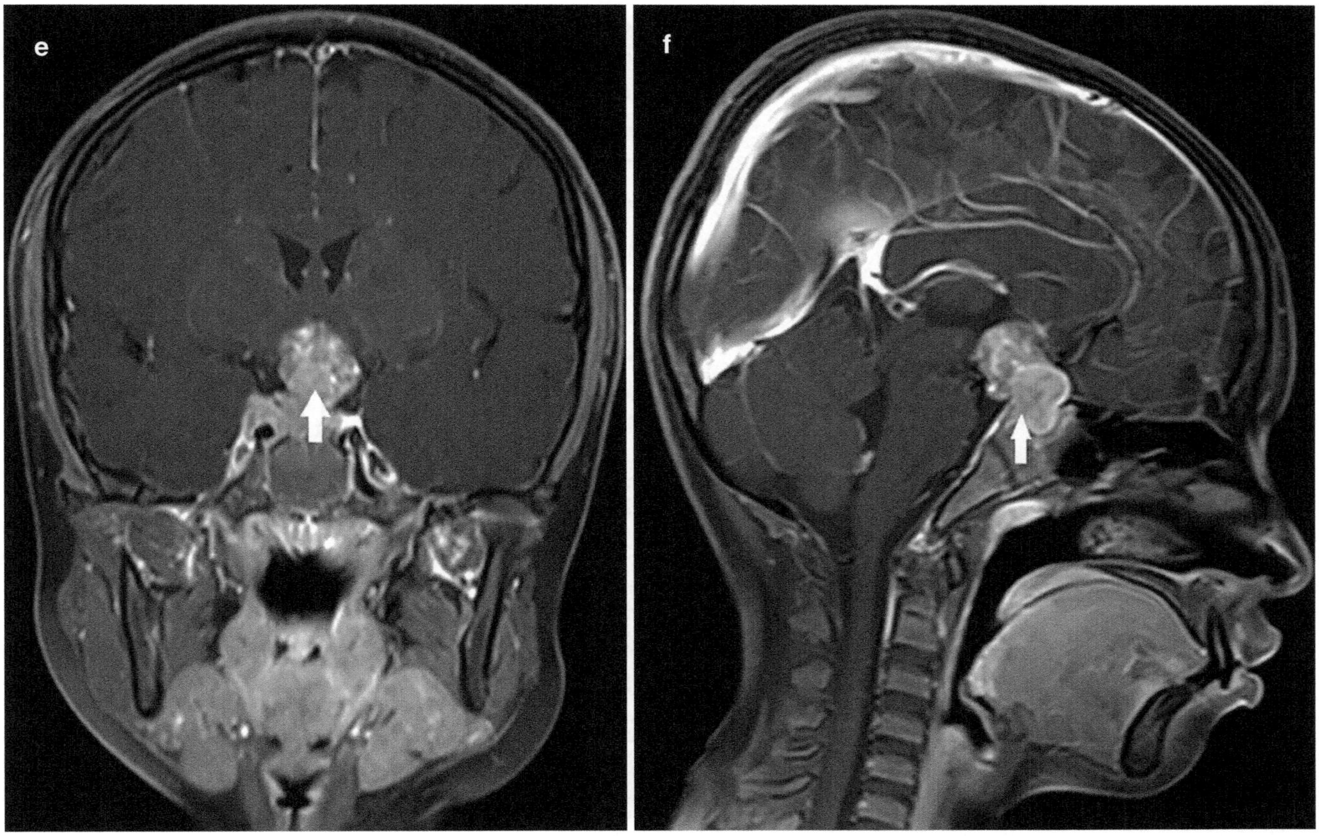

Fig. 2.28 (continued)

Imaging Findings

A-B. Coronal and Sagittal T1-weighted images demonstrate abnormal pituitary height and high signal in adenoma area (Fig. 2.29a–b).

C-D. Coronal and Sagittal contrast-enhanced T1-weighted images show adenoma with delayed enhancement, early mild enhancement, and obvious enhancement in the late stage. Preliminary diagnosis was pituitary adenoma with hemorrhage (Fig. 2.29c–d).

Discussion

Pituitary adenomas (PAs) are a common brain tumor composed of adenohypophyseal cells, but it is rare in children, accounting for less than 3% of all supratentorial neoplasms [70, 71]. Although PAs are mostly benign tumors, it may also lead to significant morbidity due to its hormonal activity, mass effect, location, and interference with normal pituitary hormone function.

PAs have different classification criteria, which can be divided into microadenoma and macroadenoma according to the size boundary of 10 mm. They are divided into functional adenoma and non-functional adenoma according to their functions. Among them, prolactinoma is the most common PA type in adults (39–50%). Non-functional PAs accounted for 23–27%. Prolactinoma is more common in older children (50%) and adolescents. Adrenocorticotropic hormone (ACTH)-secreting adenomas are most common in childhood and pre-adolescent children. The most common cause of childhood endogenous Cushing's syndrome is excessive secretion of ACTH by the pituitary gland, also known as Cushing's disease; It is usually caused by ACTH secreted by pituitary microadenoma, but rarely by macroadenoma. Cushing's disease accounts for approximately 75% of cases of Cushing's syndrome in children over 7 years of age. But in children under 7, Cushing's disease is uncommon. The adrenal etiology of Cushing's syndrome in infants is adenoma, carcinoma, or bilateral hyperplasia [72, 73].

The important tool in the localization of pituitary tumor is magnetic resonance imaging (MRI). Conventional T1WI sequence shows mild low signal; T2WI and T2WI-FLAIR sequence shows high signal. More than 90% of ACTH-producing tumors are hypoenhancing, while only about 5% are hyperenhancing after contrast infusion. Since only macroadenomas will be detectable without contrast, the latter is important. An otherwise normal-looking pituitary MRI might show a hypoenhancing lesion after contrast, usually a microadenoma. However, even with the use of contrast material, only up to approximately 50% of ACTH-producing pitu-

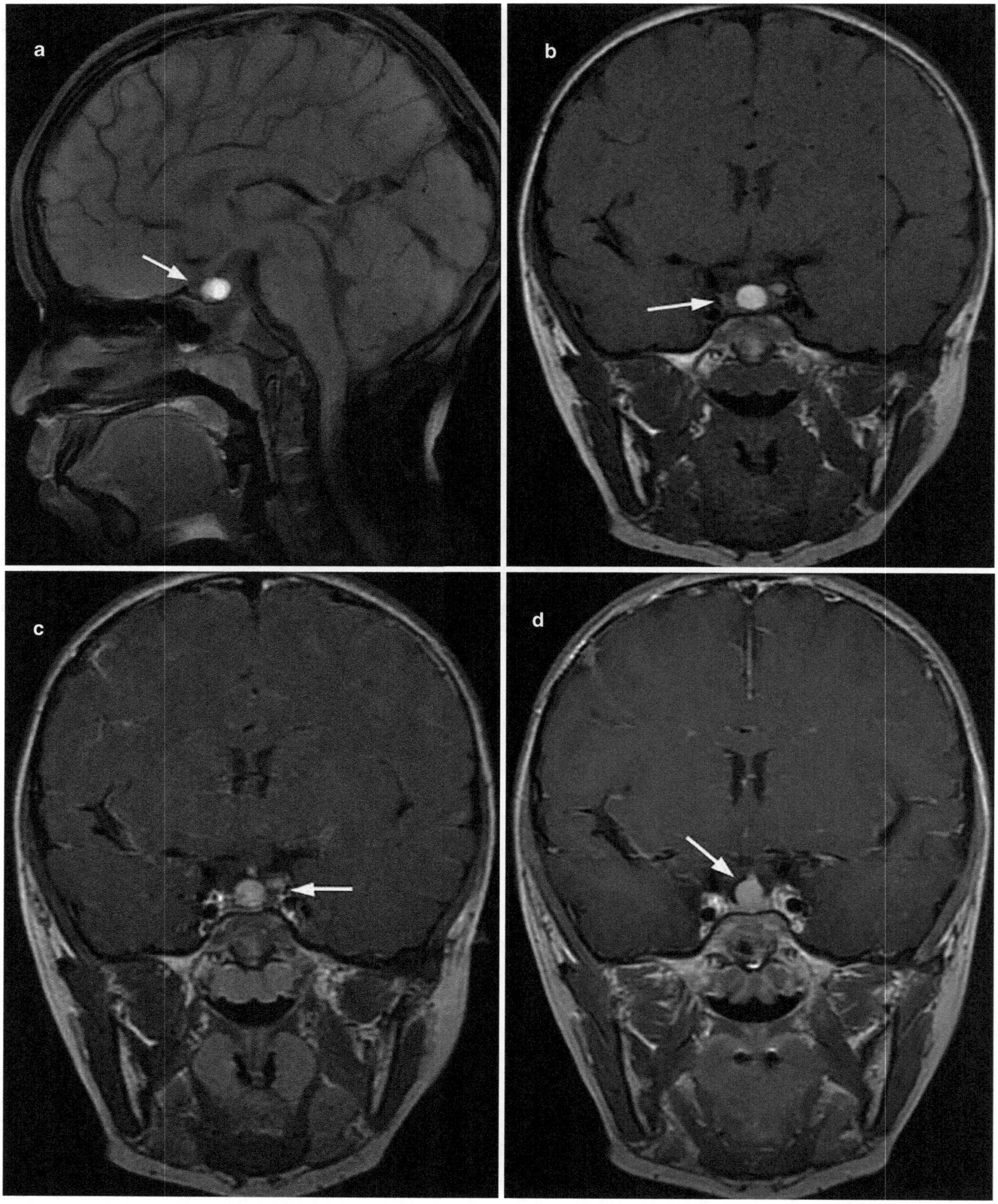

Fig. 2.29 Pituitary adenomas

itary tumors can be detected by pituitary MRI. Invasive adenomas often show unclear borders with surrounding structures, and internal signals are uneven, often accompanied by necrotic low signals. T1WI and T2WI sequence shows high signal when combined with bleeding. Enhanced scanning presents uneven enhancement. CT, more preferable than MRI, of the adrenal glands is useful in the distinction between Cushing's disease and adrenal causes of Cushing's syndrome, mainly unilateral adrenal tumors. Most patients with Cushing's disease have ACTH-driven bilateral hyperplasia, and both adrenal glands will appear enlarged and nodular on CT or MRI [74].

The disease needs to be differentiated from craniopharyngioma and Rathke cyst. Because it depends on the protein content of the cysts, the signal intensity of craniopharyngioma in MRI is highly variable. It is isointense for solid tumor portions and cyst membranes in T1-weighted images, often with a mildly heterogeneous structure. The combination of solid, cystic, and calcified tumor components is an important imaging feature. MRI before and after gadolinium applica-

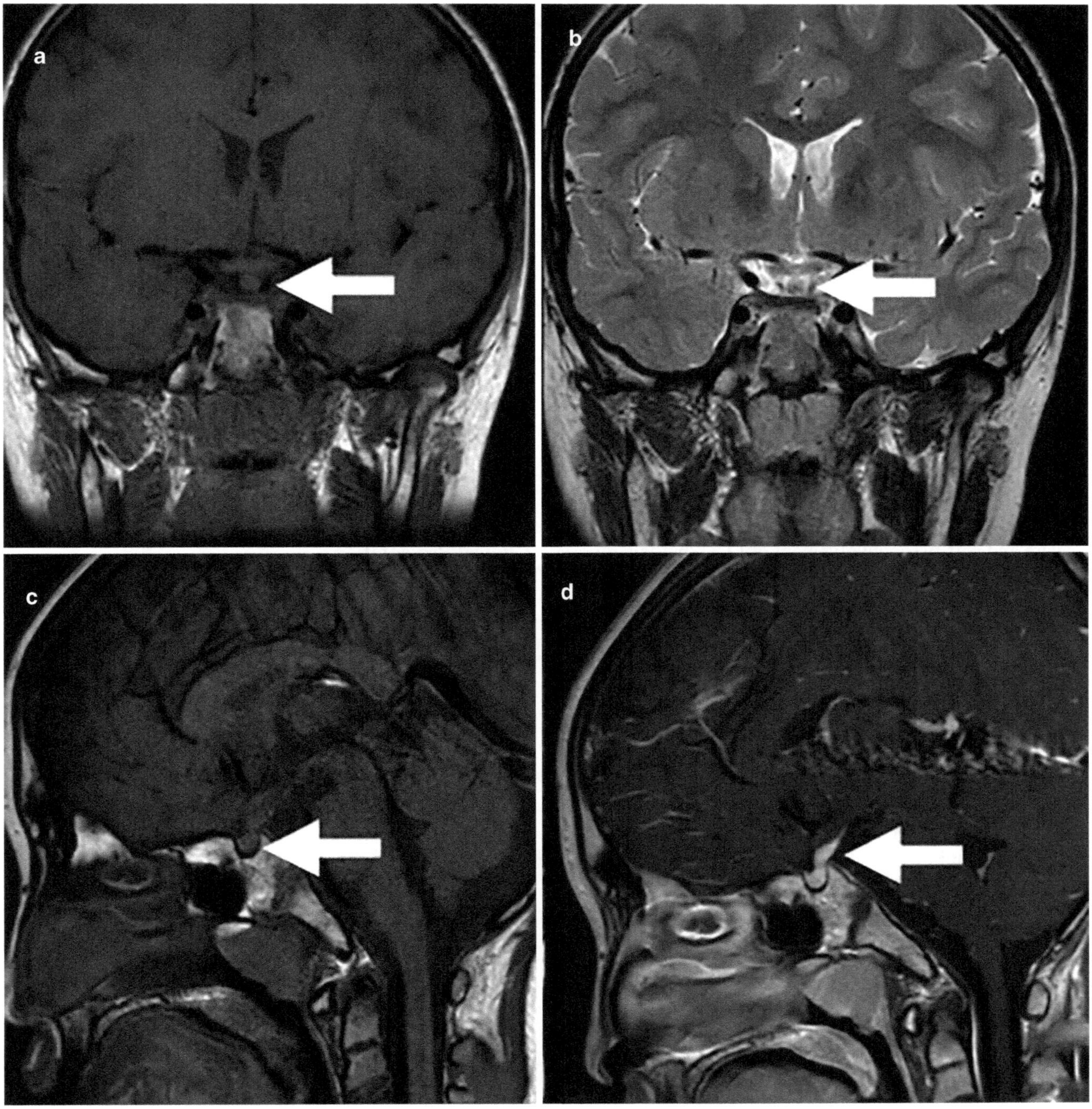

Fig. 2.30 Langerhans cell histiocytosis

tion is the standard imaging for the diagnosis of craniopharyngioma, further imaged by unenhanced CT to detect calcifications. Rathke cyst manifests itself as a smooth and intact cyst wall, and post-contrast injection demonstrates no enhancement.

Case 2.5.6 Langerhans Cell Histiocytosis

Clinical Presentation

A 13-year-old girl presented to hospital with polydipsia and polyuria. Her past medical, surgical, and family histories were negative. She had no recent trauma or traveling in the epidemic area.

Imaging Findings

A-B. Coronal T1-weighted and T2-weighted images demonstrate the nodular thickening in the pituitary stalk (Fig. 2.30a– b).

C. Sagittal T1-weighted image shows absence of the normal high signal of posterior pituitary (Fig. 2.30c).

D. Sagittal contrast-enhanced T1-weighted images shows thickening of pituitary stalk with obvious homogeneous enhancement (Fig. 2.30d).

Discussion

Langerhans cell histiocytosis (LCH) is a group of histiocytic hyperplastic diseases with unknown causes. Langerhans cell hyperplasia is the common histopathological feature, and it is a group of heterogeneous clinical diseases.

LCH is common in children and any organ can be affected, at present. There are many reports about bone and viscera and soft-tissue involvement of LCH, but few reports about pituitary invasion. The invasion of the isolated pituitary gland always leads to central diabetes insipidus (CDI), which the incidence is approximately 1:25,000 ~ 1:100,000, more in men than women. First symptom of LCH in pituitary stalk in children is central diabetes insipidus; when there is loss of hyper-intensity in the posterior pituitary and thickening of the pituitary stalk, LCH should be considered [75]. The value of MRI in the diagnosis of pituitary lesions has been recognized. MRI can show the structure of the pituitary gland clearly due to its high soft-tissue resolution. The shape, height of the pituitary gland, the width of pituitary stalk, and the characteristic posterior lobe signals can be measured and observed on sagittal and coronal images. MRI findings of LCH invasion of pituitary gland showed thickening of the pituitary stalk or occupying lesion, and equal-iso T1 and T2 signals during plain scanning. And the normal high signal of the posterior pituitary on T1WI disappears. After enhancement, the lesion enhanced gradually, and shows homogeneous high signal. Due to infiltration of the hypothalamic–pituitary axis, CDI can be the first manifestation, even before LCH is diagnosed, but the diagnosis of LCH also requires the combination of histopathology and immunohistochemical staining.

CDI is a rare symptom in children and adolescents. Most of the causes are idiopathic, while others are caused by central nervous system (CNS) disorders. LCH needs to be differentiated from lymphocytic hypophysitis, germinoma, pituitary microadenoma, and Rathke cleft cysts. (1) ymphocytic hypophysitis: Lymphocytic hypophysitis is common in females, especially during pregnancy. Patients usually present with low adrenocorticotropic hormone secretion and CDI. The pituitary has increased diffusion and symmetry, and the normal high signal of the posterior pituitary on T1WI also disappears, sometimes with the thickening pituitary stalk (2)Germinoma: Germinoma is mainly solid with some cystic changes, calcification, and hemorrhage [67]. In terms of MRI examination, germinoma shows equal or slightly higher signal on T1WI and T2WI. The enhancement scan shows obvious uniform enhancement. (3) Pituitary microadenoma: The tumor is located in the anterior pituitary lobe. The degree of early enhancement is weak during the enhancement examination and delayed enhancement. T1 sequence of high signal in posterior pituitary lobe can be existed. (4) Rathke cleft cysts: Located in front of the anterior and posterior lobes of the pituitary gland; after injection of contrast agent, the lesion shows no enhancement.

Case 2.5.7 Ectopic Posterior Pituitary Gland (EPP)

Clinical Presentation

A 6-year-old boy presented with delayed reproductive development for 3 years, history of malnutrition, no genetic metabolic disease, no adverse pregnancy record, growth hormone deficiency confirmed by stimulation tests, without diabetes, without cryptorchidism, and micropenis malformation.

Imaging Findings

A-B. Sagittal and coronal T1-weighted images demonstrate ectopia of the posterior pituitary gland located at the distal end of a truncated pituitary stalk along the median eminence of the hypothalamus (white arrow). The sella turcica and adenohypophysis are both small (red arrow) (Fig. 2.31a–b).

Discussion

Fujisawa first described the pituitary stem disruption syndrome (SITP) in 1987. Ectopic posterior pituitary gland (EPP) is congenital defect disease, and pituitary stalk inter-

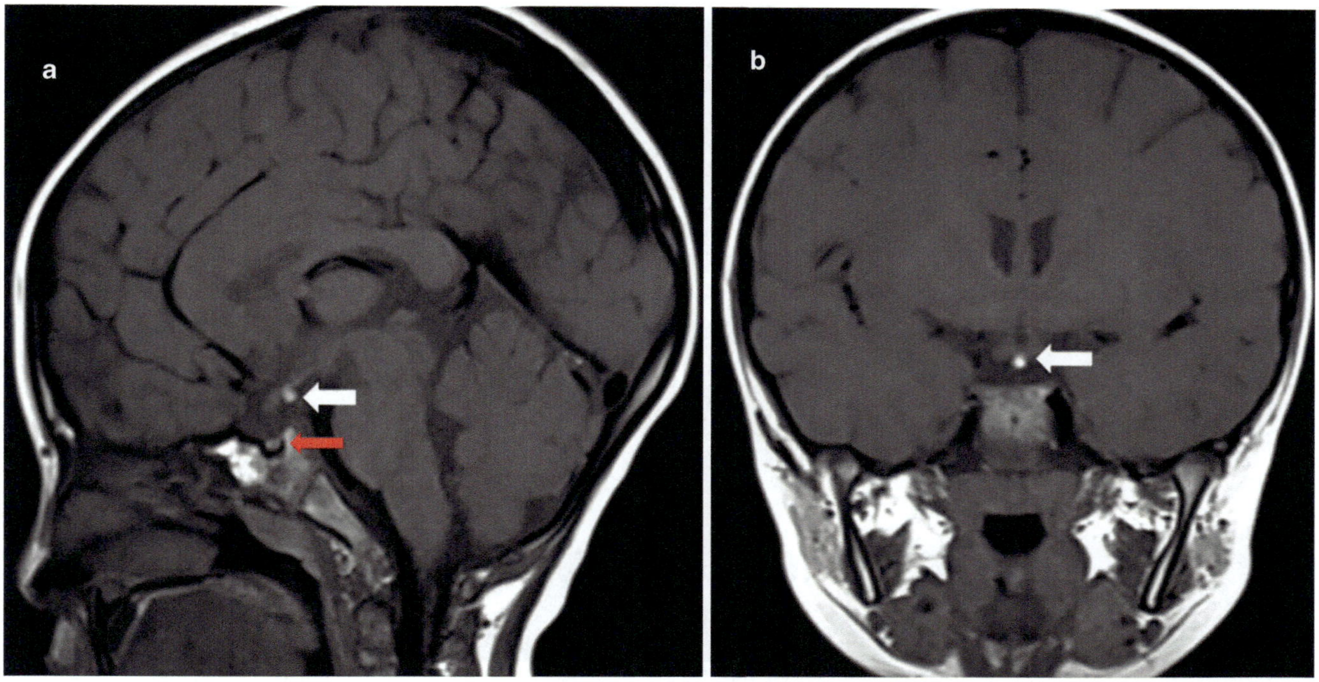

Fig. 2.31 Ectopic posterior pituitary gland (EPP)

ruption syndrome (PSIS) is the most common manifestation [76]. The pituitary stalk becomes thinner or congenitally absent, and the posterior pituitary is ectopic. The hormone secreted from the hypothalamus cannot be transported to the normal post-hypophysis via the pituitary stalk. The pathophysiology of EPP is not fully understood, but chromosomal microdeletions and perinatal asphyxia have some established role in the literature as primary miscreants [77], including congenital causes and acquired causes. PSIS can be seen in newborns, children, and adults. The main clinical manifestations are growth retardation, microsomia, hypotrichosis, usually, lagging behind the normal body height, bone age hysteresis on X-ray picture, feature immature, cunnus immature, and small testicles and penis. Adults usually have thyroid hypofunction. Nawaz Atif et al. [78] reported a case of pituitary stalk interruption syndrome presenting in a euthyroid adult with short stature.

Because the pituitary is very small, it requires special scanning method and sequence. For the diagnosis of ectopic posterior pituitary gland (EPP), plain scan of sagittal and slice coronal T1WI are the best methods, because the ectopic posterior pituitary showed high signal intensity on T1WI. But for displaying the pituitary stalk, the enhanced T1WI is better than the plain scans, because the pituitary stalk can be enhanced obviously early. The EPP has diagnostic criteria of MRI. It has three items: first, the absence of pituitary stalk; second, no short T1 signal intensity of posterior pituitary in the hypophysial fossa; third, we can see the high signal of the ectopia posterior pituitary in the infundibular recess or the median eminence. Although the imaging performance is simple, differential diagnosis is still needed. Sella turcica, the pituitary fossa, was occupied by cerebrospinal fluid signals, but there was no disruption of the pituitary stalk and heterotopia of hypophysis in the posterior lobe. But the final diagnosis requires a combination of the following: clinical manifestation and laboratory examination. MR is the most effective imaging methods for its final diagnosis.

Early diagnosis and treatment is very important, especially height and gonadal development. If the time of diagnosis and treatment is delayed, it does not just affect growth, but it has a serious impact on the patient's personality and social psychology.

2.6 Brain Stem Tumors

Case 2.6.1 Brainstem Glioma

Clinical Presentation

A 7-year-old girl was sent to neurosurgery for a sudden headache. The right limb weakness occurred half a month

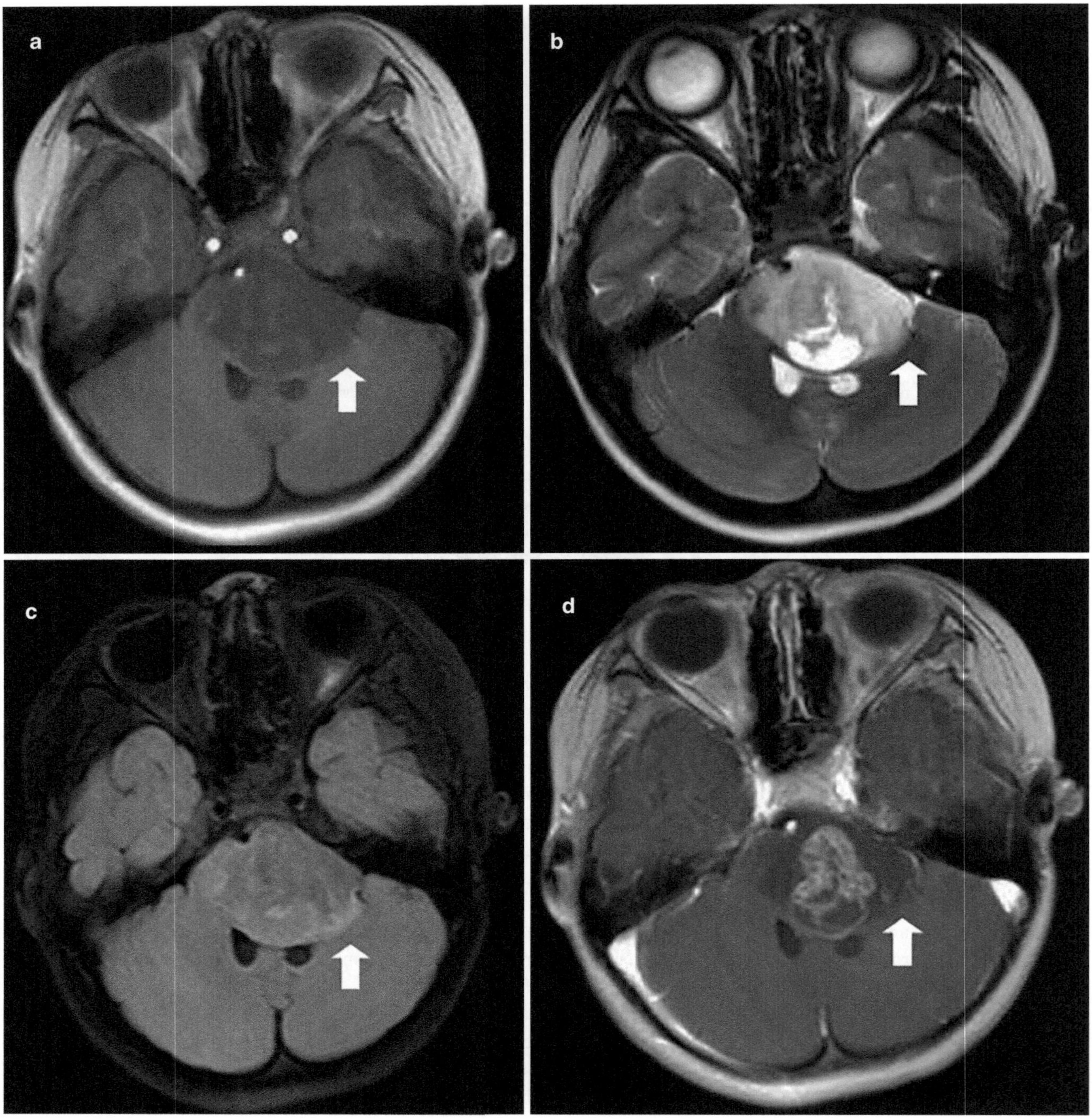

Fig. 2.32 Brainstem glioma

ago and was not taken seriously. Her past medical, surgical, and family histories were negative. She had no recent trauma or traveling in the epidemic area.

Imaging Findings

A. Axial T1-weighted images demonstrate a mass in the pontine, inhomogeneous hypointensity (Fig. 2.32a).

B-C. The signal inhomogeneity of the mass can be shown more clearly on axial T2-weighted and T2-FLAIR images (Fig. 2.32a–c).

D. Axial contrast-enhanced T1-weighted image shows the tumor was obviously inhomogeneous enhanced, surrounding by obvious edema (Fig. 2.32d).

Discussion

Brainstem gliomas mainly refer to tumors from neuroectoderm that occur in brain cadres. They are more common in children, accounting for 15–20% of all brain tumors in children [79]. The brainstem is mainly divided into three parts: pons, midbrain, and medulla oblongata. The location of glioma in brainstem involves more than two parts. The incidence rate of glioma is the highest in the medulla oblongata, followed by the pons and midbrain. Brainstem gliomas can be simply divided into two categories: diffuse brainstem gliomas (most commonly in the pons) and focal brainstem gliomas (mostly in the midbrain and medulla oblongata). In the literature, the brainstem tumors are classified into four categories obtained by Jin B et al. [80]: The first category is diffuse brainstem gliomas; the second type is focal glioma, which is characterized by focal and inherent tumor, which can be cystic or solid; The third type is exophytic tumor, which originates from the glial tissue under the smothering membrane of the fourth ventricle, and most of them grow dorsal and lateral, The fourth type is cervical medullary glioma.

The main factors affecting patients with brainstem gliomas include the diameter of brainstem gliomas, whether there are necrotic foci, whether there is cystic degeneration, whether there is midline growth across brainstem axis, etc. Through the analysis of these pathological factors, the tumor development degree of patients can be judged. Gliomas with a diameter less than 2 cm belong to low-grade gliomas, which can be treated with conservative methods in the early stage. For gliomas larger than 2 cm, surgical treatment should be advocated in the early stage, so as not to miss the best treatment opportunity. Through the analysis of relevant pathological factors, we can guide patients to symptomatic treatment and effective prognosis, so as to improve patients' condition.

In view of the absence of skull artifacts and multidirectional imaging features, MR is the best method for the diagnosis and accurate localization of gliomas at present, which is of great help to the formulation of treatment plans and follow-up. Characteristic MR manifestations of brainstem gliomas were expansive growth, mostly substantial, most clearly displayed on T2-weighted images, for obvious high signal, low signal, or low mixed signal on T1-weighted images. After injection of GD-DTPA, most lesions increased significantly, but a few did not. The enhancement modes were diffuse and nodular, with a ring along the edge of the tumor or the necrotic area of the cyst. Tumor margin is more clear, surrounding brain tissue edema is more light or not obvious, small cystic change or small hemorrhage can occur inside the tumor, the tumor grows forward and embeds the basilar artery, some brainstem gliomas can be located near the midbrain aqueduct, although small, but can cause pressure on the midbrain aqueduct, and secondary hydrocephalus. Compared with CT, MRI can better define the nature, location, and scope of space-occupying lesions.

Brainstem glioma should be differentiated from the following non-neoplastic diseases. Vascular malformations are mainly manifested in mixed signals on T1WI and T2WI, such as empty blood vessels and subacute hemorrhagic products such as orthoferric hemoglobin and hemosiderin, which can be clearly diagnosed. Acute disseminated encephalomyelitis is caused by vaccination or virus infection. It affects the white matter of supratentorial and cerebellum besides brainstem. It can be diagnosed according to the multiple and inducing factors of the lesion. Demyelinating lesions are mainly symmetrical and supratentorial. Central pontine myelin destruction is rare in infants and children. It is common in adults. Most of them have a history of hyponatremia and alcoholism, which is not difficult to identify [81].

Case 2.6.2 Pilocytic Astrocytoma

Clinical Presentation

A 6-year-old boy presented to our pediatric department with left limb weakness for about 5 days. He collapsed frequently and began to appear astasia afterward. No history was presented, and family history was unremarkable.

Imaging Findings

A-B. Axial T2-weighted and T1-weighted images demonstrate a predominantly cystic-solid lesion is found in the brainstem, hyperintense to the gray matter on T2WI and hypointense but a little hyperintense to the cerebrospinal fluid (CSF) on T1WI (Fig. 2.33a–b).

C. Axial T2- FLAIR shows that the cystic fluid does not suppress completely and the solid part appears hyperintense (Fig. 2.33c).

D. On contrast-enhanced T1WI, the lesion exhibits ring-like enhancement (Fig. 2.33d).

Discussion

Pilocytic astrocytoma (PA) was classified as a WHO grade I localized astrocytoma in the 2016 WHO Classification of Tumors of the Central Nervous System [82]. It is a slow-growing glioma typically occurring in young patients [83, 84].

PA accounts for 5.4% of all gliomas and is the most common primary gliomas in children and young adults during the first two decades of life and makes up about 17.6% of all childhood primary brain tumors and 85% of posterior fossa astrocytomas in that age group [83, 85]. Over 80% of PAs arise under 20 and the peak incidence ranges from 5 to 15 years [86].

Genetically, PAs can be syndromic, namely that some can develop in neurofibromatosis type 1 (NF-1), or sporadic, and they have different gene mutations. Nearly all sporadic PAs are characterized by the presence of the fusion of *BRAF* gene, which causes the activation of MEK signaling cascade and then leads to the increased cell proliferation [83, 87]. But

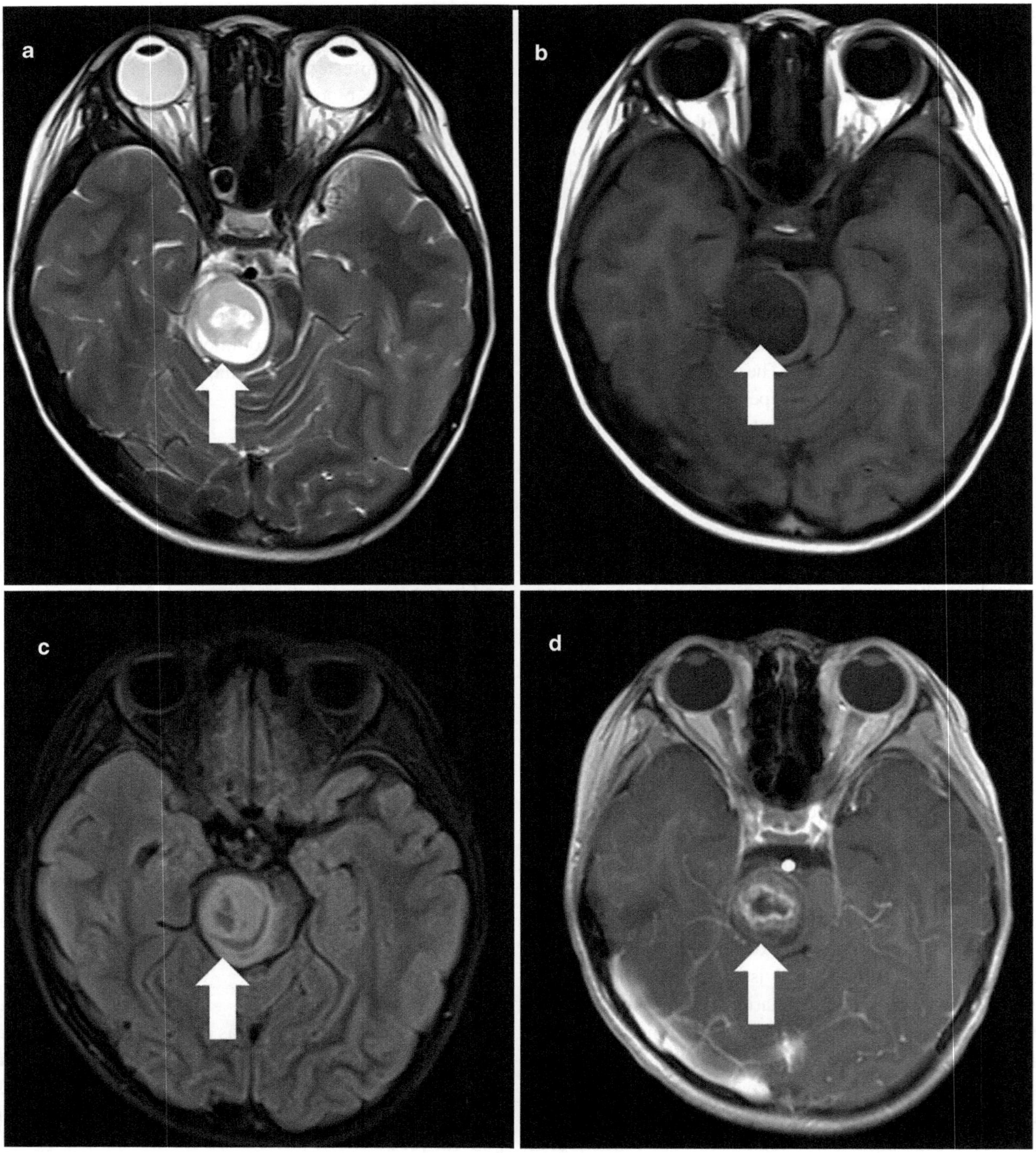

Fig. 2.33 Pilocytic astrocytoma

NF-1 associated PAs have the mutation of *NF1*gene, hence activation RAS and MARK pathways and consequent occurrence of PA [83].

About 60% of all PAs occur in the cerebellum and could cause symptoms such as headache, morning nausea, and vomiting. Some patients can also present with ataxia, dysdiadochokinesia, etc. [83, 85, 86].

The optic nerve/chiasm and hypothalamus/third ventricle is the second most common site for PAs. They often present with visual loss, proptosis, or diencephalic syndrome [86]. The third preferred site of PA is the pons and medulla, and sometimes the tectum, where aqueductal stenosis and neurological deficits, such as hemiparesis, can be the clinical manifestations [85, 86].

The imaging findings differ due to its location. Most brainstem and cerebellar PAs are round and well-circumferential. The typical imaging finding is a nonenhancing cyst with an enhancing mural nodule [84, 85]. On CT and MR scans, the cystic portion is hypoattenuated and slightly hyperintense to CSF on T1WI and T2WI, respectively, and it often does not suppress completely on FLAIR. The solid portion often shows isodense on CT, iso/hypointense on T1WI, and iso/hyperintense on T2WI/FLAIR and presents with intense but heterogeneous enhancement in many cases [88–90]. The cyst wall enhances from none to moderate [86].

When PAs happen in the optic nerve, chiasm, third ventricle, and tectum, they tend to be solid, infiltrating, and less well-marginated [85, 86]. And the enhancement of the PAs varies from none to striking [86].

The PAs need to be differentiated from medulloblastoma, ependymoma, and hemangioblastoma when found in the posterior fossa and pilomyxoid astrocytoma when occurring in the hypothalamic region [85, 86]. The prognosis of PA is good, and 10-year survival often exceeds 90% after resection of the tumors [83, 86].

Case 2.6.3 Hemangioblastoma

Clinical Presentation

A 2-year-old girl was admitted to the department of neurosurgery 2 days ago, due to unsteady walking, ataxia, dizziness, and vomiting. Her medical and family history was unremarkable. She had no recent trauma either.

Imaging Findings

A. Axial T1-weighted image demonstrates a slight hypointense mass originating from the dorsal pontine and protruding into the fourth ventricle (Fig. 2.34a).

B-C. Axial T2-weighted and T2- FLAIR show hypointense in the central region of the mass (Fig. 2.34a–c).

D. Axial contrast-enhanced T1-weighted image shows the mass with obvious homogeneous enhancement (Fig. 2.34d).

Discussion

Hemangioblastomas of the central nervous system (CNS) are rare histologically benign vascular tumors that can occur throughout the neural axis [91]. HBs are most common in the cerebellum, followed by the spinal cord and brainstem. They can occur sporadically or in the context of von Hippel–Lindau disease (VHL) which is an autosomal dominant tumor syndrome that affects multiple organ systems. Brainstem HB (BSH) is a hemangioblastoma that originates in the brainstem and frequently occurs in the medulla oblongata. Hemangioblastoma accounts for 5–15% of intracranial HBs [92], usually occurring in adults, but is extremely rare in children with an incidence rate of less than 1 per 1,000,000 [93]. According to location and multiplicity, hemangioblastoma is associated with significant irreversible neurological deficits.

The main clinical manifestations of BSH patients are headache, dizziness, vomiting, paresthesia, pyramidal sign, and cranial nerve deficit. Pathologically, BSH is the same as HBs that originate elsewhere in CNS. According to reports, 64% of pediatric HBs were associated with VHL disease, which was much higher than reports of adult HBs, of which 3–25% of CNS HBs were associated with VHL disease [93]. Hemangioblastoma in childhood is highly indicative of VHL disease. Early diagnosis and appropriate treatment will lead to improved clinical results. Although HBs are histologically benign tumors, they may recur during long-term follow-up [82].

Hemangioblastoma is divided into two types: cystic-solid and solid, most of which (about 70%) are cystic-solid tumors. However in BSH patients, solid tumors accounted for the majority, and cystic-solid accounted for only about 20%. According to the relationship between the tumor and the brainstem parenchyma, these tumors can be divided into two types: intrabrainstem and extrabrainstem. Generally, those tumors with huge volume and rich blood supply belonged to the extrabrainstem type. The clinical manifestations of BSH are diverse and lacking in characteristics, mainly relying on imaging examination for diagnosis, especially MRI. On MRI, the characteristic manifestations of BSH include the following: (1) The solid components show obvious uniform enhancement. (2) The tumor has features with large cysts and small nodules. (3) There is a serpentine, distorted strip-like signal-free area in or around the tumor. (4) Diffusion-weighted imaging (DWI) technique in MRI can also be used as an identification method. In solid hemangioblastoma, DWI is mostly hypointense or a little isointense, and the apparent diffusion

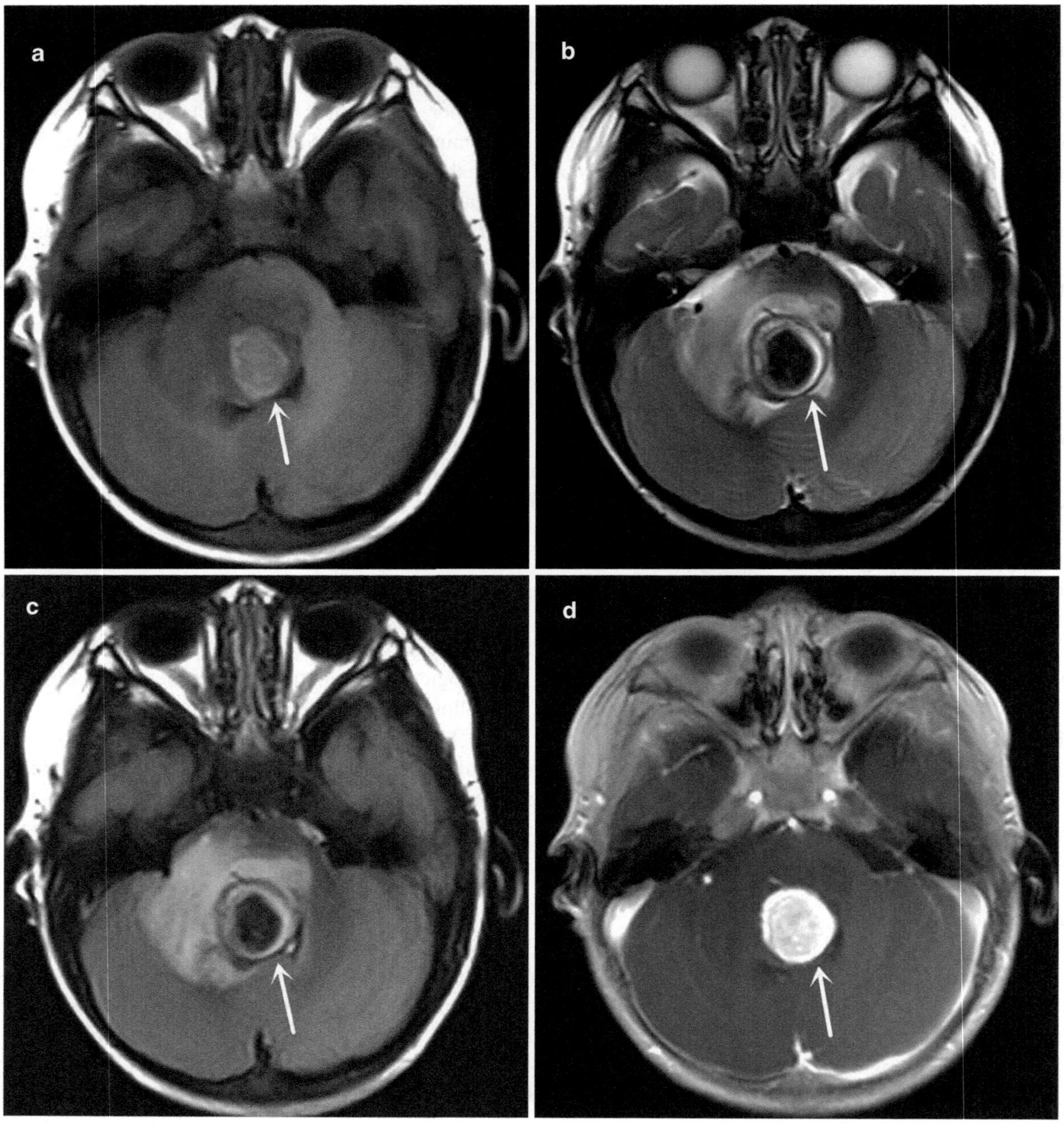

Fig. 2.34 Hemangioblastomas

coefficient (ADC) value is high, while the DWI of other blood-rich tumors in the posterior fossa often shows high signal or iso-signal intensity, and the ADC value is low.

BSH needs to be differentiated from choroid plexus papilloma and medulloblastoma. (1) Choroid plexus papilloma often occurs in the ventricles, usually causing hydrocephalus. (2) Medulloblastoma often occurs in the cerebellar vermis, more common in children, which is easy to spread with cerebrospinal fluid. The tumor has obvious enhancement and demonstrates restricted diffusion on DWI.

2.7 Metastatic Tumor

Clinical Presentation

A 4-year-old girl presented with head mass for more than 5 months, lower limb pain for more than 1 month, and retroauricular lymphadenectasis for 1 week. A mass with a diameter of about 5.0 cm was found in the abdomen. The left renal malignant rhabdoid tumor was confirmed by pathology.

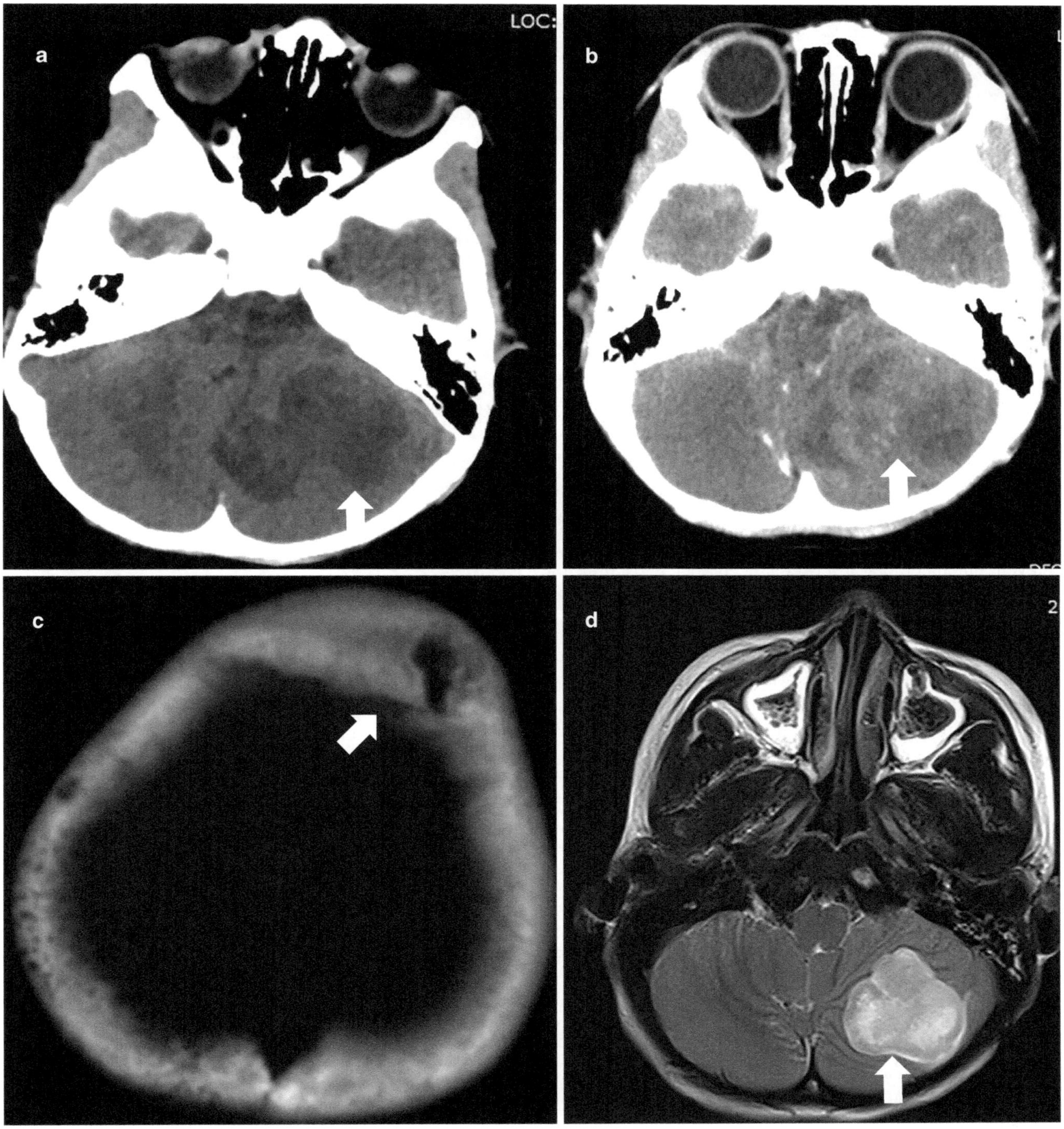

Fig. 2.35 Metastatic tumor

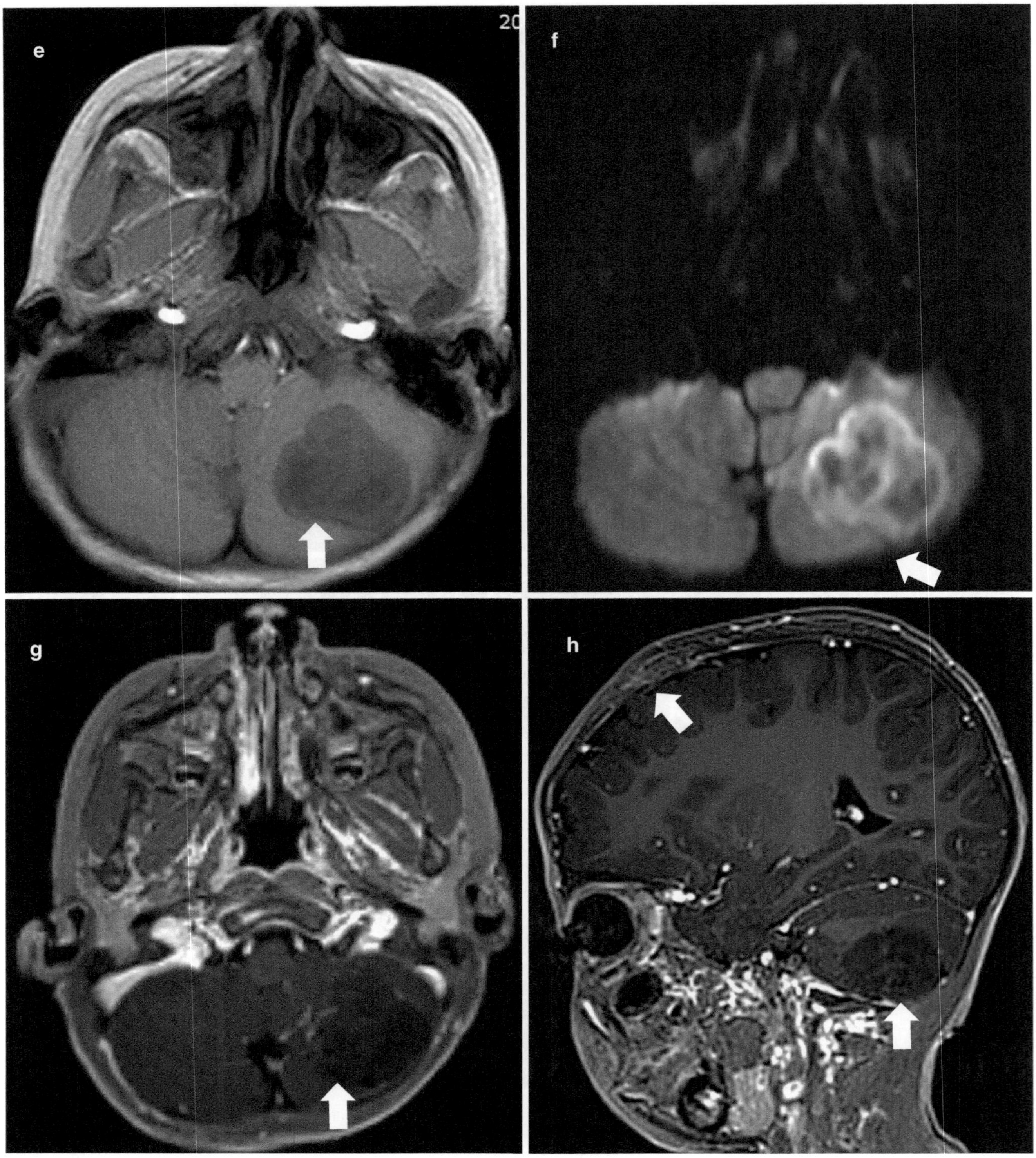

Fig. 2.35 (continued)

Imaging Findings

A. Axial CT ordinary scan showed a round hemispheric mass in the left cerebellum, with heterogeneous density and cystic degeneration (Fig. 2.35a).
B. The CT enhanced scan showed that the mass was heterogeneous enhancement with incomplete ring enhancement; (Fig. 2.35b).
C. CT bone window showed multiple bone destruction areas in skull (Fig. 2.35c).
D. Axial T2-weighted image demonstrate round-like, heterogeneous, long T2 signal lesion in the left cerebellum (Fig. 2.35d).
E. Axial T1-weighted image shows the mass with heterogeneous hypointense (Fig. 2.35e).

F. Axial DWI shows a hyperintense lesion with low ADC value, representing restricted diffusion (Fig. 2.35f).

G-H. Contrast-enhanced T1-weighted images demonstrate ring enhancement in the lesion of the left cerebellum and heterogeneous enhancement in the skull masses (Fig. 2.35g–h).

Discussion

Brain metastases are rare in children. Germ cell tumors, sarcomas, and neuroblastomas are common offenders. Ewing sarcoma and soft-tissue sarcoma, followed by osteosarcoma, are the main primary tumors that metastasize to the brain [88].

The nature of children's brain tumors is very different from that of adults. Children's brain tumors cannot be regarded as the "miniature" of adult brain tumors, and they are different in clinical manifestations and treatment. The main symptoms of brain metastases in children were increased intracranial pressure, mental symptoms, and meningeal irritation. Depending on the site of the lesion, there may also be focal localized signs, such as hemiplegia, aphasia, dysesthesia, nystagmus, and ataxia. Physical examination is often associated with motor and sensory impairment, speech impairment, and visual papilledema.

In the pediatric population, brain metastasis generally follows extensive systemic metastasis and disease progression. Intraparenchymal brain metastases constitute more than 50% of all intracranial metastatic disease and are thought to result from hematogenous dissemination. Intracranial metastases may also originate from the direct extension of cranial or dural lesions. Brain seeding is common in patients with leukemia.

The imaging studies used to identify brain metastases varied. At present, CT scans were used most frequently closed followed by MRI. Most brain metastases were supratentorial or involved both supratentorial and infratentorial regions. Most of brain metastatic tumors are located in the gray matter, involving the temporal, frontal, parietal, and occipital lobes, and the cerebellum. It can develop as extension from leptomeningeal spread through the Virchow-Robin spaces. These features are similar to those described in adults. Solitary metastases, hemorrhagic metastases, cerebellar metastases, and dural metastasis may present in children. CT plain scan shows multiple or single round or quasi-circular intracranial lesions with high, medium, low, or mixed density, solid nodules with small tumors, and necrosis with irregular rings in the middle of large tumors. Enhanced scan shows nodular and circular enhancement. The main manifestations of brain metastases on MR are multiple or single round-like abnormal signal foci in brain parenchyma, no cystic necrosis or hemorrhage foci, equal or low signal on T1WI, slightly high or high signal on T2WI, and equal signal on a few lesions. If cystic necrosis occurs, low signal on T1WI, high signal on T2WI, mixed (short, long) T1 signal and mixed (long, short) T2 signal on hemorrhage, irregular hemosiderin ring with different thickness, or incomplete on T2WI image are seen. Enhanced scan shows that 85% of the cases found more lesions than plain scan, which could significantly improve the sensitivity. Enhanced images with uniform nodules or rings are most common.

Differential diagnosis. Single brain metastatic tumor is easily confused with malignant glioma in the brain. Gliomas are mostly located in the white matter of deep brain with unclear margins, uneven wall thickness and nodules, and relatively mild peritumoral edema, which may involve the corpus callosum [89]. Brain abscess has necrosis and liquefaction in the center of a few large brain metastatic tumors, but its periphery is often zigzag. Patients with brain abscess have fever, and other parts of the body have a history of trauma or infection. CT or MRI shows that the enhancement scan of brain abscess shows circular enhancement and more uniform thin-walled and nonwalled nodules. The peripheral edema is mainly mild to moderate flaky edema. It shows high signal on DWI and low signal on ADC, suggesting limited diffusion. Cerebral cysticercosis is characterized by increased intracranial pressure. There was past history of contact with livestock or eating "rice pork." CT or MRI shows diffuse uneven distribution of small brain edema, with circular or semi-circular calcification, scattered in multiple, some visible cephalic ganglia. Brain tuberculosis is a granulomatous lesion formed by tuberculosis bacilli in the central nervous system, often secondary to tuberculosis in other parts of the body. In addition to the symptoms of cranial hypertension and epilepsy, patients often have systemic symptoms such as fever, night sweat, and emaciation. CT or MRI shows single or multiple round lesions with obvious peripheral enhancement.

The prognosis of pediatric patient with brain metastatic tumor is poor because the disease is very advanced when diagnosed. Treatment only improved survival marginally [90].

2.8 Meningiomas

Clinical Presentation

A 9-year-old boy presented with headache for more than 6 months, accompanied by vomiting and lower limb spasm. Recently, he had a headache and vomiting symptoms increased. He had poor diet and weight loss since the onset of the disease. There was no history of fever or head trauma.

Imaging Findings

A. Axial T1-weighted image demonstrates a heterogeneous mass in the right frontal lobe, beside the cerebral falx. Obvious high signal can be seen at the edge of the mass (Fig. 2.36a).

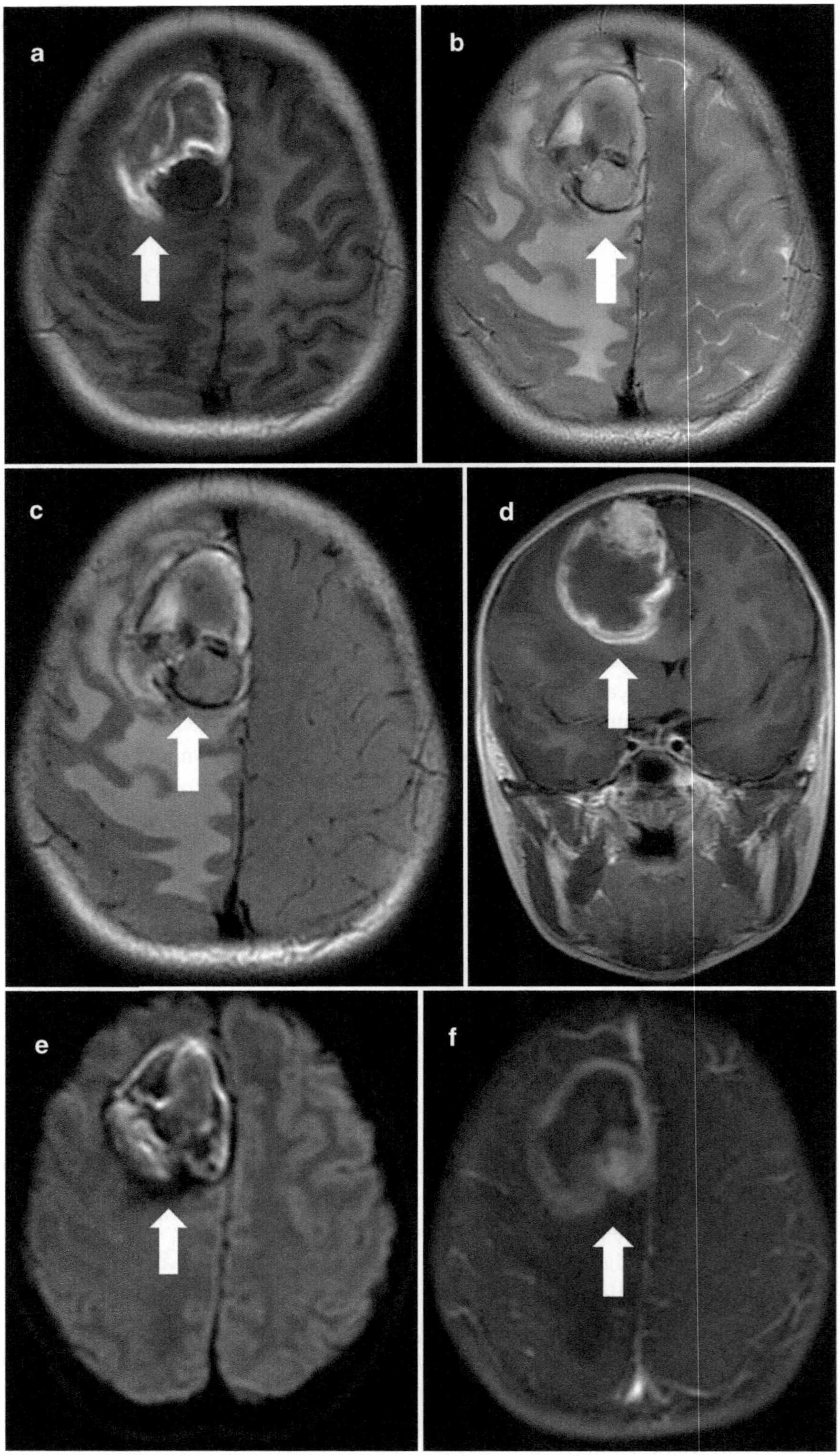

Fig. 2.36 Meningiomas

B-C. T2 hyperintense perilesional edema in adjacent brain parenchyma was best depicted on FLAIR (Fig. 2.36a–c).

D. Coronal T1-weighted image shows a well-defined mass in the right frontal lobe with a broad-based attachment on the cerebral (Fig. 2.36d).

E. Diffusion-weighted image shows the mass with heterogeneous hyperintense (Fig. 2.36e).

F. Contrast-enhanced T1-weighted image demonstrates remarkably annular heterogeneous enhancement (Fig. 2.36f).

Discussion

Meningiomas are extracranial tumors which originate from the epithelial cells in the dura or arachnoid cap cells. The incidence rate is only lower than that of glioma, accounting for about 15–20% of intracranial tumors and a higher incidence noted in females at the age of 40–60. Pediatric meningiomas are exceedingly rare but tend to be more aggressive than their adult counterparts. Neurofibromatosis Type 2 has been shown to increase the risk of developing meningioma. They are classified based on morphologic criteria by the World Health Organization (WHO) into three groups. Nearly 90% are grade I (benign), 10% are grade II (borderline), and less than 3% are grade III (malignant).

Meningiomas most commonly occur where arachnoid cap cells are most numerous, such as where the arachnoid granulations are concentrated along the dural venous sinuses. Of all the tumors, 50% are located along the skull base, 40% along the calvarial convexity, 10% along the falx and parasagittal region, and a small fraction within the ventricle. Meningiomas are generally considered benign, solitary, and slow-growing lesions with an indolent clinical course. The tumors cause different clinical symptoms depending on location. The patient will present with intracranial hypertension and peritubular reactive vasogenic edema when the tumor is large or growing rapidly. Meningiomas in the cavernous sinus can involve both the oculomotor and trigeminal nerves, leading to eye movement disorders and facial paralysis; because of their location in the optic nerve sheath they will not only have the appearance of exophthalmos and visual field defects, but also have the symptoms of painless progressive vision loss and papillary edema. In addition to cranial osteomatoid hyperplasia, some patients also present pupil changes, vomiting, and other manifestations. However, with increasing cranial imaging such as CT or MRI, incidentally discovered meningiomas are becoming more frequent.

Typical CT features include a sharply equal or slightly high-density well-defined lobular mass with a broad-based dural attachment on unenhanced CT, which demonstrates homogeneous enhancement following contrast and obvious extracranial tumor-occupying effect. CT also demonstrates the bony changes including hyperostosis, osteolysis, and, in the setting of an anterior skull base, meningioma. Intratumoral calcification is commonly seen on CT as their slow growth rate. Edema belt may appear around the tumor of malignant meningiomas, or large areas of bone destruction may occur in the skull corresponding to the tumor.

On MRI, meningiomas are usually hypo -to isointense relative to cerebral cortex on T1-weighted sequences and iso- to hyperintense on T2-weighted sequences. After T1 contrast sequence, meningiomas typically show avid, homogeneous enhancement. The presence of intratumoral cysts, hemorrhage, or necrosis produces a heterogeneous appearance and may be associated with aggressive behavior of the tumor. A dural tail is usually seen on contrast imaging but the sign is not specific, as other dural neoplasms can also demonstrate this finding. On MRS, meningiomas show increased choline peak with significant reduction in the NAA and creatine levels, small alanine peak.

Differential diagnoses of the meningiomas are lymphomas, solitary fibrous, dural metastases (e.g., from lung, breast, or prostate primaries), etc. MRI is the modality of choice for diagnosis. Imaging features which distinguish meningiomas from other intracranial tumors are whether the location of the tumor is connected to the dura. The signal or density of metastatic tumor is more heterogeneity, and hemorrhage is more commonly seen, although the tumor can be close to the surface of the brain, but meninges thickening is not seen much. Solitary fibroma is originated from non-meningeal epithelial tissue tumor, and its density and signal are similar to meningioma, and it rarely causes meningeal thickening and "dural tail sign."

2.9 Hematologic Malignancies

Case 2.9.1 Primary Central Nervous System Lymphomas

Clinical Presentation

A 15-year-old boy patient presented with intermittent headache for 2 months and sustained headache for 5 days. He was conscious but a bit slow to respond, the muscle strength of the limbs was V grade, and the muscle tension was normal.

Imaging Findings

A. Axial T1-weighted image demonstrates a hypointense mass in the right cerebellar hemisphere (Fig. 2.37a).
B-C. Axial T2-weighted and T2-FLAIR show hyperintensities in the central edge of the mass (Fig. 2.37b–c).
D. Axial DWI shows a hyperintense lesion with low ADC value, representing restricted diffusion (Fig. 2.37d).
E-H. Native T1 and contrast-enhanced T1-weighted images demonstrate remarkably homogeneous enhancement of the lesion (Fig. 2.37e-h).

Discussion

Primary central nervous system lymphoma (PCNSL) represents up to 5% of all primary central nervous system (CNS) malignancies. The vast majority of PCNSLs are a subtype of non-Hodgkin's lymphoma (NHL) and is usually large cell or immunoblastic type.

The epidemiology and clinical presentation vary depending on the invading sites and the immune status of the patient. The main clinical symptoms were cognitive disorder, numbness, disorder of consciousness, etc.

Regarding the location of the lesions, most patients showed invasion of supratentorial, and some patients have infratentorial lesions. The absence of necrosis in the corpus callosum is not a frequent finding but is rather specific and thus highly suggestive of lymphoma. The vast majority will have at least one intra-axial lesion contacting the surface of either ventricular or pial [94].

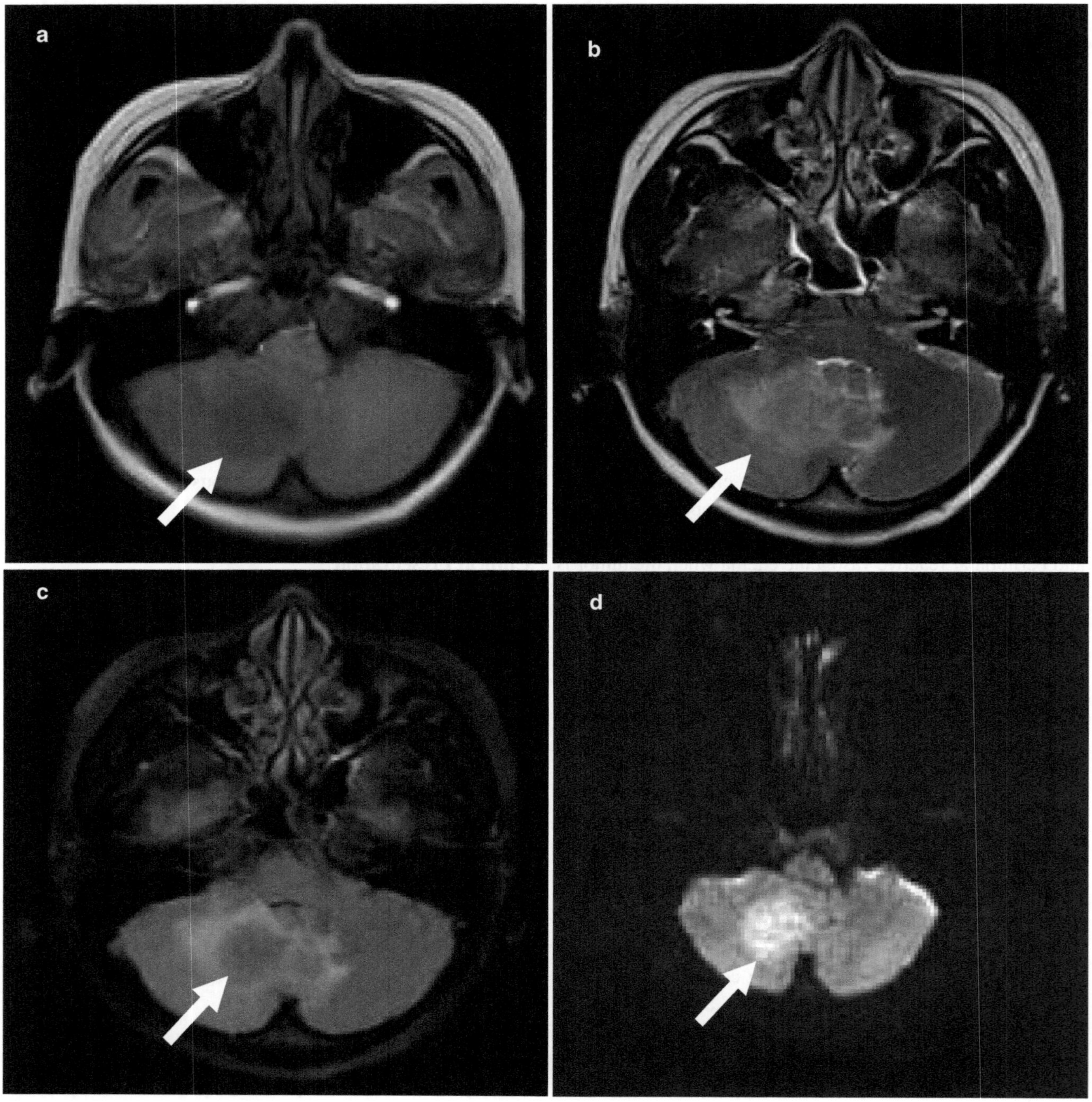

Fig. 2.37 Primary central nervous system lymphomas

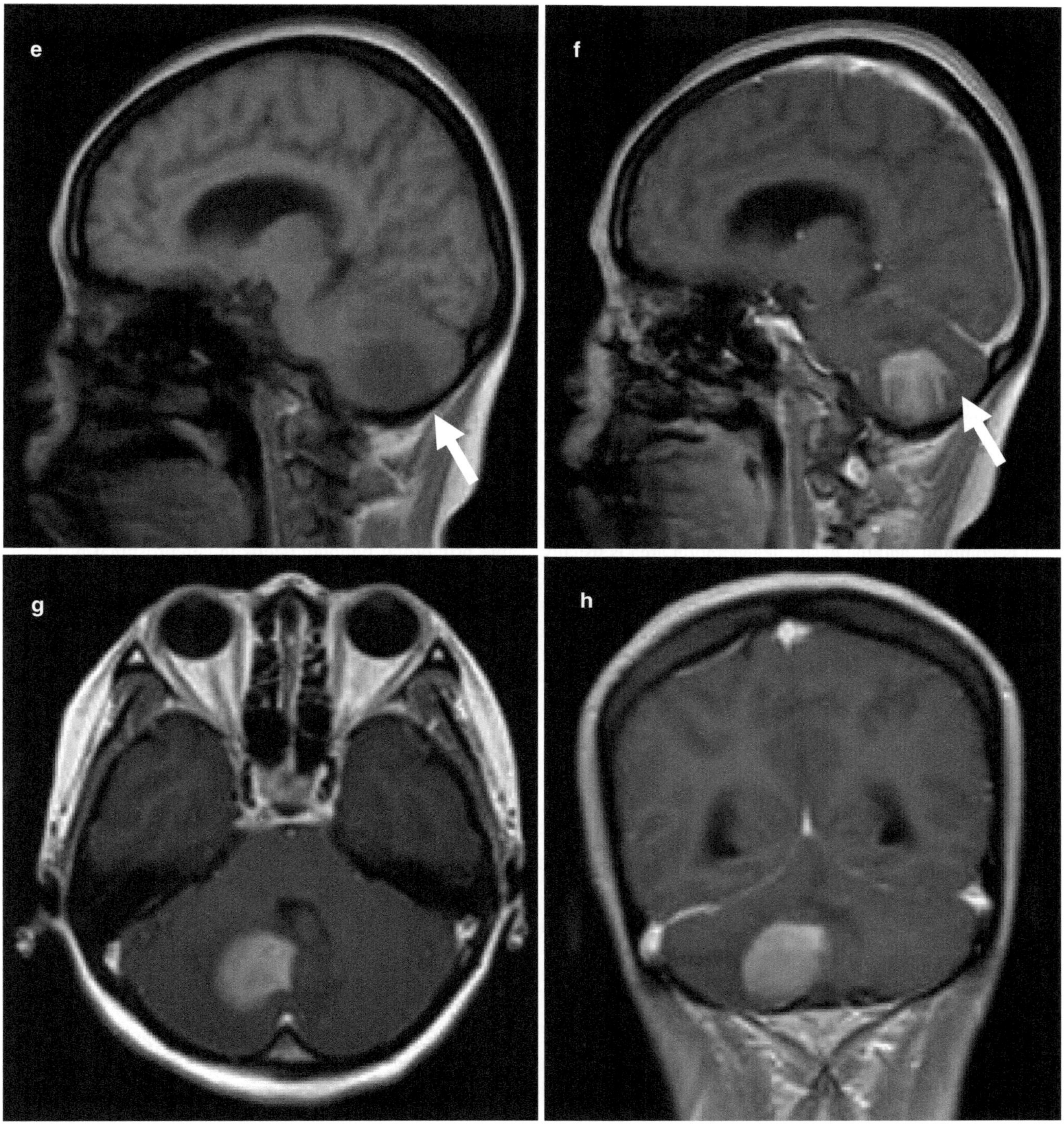

Fig. 2.37 (continued)

The signal features in MRI conventional sequences varied depending on the tissue characteristics, but some of them should point to this diagnostic possibility. Indeed, PCNSL tissues are with high cell density, high nuclear/cytoplasmic volume ratio, enriched in reticular fibers, and small stromal components. Therefore, they will show iso- or hypointensity on T1WI, and iso- or relative hyperintensity, or even hypointensity on T2WI. The highly cellular nature of these tumors usually results in restricted diffusion within lesions. Furthermore, the perilesional white matter signal change is common in CNS lymphoma. After contrast injection, these usually present strong homogeneous enhancement. PCNSL would also develop characteristic "incision," "angular," or "fist" signs on enhanced MRI, which would be helpful for the diagnosis of PCNSL. Apart from these, linear enhancement along the periventricular area strongly suggests PCNSL [95]. Cystic degeneration and necrosis is less common in PCNSL, and ring enhancement is also rarely seen.

It needs to be differentiated from glioblastoma multiforme. In glioblastoma multiforme, necrotic cystic degeneration is common, and the cystic degeneration area is usually large and irregular, with obvious peritumoral edema.

And the cases with multiple lesions should be differentiated from metastatic tumors. Most intracranial metastatic tumors occur in the subcortical region, with significant peritumor edema. The signal features in MRI showed hyperintensity on T2WI, with obvious annular or nodular enhancement [96].

Case 2.9.2 Leukemic Brain Invasion

Clinical Presentation

A 5-year-old boy was diagnosed with leukemia for 2 years and 6 months, now manifested as headache, right limb motor disorder, and memory deterioration. The cerebrospinal fluid examination (CSF) WBC was 5/μL.

Imaging Findings

A-C. Axial MR images demonstrate a lesion In the left basal ganglia, heterogeneously hyper- to isointense on T2WI, Hypo-/isointense to brain on T2- FLAIR and T1WI, no edema around the lesion (Fig. 2.38a–c).

D-E. Axial DWI and ADC map show a hypointense lesion with high ADC value, representing no restricted diffusion (Fig. 2.38d–e).

F. Contrast-enhanced T1-weighted image demonstrates the lesion without enhancement (Fig. 2.38f).

Discussion

Leukemic brain invasion is one of the common complications of acute leukemia. Its prognosis is poor, and the recurrence rate is high. It is one of the common lethal factors of leukemia. The incidence of brain invasion in acute lymphoblastic leukemia is higher than that in other parts of acute lymphoblastic leukemia. Leukemic brain invasion can be seen in all stages of leukemia, and its invasion mode and location is diverse and can locally or diffusely invade the pia mater, dura mater, and brain parenchyma and invade the skull to cause skull damage [97]. Invasion of venous sinus resulted in venous sinus embolism.

The clinical manifestations of leukemic brain invasion are varied due to the different location and scope of invasion. Most patients are mainly affected by meningeal or cerebral parenchyma, such as headache, nausea, vomiting, and so on. Facial paralysis, visual impairment, hearing impairment, and other cranial nerve involvement can also occur. Its clinical manifestations are not specific, and are similar to those of infection, bleeding, and other tumors. Diagnostic criteria for brain invasion in leukemia (NCCN2017 guidelines) [98] are (CSF) WBC $\geq$ 5/μL in cerebrospinal fluid examination during the course of diagnosis or treatment, and there are morphologically identifiable primordial lymphoid cells in cerebrospinal fluid. The imaging findings of leukemic brain invasion were as follows [99]: (1) leukemias infiltrate pia mater, CT can see sulcus and cistern disappears, strip low density foci are seen, corresponding MRI shows T1WI equal or low signal intensity, T2WI/FLAIR shows high signal intensity, and gyrus swelling is seen. The DWI showed a slightly higher signal, enhanced obviously after enhancement. After the leukemia cells invade the superficial pia mater, they extend around the vessels along the Virchow-Robin space and enter the intracranial by destroying the pia mater to form a mass, that is, a "green tumor." Green tumor can infiltrate the orbit, can cause the destruction of skull, infiltrate the eye muscle to make it thicker, invade optic nerve, and so on, especially in children. (2) Dura mater involvement, involving forehead plate barrier, soft-tissue density focus on CT, soft-tissue signal focus on MRI, and obvious enhancement after enhancement. (3) Brain parenchyma infiltration, often multiple masses; MRI showed TIWI low signal intensity, T2WI/FLAIR high signal intensity, DWI high signal intensity, no obvious space-occupying effect, enhanced after enhancement, and often complicated with bleeding. The sensitivity and specificity of MRI were higher than those of CT. The leukemic brain invasion should be distinguished from the following diseases: (1) Cerebral hemorrhage: The MRI findings of leukemia are intracranial space occupying, and the enhancement is obvious after enhancement. However, there was no enhancement after enhancement of cerebral hemorrhage. (2) Meningitis: Meningeal leukemia and meningitis have similar manifestations, but the clinical manifestations are different. Cerebrospinal fluid examination can be used to

Fig. 2.38 Leukemic brain invasion

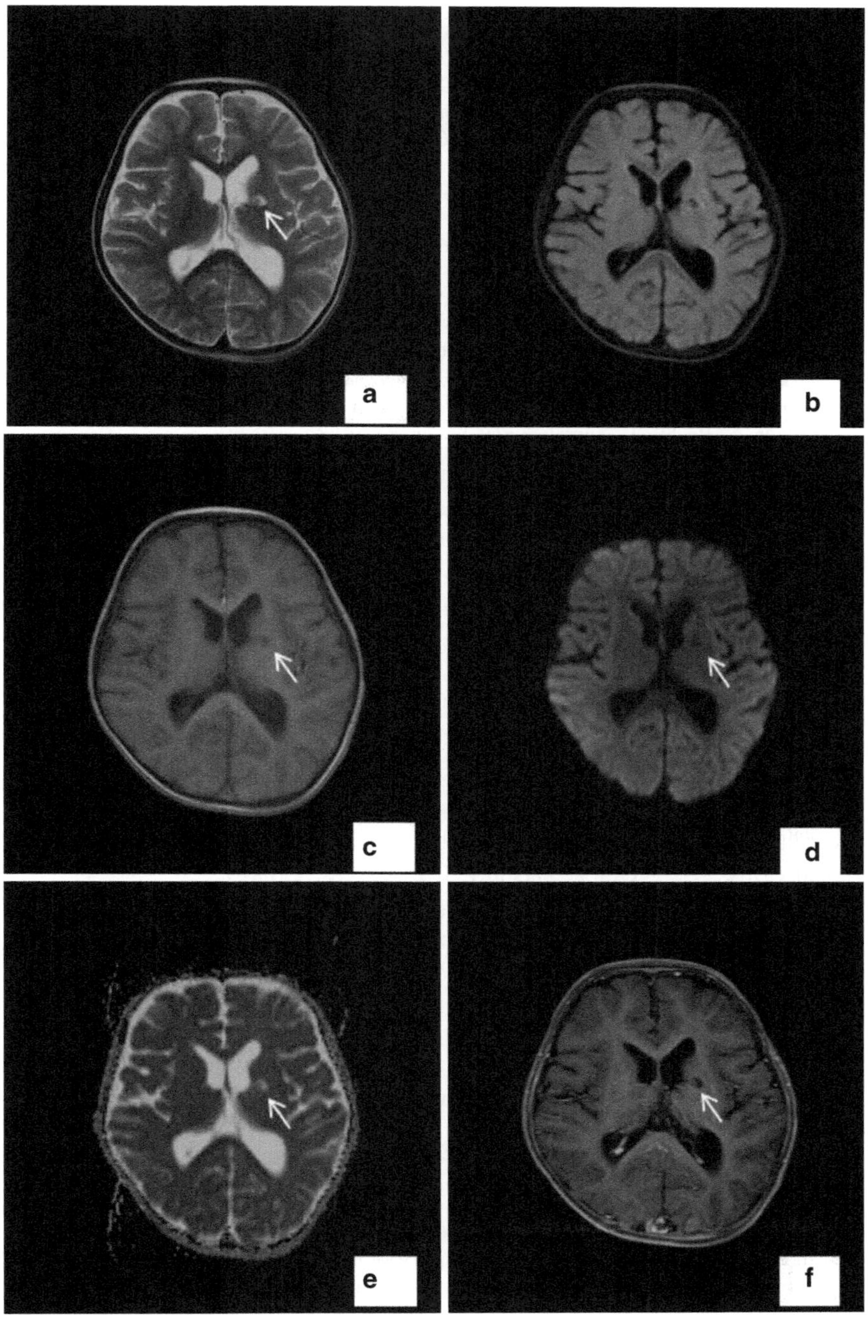

distinguish. (3) White matter lesions caused by chemotherapy or drugs: MRI findings of white matter lesions caused by chemotherapeutic drugs are flake signal abnormalities, enhanced scan has no obvious enhancement, and leukemia is mainly cerebral parenchyma space occupying. The signal enhancement was obvious. (4) Metastasis: It showed low signal intensity on T1WI. After enhancement, most of them showed nodular enhancement; edema around the tumor was obvious, so it was easy to distinguish.

The 5-year event free survival rate of childhood acute leukemia (event free survival, EFS) has reached 80%. The total 5-year overall survival rate (overall survival, OS) is also close to 90 percent.

At present, recurrence, especially leukemia brain invasion, is still one of the main reasons for the failure of leukemia treatment. It is very important to realize the early diagnosis of leukemia brain invasion and effective intervention to prolong the survival time of leukemia patients.

References

1. Ostrom QT, Gittleman H, Liao P, Rouse C, Chen Y, et al. CBTRUS statistical report: primary brain and central nervous system tumors diagnosed in the United States in 2007–2011. Neuro Oncol. 2014;16 Suppl 4:iv1-63.
2. Burkhard C, Di Patre PL, Schuler D, Schuler G, Yasargil MG, et al. A population-based study of the incidence and survival rates in patients with pilocytic astrocytoma. J Neurosurg. 2003;98:1170–4.
3. Sato K, Rorke LB. Vascular bundles and wicker works in childhood brain tumors. Pediatr Neurosci. 1989;15:105–10.
4. Giannini C, Scheithauer BW, Burger PC, Brat DJ, Wollan PC, et al. Pleomorphic xanthoastrocytoma: what do we really know about it? Cancer. 1999;85:2033–45.
5. Ajlana A, Rechtb L. Supratentorial low-grade diffuse astrocytoma: medical management. Semin Oncol. 2014;41(4):446–57.
6. Morana G, Bottoni G, Mancardi MM, Verrico A, Piccardo A. Seizure-induced increased 18F-DOPA uptake in a child with diffuse astrocytoma and transient brain MRI abnormalities related to status epilepticus. Clin Nucl Med. 2018;43(5):e149–50.
7. Gahramanov S, Varallyay C, Tyson RM, et al. Diagnosis of pseudoprogression using MRI perfusion in patients with glioblastoma multiforme may predict improved survival. CNS Oncol. 2014;3(6):389–400.
8. Ion-Mărgineanu A, Van Cauter S, Sima DM, et al. Classifying glioblastoma multiforme follow-up progressive vs. responsive forms using multi-parametric MRI features. Front Neurosci. 2016;10:615.
9. Anwar SSM, Baig MZ, Laghari AA, et al. Accuracy of apparent diffusion coefficients and enhancement ratios on magnetic resonance imaging in differentiating primary cerebral lymphomas from glioblastoma. Neuroradiol J. 2019;32(5):328–34.
10. Sener RN. Diffusion MR imaging of giant cell tumors in tuberous sclerosis. J Comput Assist Tomogr. 2003;27(3):431–3.
11. Baron Y, Barkovich AJ. MR imaging of tuberous sclerosis in neonates and young infants. AJNR Am J Neuroradiol. 1999;20(5):907–16.
12. Braffman BH, Bilaniuk LT, Naidich TP, et al. MR imaging of tuberous sclerosis: pathogenesis of this phakomatosis, use of gadopentetate dimeglumine, and literature review. Radiology. 1992;183(1):227–38.
13. Nishio S, Morioka T, Suzuki S, et al. Subependymal giant cell astrocytoma: clinical and neuroimaging features of four cases. J Clin Neurosci. 2001;8(1):31–4.
14. Panigrahy A, Bluml S. Neuroimaging of pediatric brain tumors: from basic to advanced magnetic resonance imaging (MRI). J Child Neurol. 2009;24(11):1343–65.
15. Bulakbasi N, Kocaoglu M, Ors F, et al. Combination of single-voxel proton MR spectroscopy and apparent diffusion coefficient calculation in the evaluation of common brain tumors. AJNR Am J Neuroradiol. 2003;24(2):225–33.
16. Chassoux F, Rodrigo S, Mellerio C, et al. Dysembryoplastic neuroepithelial tumors: an MRI-based scheme for epilepsy surgery. Neurology. 2012;79(16):1699–707.
17. Chassoux F, Daumas-Duport C. Dysembryoplastic neuroepithelial tumors: where are we now? Epilepsia. 2013;54(Suppl 9):129–34.
18. Louis DN, Perry A, Reifenberger G, et al. The 2016 World Health Organization classification of tumors of the central nervous system: a summary. Acta Neuropathol. 2016;131(6):803–20.
19. Richardson AM, Armstrong VL, Gernsback JE, Gultekin SH, Komotar RJ. Central neurocytoma: rare presentation in fourth ventricle and review of literature. World Neurosurg. 2019;123: 357–61.
20. Ma Z, Yan H, Shi H, et al. The typical and atypical MR imaging findings of central neurocytomas: report on eighteen cases and review of the literature. Clin Neurol Neurosurg. 2016;146:18–23.
21. Tlili-Graiess K, Mama N, Arifa N, et al. Diffusion weighted MR imaging and proton MR spectroscopy findings of central neurocytoma with pathological correlation. J Neuroradiol. 2014;41:243–50.
22. Delgado-López PD, Corrales-García EM, Alonso-García E, et al. Central nervous system ependymoma: clinical implications of the new molecular classification, treatment guidelines and controversial issues. Clin Transl Oncol. 2019;21:1450–63.
23. Hübner JM, Kool M, Pfister SM, et al. Epidemiology, molecular classification and WHO grading of ependymoma. J Neurosurg Sci. 2018;62(1):46–50.
24. Nowak J, Seidel C, Pietsch T, et al. Systematic comparison of MRI findings in pediatric ependymoblastoma with ependymoma and CNS primitive neuroectodermal tumor not otherwise specified. Neuro-Oncology. 2015;17(8):1157–65.
25. Khilji MF, Hamid RS, Qureshi A. Supratentorial extraventricular anaplastic ependymoma in a child. BMJ Case Rep. 2014;2014:bcr2014203750.
26. Elsharkawy AE, Abuamona R, Bergmann M, et al. Cortical anaplastic ependymoma with significant desmoplasia: a case report and literature review. Case Rep Oncol Med. 2013;2013:354873.
27. Yan S, Lixia Q. Magnetic resonance imaging analysis and differential imaging of ependymoma in different parts of the screen. J Pract Med Imaging. 2012;06:344–7.
28. Wang Y, Zou L, Gao B. Intracranial germinoma: clinical and MRI findings in 56 patients. Childs Nerv Syst. 2010;26(12):1773–7.
29. Li J, Zhang XY, Wang B, et al. MRI and MR spectroscopy findings of the evolution of an intracranial germinoma: a case report. Oncol Lett. 2015;10(2):1194–6.
30. Robles FM, Gonzalo GI, De Las Casas Quispe AC, et al. Fetal intracranial immature teratoma: presentation of a case and a systematic review of the literature. J Matern Fetal Neonatal Med. 2017;30(10):1139–46.
31. Nariai H, Price DE, Jada A, et al. Prenatally diagnosed aggressive intracranial immature teratoma-clinicopathological correlation. Fetal Pediatr Pathol. 2016;35(4):260–4.
32. Thakran A, Rao S, Sreenivas M, et al. Massive congenital intracranial immature teratoma: an autopsy report. Indian J Pathol Microbiol. 2012;55(2):272–4.
33. Athale UH, Duckworth J, Odame I, Barr R. Childhood atypical teratoid rhabdoid tumor of the central nervous system: a meta-analysis of observational studies. J Pediatr Hematol Oncol. 2009;31(9):651–63.
34. Wangchun D, Hongsheng L, Xiwen C, Sihui Z, Qianqian W, Yuankai C, Zhenqing L. Imaging findings of atypical teratoid/rhabdoid tumor of central nervous system with clinical correlation. Chin J Radiol. 2017;8:612–5.
35. Echevarria ME, Fangusaro J, Goldman S. Pediatric central nervous system germ cell tumors: a review. Oncologist. 2008;13(6): 690–9.
36. Shibamoto Y, Takahashi M, Sasai K. Prognosis of intracranial germinoma with syncytiotrophoblastic giant cells treated by radiation therapy. Int J Radiat Oncol Biol Phys. 1997;37(3):505–10.
37. Ho DM, Liu HC. Primary intracranial germ cell tumor. Pathologic study of 51 patients. Cancer. 1992;70(6):1577–84.
38. Goyal N, et al. Mature teratoma in association with neural tube defect (occipital encephalocele): series of four cases and review of the literature. Pediatr Neurosurg. 2012;48(2):67–72.
39. Fujimaki T, et al. CT and MRI features of intracranial germ cell tumors. J Neuro-Oncol. 1994;19(3):217–26.
40. Smith AB, Rushing EJ, Smirniotopoulos JG. From the archives of the AFIP: lesions of the pineal region: radiologic-pathologic correlation. Radiographics. 2010;30(7):2001–20.
41. Dahiya S, Perry A. Pineal tumors. Adv Anat Pathol. 2010;17(6):419–27.
42. Jouvet A, et al. Pineal parenchymal tumors: a correlation of histological features with prognosis in 66 cases. Brain Pathol. 2000;10(1):49–60.

43. Borit A, Blackwood W, Mair WG. The separation of pineocytoma from pineoblastoma. Cancer. 1980;45(6):1408–18.
44. Schild SE, et al. Pineal parenchymal tumors. Clinical, pathologic, and therapeutic aspects. Cancer. 1993;72(3):870–80.
45. Chun C, Haixia B, Fulin Z, et al. Clinicopathological characteristics of the choroid plexus papilloma: a report of 13 cases. Fudan Univ J Sci. 2013;40(5):579–83.
46. Brat DJ, Parisi JE, Kleinschmidt-DeMasters BK, et al. Surgical neuropathology update: a review of changes introduced by the WHO classification of tumours of the central nervous system, 4th edition. Arch Pathol Lab Med. 2008;132:993–1007.
47. Feng G, Zheng L, Yane Z, et al. MRI finds of atypical choroid plexus papilloma. J Med Imaging. 2012;22(7):1056–9.
48. Tianmei L. Choroid plexus papillary carcinoma in infant: case report. Chin J Med Imaging Technol. 2019;35(4):585.
49. Xinyi H, Ding M, Peiyi G. Imaging features of medulloblastoma in children. Radiol Pract. 2015;30(6):670–2.
50. Ping M. CT and MRI manifestations of cerebellar pilocytic astrocytoma in children. J Med Imaging. 2017;27(9):1803–6.
51. Weiping H, Linbo C, Xiao X, et al. Treatment and prognosis of Pilomyxoid astrocytoma in 11 cases. Guangdong Med J. 2017;38(1):49–52.
52. Barton VN, Donson AM, Birks DK, et al. Insulin-like growth factor 2 mRNA binding protein 3 expression is an independent prognostic factor in pediatric pilocytic and pilomyxoid astrocytoma. J Neuropathol Exp Neurol. 2013;72(5):442–9.
53. Sai DU, Jun-hong GUAN, Yue LI. Yolk sac tumor in fourth ventricle (report of one case and review of literature). J Clin Neurosurg. 2020;17(3):339–42.
54. Wei S, Hao L, Rui Z. Treatment experience of atypical teratoid/rhabdoid tumors of the central nervous system in infants. Chin J Neurosurg. 2016;32(4):349–52.
55. Schrey D, Carceller LF, Malietzis G, et al. Multimodal therapy in children and adolescents with newly diagnosed atypical teratoid rhabdoid tumor: individual pooled data analysis and review of the literature. J Neuro-Oncol. 2016;126(1):81–90.
56. Müller HL. Craniopharyngioma. Endocr Rev. 2014;35(3):513–43.
57. Gabel BC, Cleary DR, Martin JR, et al. Unusual and rare locations for craniopharyngiomas: clinical significance and review of the literature. World Neurosurg. 2017;98(2):381–7.
58. Prieto R, Pascual JM, Barrios L. Topographic diagnosis of craniopharyngiomas: the accuracy of MRI findings observed on conventional T_1 and T_2 images. Am J Neurdiol. 2017;38(11):2073–80.
59. Aihara Y, Chiba K, Eguchi S, et al. Pediatric optic pathway/hypothalamic glioma. Neurol Med Chir (Tokyo). 2018;58(1):1–9.
60. Rasool N, Odel JG, Kazim M. Optic pathway glioma of childhood. Curr Opin Ophthalmol. 2017;28(3):289–95.
61. Beres S, Avery R. Optic pathway gliomas secondary to Neurofibromatosis type 1. Semin Pediatr Neurol. 2017;24(2):92–9.
62. Harrison VS, Oatman O, Kerrigan JF. Hypothalamic hamartoma with epilepsy: review of endocrine comorbidity. Epilepsia. 2017;58(Suppl 2):50.
63. Fuller CE, Jones D, Kieran MW. New classification for central nervous system tumors: implications for diagnosis and therapy. Am Soc Clin Oncol Educ Book. 2017;37:753–63.
64. Burcher GC, Liang H, Rebecca L, Helen Cross J, Tisdall M, Varadkar S, Spoudeas HA, Caredda E, Bennett S, Heyman I. Neuropsychiatric profile of paediatric hypothalamic hamartoma: systematic review and case series. Dev Med Child Neurol. 2019;61(12):1377–85.
65. Striano S, Striano P. Clinical features and evolution of the gelastic seizures-hypothalamic hamartoma syndrome. Epilepsia. 2017;06(58 Suppl 2):12–5.
66. Gadgil N, Lam S, Pan I-W, LoPresti M, Wagner K, Ali I, Wilfong A, Curry DJ. Staged magnetic resonance-guided laser interstitial thermal therapy for hypothalamic hamartoma: analysis of ablation volumes and morphological considerations. Neurosurgery. 2020;86(6):808–16.
67. Celik O, Ozyurt S, Saglican Y. Suprasellar germinoma with hypopituitarism in an 18-year old man: a case report and review of literature. Clin Neurol Neurosurg. 2020;196:106026. https://doi.org/10.1016/j.clineuro.2020.106026.
68. Kyritsis AP. Management of primary intracranial germ cell tumors. J Neuro-Oncol. 2010;96(2):143–9.
69. Kim JW, Kim WC, Cho JH, et al. A multimodal approach including craniospinal irradiation improves the treatment outcome of high-risk intracranial nongerminomatous germ cell tumors. Int J Radiat Oncol Biol Phys. 2012;84(3):625–31.
70. Personnier C, Cazabat L, Bertherat J, et al. Clinical features and treatment of pediatric somatotropinoma: case study of an aggressive tumor due to a new AIP mutation and extensive literature review. Horm Res Paediatr. 2011;75(6):392–402.
71. Aghi MK, Blevins LS. Introduction to pituitary adenomas. Neurosurg Clin N Am. 2019;30(4):xiii.
72. Honegger J, Nasi-Kordhishti I, Giese S. Pituitary adenomas. Nervenarzt. 2019;90(6):568–77.
73. Walz PC, Drapeau A, Shaikhouni A, et al. Pediatric pituitary adenomas. Childs Nerv Syst. 2019;35(11):2107–18.
74. Stratakis CA. Cushing syndrome in pediatrics. Endocrinol Metab Clin N Am. 2012;41(4):793–803.
75. Zhou W, Rao J, Li C. Isolated Langerhans cell histiocytosis in the hypothalamic-pituitary region: a case report. BMC Endocr Disord. 2019;19(1):143.
76. Fatima T, Hussain Chandio S, Muzaffar K, Mumtaz H, Jahan N. Pituitary stalk interruption syndrome. Cureus. 2020;12(9):e10518.
77. Zhang W, Qian F, Lu G, Wu Y, Li R, Xia L, Zhao R, Lin Y, Gu M, Chen W. Pituitary stalk interruption syndrome: a rare case report and literature review. Medicine (Baltimore). 2020;99(50):e23266.
78. Atif N, Muhammad A, Jehanzeb S. Pituitary stalk interruption syndrome presenting in a euthyroid adult with short stature. Radiol Case Rep. 2018;13:503–6.
79. Yashar M, Morteza ST, Farhad N, et al. Brainstem glioma: prediction of histopathologic grade based on conventional MR imaging. Neuroradiol J. 2018;31(1):10–7.
80. Biao J, Yu G, Yun F, et al. MRI diagnosis of brainstem glioma in children. Radiol Pract. 2000;15(3):193–5.
81. Tina YP, Mehmet K, Sridhar V, et al. MRI as a central component of clinical trials analysis in brainstem glioma: a report from the Pediatric Brain Tumor Consortium (PBTC). Neuro Oncol. 2011;13(4):417–27.
82. Siller S, Szelenyi A, Herlitz L, et al. Spinal cord hemangioblastomas: significance of intraoperative neurophysiological monitoring for resection and long-term outcome. J Neurosurg Spine. 2017;26(4):483–93.
83. Louis DN, Otmar OD, Webster WK, et al. WHO classification of tumours of the central nervous system, revised 4th edition. Lyon: International Agency for Research on Cancer; 2016. p. 80–9.
84. Barkovich AJ, Raybaud. Pediatric neuroimaging. 6th ed. China: Wolters Kluwer; 2019. p. 726–9.
85. Coley BD. Caffey's diagnostic imaging. 13th ed. China: Elsevier; 2019. p. 348–9.
86. Barkovich AJ. Diagnostic imaging pediatric neuroradiology. 2nd ed. Canada: Elsevier; 2015. p. I-4-6-9.
87. AlRayahi J, Zapotocky M, Ramaswamy V, et al. Pediatric brain tumor genetics: what radiologists need to know. Radiographics. 2018;38:2102–22.
88. Kumar RS, Rotondo RL. Pediatric brain metastases. 2018;
89. Udaka YT, et al. Pediatric brain tumors. Neurol Clin. 2018;36(3):533–56.
90. Stefanowicz J, Iżycka-Świeszewska E, Szurowska E, et al. Brain metastases in paediatric patients: characteristics of a patient series and review of the literature. Folia Neuropathol. 2011;49: 271–81.

91. Giammattei L, Messerer M, Aghakhani N, et al. Surgical resection of medulla oblongata hemangioblastomas: outcome and complications. Acta Neurochir. 2016;158(7):1333–41.
92. Ma D, Wang Y, Du G, et al. Neurosurgical management of brainstem hemangioblastomas: a single-institution experience with 116 patients. World Neurosurg. 2015;84(4):1030–8.
93. Cheng J, Liu W, Hui X, et al. Pediatric central nervous system hemangioblastomas: different from adult forms? A retrospective series of 25 cases. Acta Neurochir. 2017;159(9):1603–11.
94. Yap Kelvin K, Tom S, Elaine L, et al. Magnetic resonance features of primary central nervous system lymphoma in the immunocompetent patient: a pictorial essay. J Med Imaging Radiat Oncol. 2012;56:179–86.
95. Gang C, Jianning Z. Imaging features (CT, MRI, MRS, and PET/CT) of primary central nervous system lymphoma in immunocompetent patients. Neurol Sci. 2019;40:535–42.
96. Qiang L, Lu W, Feiping L, et al. [Magnetic resonance imaging features for primary brain lymphoma]. Zhong Nan Da Xue Xue Bao Yi Xue Ban. 2018;43:1118–22.
97. Hannon M, Wilde L, Nwaoduah N, Kasner M. Chronic myelomonocytic leukemia with central nervous system involvement. Leuk Lymphoma. 2018;59(9):2267–8.
98. Brown PA, Shah B, Fathi A, et al. NCCN Guide—lines insights: acute lymphoblastic leukemia, Version 1.2017. J Natl Compr Cancer Netw. 2017;15(9):1091.
99. Liang Z, Huang S, Zhou J, Yuan D. MRI findings of central nervous system invasion in leukemia. Imaging Diagn Interv Radiol. 2015;24(03):199.
100. Qingshi H, Dong Z, Long P, et al. Clinical data analysis of 112 cases of subatentorial brain tumors in children. Chin J Neurosurg. 2013;29(6):572–4. https://doi.org/10.3760/cms.j.issn.1001-2346.2013.06.01.
101. Yongti Z, Shixiang S, Xianyong S. MR diagnosis and pathological analysis of the pilocytic astrocytoma. Chin J CT MRI. 2018;16(1):144–1461.
102. Wangchun D, Hongsheng L, Xiwen C, et al. Imaging findings of atypical teratoid/rhabdoid tumor of central nervous system with clinical correlation. Chin J Radiol. 2017;51(8):612–5.
103. Yong Z, Jingliang C, Ruiping Z, et al. Whole-tumor histogram analysis of apparent diffusion coefficient maps in grading diagnosis of ependymoma. Chin J Radiol. 2018;52(10):751–5.
104. Huang RY, Bi WL, Brent G, et al. Imaging and diagnostic advances for intracranial meningiomas. Neuro Oncol. 2019;21(Supplement_1):i44–61.
105. Garcia CR, Slone SA, et al. Initial management of meningiomas: analysis of the National Cancer Database. Cancer Epidemiol. 2019;60:16–22.
106. Hwang K, Joo J-D, Kim Y-H, et al. Risk factors for preoperative and late postoperative seizures in primary supratentorial meningiomas. Clin Neurol Neurosurg. 2019;180:34–9.

Intracranial Infection

3

Xinzi Li, Mengjie Zhang, Guifen Zheng, Xin Li, and Jing Chen

Intracranial inflammatory disorders are common in children, including infection and immune-associated encephalitis. Common intracranial infectious encephalitis pathogens include bacteria, viruses, fungi, tuberculosis, parasites, and other pathogens. Immune-associated encephalitis is becoming more common due to its underlying abnormal immune response in the central nervous system. Some immune-associated encephalitis are associated with antibodies against cell surface antigens, which include NMDAR, MOG, AQP4, etc. CT and MRI examinations can assist clinicians to determine the location and extent of the lesions, follow up the evolution of the lesions, find out the complications, observe the treatment effect, and give a qualitative diagnosis in certain cases. MRI is much more effective than CT and has become the preferred method for the examination of inflammatory disorders in children.

3.1 Congenital Intracranial Infection

Case 3.1 Congenital Intracranial Infection

Clinical Presentation

A 21-day-old girl presented with mental retardation and feeding refuse for 1 day. The serous cytomegalovirus antibody detections of her and her mother are both positive.

Imaging Findings

A. Axial non-contrast CT image shows bilateral periventricular hypoattenuating lesions (arrow head) and multiple subependymal calcifications (arrow) (Fig. 3.1a).
B. The slightly proximal level of the Fig.3.1a in the same patient (Fig. 3.1b).

X. Li · M. Zhang · G. Zheng · J. Chen
Department of Radiology, Tianjin Children's Hospital (Children's Hospital of Tianjin University), Tianjin, P.R. China

X. Li (✉)
Tianjin Second People's Hospital (Tianjin Institute of Hepatology), Tianjin, P.R. China

Discussion

The organisms involving intrauterine central nervous system infection can be summarized as a term of TORCH, a mnemonic acronym, including toxoplasma gondii, rubella virus, cytomegalovirus (CMV), herpes virus, and other organisms, such as Syphilis, lymphocytic choriomeningitis virus, parvovirus B19, human immunodeficiency virus and zika virus which is recently reported [1]. Transmission of infection to the fetus occurs via placenta. CMV and rubella virus are the most common TORCH infections, and CMV is the most common cause of infectious hearing loss. Rubella virus display a central nervous system predilection, and the central nervous system involvement of the afflicted infants can be encephalitis [2].

The pathophysiology of the central nervous system in utero infection is significantly different from elder children and adults. The manifestations and prognosis of these infections vary greatly, which depend on the gestational age of the fetus at the outset of infection and the virulence. The mature brain responds to infectious injury by gliosis and lacking of functional plasticity. In contrast, the developing brain typically appears little immune-mediated inflammatory response with minimal gliosis because of immature immune system of fetus. Infections in the first two trimesters are usually characterized by interference of the normal developing processes and resulting in kinds of congenital malformations, while those in the third trimester may cause destructive lesions. Although during the last trimester, the destructions are more frequent, whereas the functional plasticity can be continued to infancy and early childhood. Newborns and infants with TORCH infection usually have neurodevelopmental sequela including mental retardation, epilepsy, vision and hearing loss. Affected patients are typically microcephalic with diminished white matter, ventriculomegaly, lissencephaly, pachygyria, polymicrogyria, delay myelin maturation, and astrogliosis.

The imaging finding of multiple subependymal and subcortical calcifications foci is a characteristic feature of TORCH infections. In general, TORCH-related intracranial

H. Liu, X. Zhang (eds.), *Pediatric Neuroimaging*, https://doi.org/10.1007/978-981-16-7928-5_3

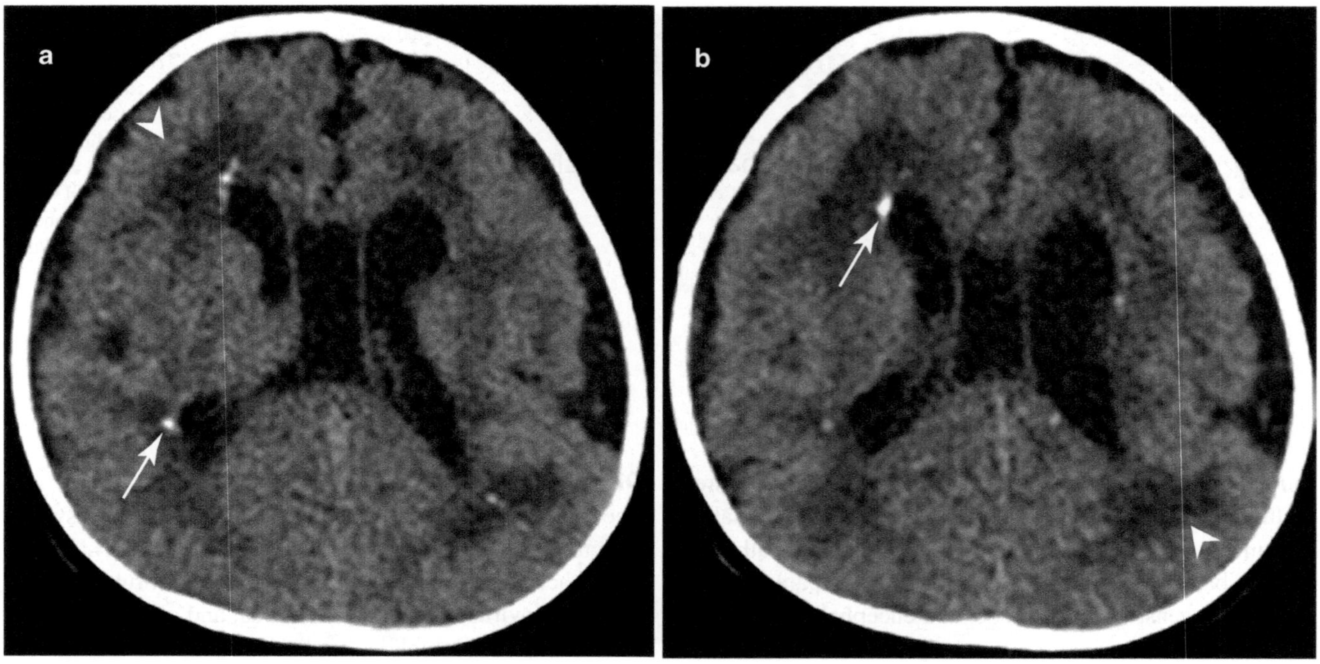

Fig. 3.1 Congenital intracranial infection

calcifications are identified in the neonatal period, while the intracranial calcified foci caused by some pathogens could not be found until later in life, such as HIV congenital infection. Intracranial calcifications can appear anywhere. Distribution and morphology of CMV calcified foci are variable with a preference of periventricular or subependymal in location. By comparison, toxoplasmosis calcifications have a tendency of relatively peripherally located.

The necrosis can occur in any part of the neuroaxis and the calcifications of the necrotic areas, which characteristic locations are basal ganglia, periventricular region, and cerebral cortex. White matter involvement of bilateral parietal, temporal and occipital regions with dilatation of the lateral ventricles is prevalent.

CT is sensitive for detecting intracranial calcification which demonstrates variable appearance on conventional MRI. However, the performance of susceptibility-weighted imaging (SWI) could not only promote the detection of calcification but also minimize unnecessary radiation exposure in neonates. The appearance of calcification on the phase images is depending on the handedness of the MRI systems from different vendors. Generally, the dimension of the calcifications is consistent with the duration of infection that can be detected by CT manifesting as hyper-density areas. Abnormal hypo-density of focal white matter corresponding to anomalous T2 hyperintensity on MR imaging [3–5].

It is important to note that the imaging findings of certain endocrine or metabolic disorders may mimic TORCH infection, such as the Aicardi–Goutières syndrome and the Baraitser–Reardon syndrome [4, 6]. The progressive course of diseases and negative serology for TORCH infections contribute to the differential diagnosis. Infants with tuberous sclerosis complex are distinguished from congenital infections by the ash leaf spot of the skin, cortical tubers, and subependymal giant cell astrocytoma. Cerebrovascular malformation is another cause of intracranial calcification, often with hemorrhage or thrombosis, may be found in any part of the brain. Finding of the markedly enhanced malformed vessel is the typical feature that differs from TORCH infection [7, 8].

3.2 Acquired Intracranial Infection

Case 3.2.1 Virus Infection

Clinical Presentation

A 6-year-old boy presented with fever for 7 days and seizures 3 times. Physical examination showed extremity hypertonia and nuchal rigidity. The CSF examination showed increased pressure and WBC with lymphocytes as the main parts.

Imaging Findings

A. Axial T1-weighted image demonstrates slightly low signal intensity in the bilateral parietal and frontal lobes (Fig. 3.2a).
B. Axial T2-weighted image shows abnormal high signal intensity corresponding to the lesions in Fig.3.2a (Fig. 3.2b).

C. The lesions in the bilateral parietal and frontal lobes are more obvious on the T2WI-FLAIR image (Fig. 3.2c).
D. Additional abnormal hyperintense in the corpus callosum could be demonstrated on the axial DWI (Fig. 3.2d).

Discussion

Viral encephalitis is one of the most common infectious diseases of the central nervous system in pediatrics. Associated pathogenic viral species could be up to 100 whereas pathogenic agents could be identified for only a few patients. Enteroviruses, arboviruses, and herpes simplex virus are the most common pathogens [9]. Most viruses affect the central nervous system through hematogenous dissemination. The clinical manifestations typically include fever, headache, vomiting, seizures, and lethargy that depending on the affected areas of the brain [10].

Neuronal degeneration and inflammation are the main pathological features of central nervous system infected by

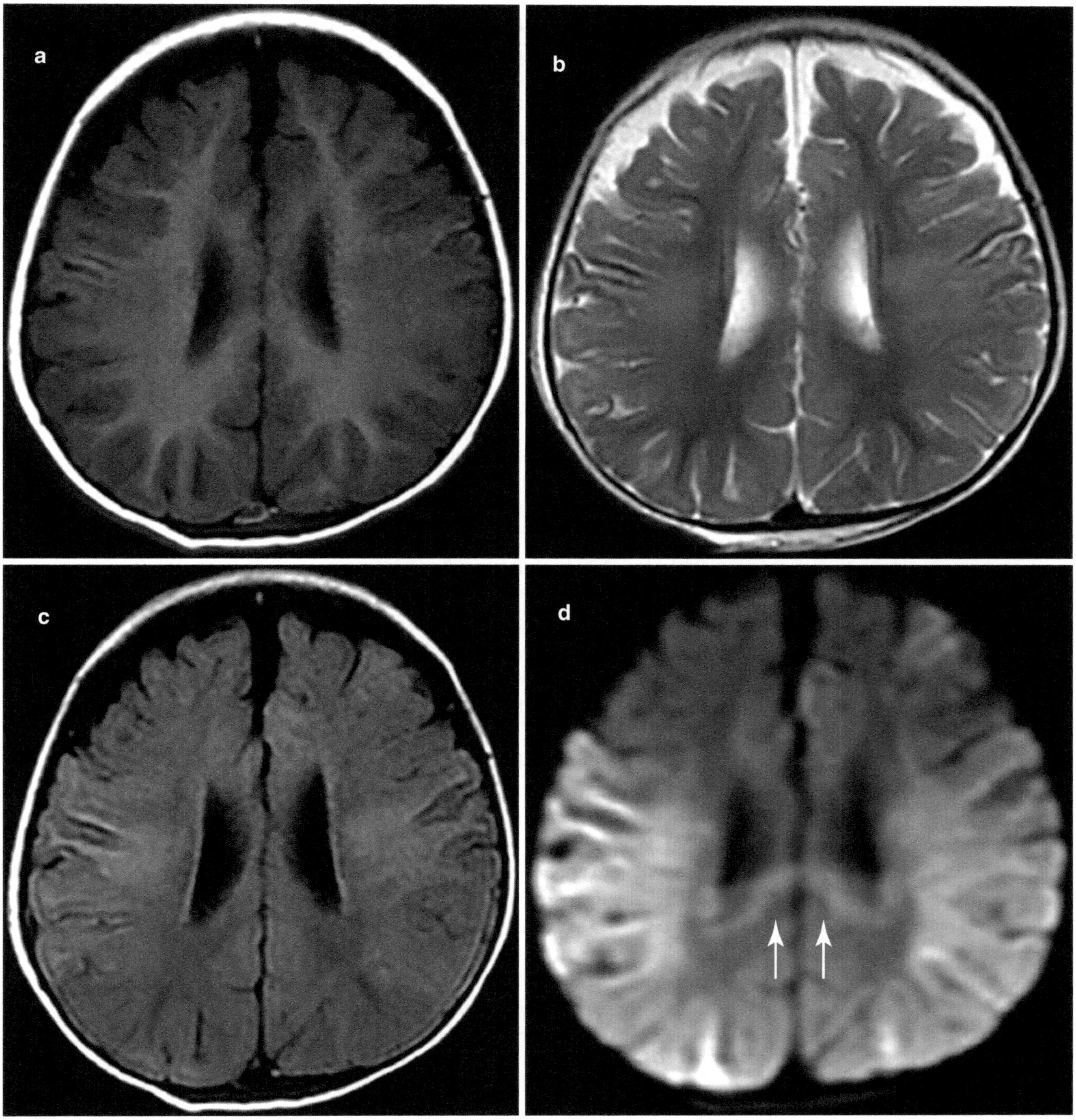

Fig. 3.2 Virus infection

viruses. It can be symmetrically or asymmetrically involving the regions of unilateral or bilateral gray matter, subcortical white matter, hypothalamus, and basal ganglia. The neuroimaging findings may show overlap that is similar to the manifestations of viral encephalitis. However, some kinds of viral encephalitis have predilections for specific locations of brain involvement. Encephalitis caused by herpes simplex virus type I typically begins in bilateral temporal lobes. Encephalitis caused by mumps virus and Japanese encephalitis virus usually affects the basal ganglia regions [9, 11].

MRI is more sensitive than CT in detecting encephalitis lesions. It shows abnormal slightly T1 and T2 prolongation without well-circumstance on MRI, which is more obvious on FLAIR imaging as hyperintensity. Diffusion-weighted Imaging is more excellent in showing restricted diffusion early in the course of viral encephalitis before abnormalities are detected on other sequences. Most of the lesions show no enhancement after gadolinium administration, whereas a few of them could present linear or gyri-like enhancement [12, 13]. The appearance of enhancement correlates with duration and severity of the disease. In the course of encephalitis, almost all viruses induce the increase of water content of the affected regions of the brain. Mild mass affection may exist due to the enlarged extent of lesions. The presence of hemorrhage of the lesions may also be seen [8, 11].

Viral encephalitis should be differentiated from metabolic or toxic diseases and parainfectious encephalitis, such as acute disseminated encephalitis (ADEM). ADEM is a relatively common kind of pediatric demyelinating disease, which usually occurs after viral infection or vaccination. ADEM is a multifocal, but usually monophasic and self-limiting process with multiple asymmetrical lesions involving bilateral white matter of the cerebrum. Meanwhile, hypothalamus, basal ganglia, brain stem, cerebellum, and spine can also be involved. It shows hyperintensity on T2 and FLAIR imaging without an obvious mass effect. The enhancement degree is varied after the administration of contrast material. X-linked adrenal leukodystrophy is a kind of sex-linked recessive hereditary disease resulting from the mutation of ABCD1 gene that codes for a peroxisomal membrane protein, resulting in the accumulation of very long-chain fatty acids in the nervous system, adrenal. The pathological feature of neural system is characterized mainly by the inflammatory demyelination of the cerebrum. Affected patients are almost exclusively boys, who usually present between age 5 and 12 years, with learning difficulties, impaired visuospatial acuity, and progressive disturbance in gait. Most of affected patients have predominant callosal splenium, peritrigonal white matter, and posterior thalami involvement early in the course. And then the lesions extend into the central parietal and occipital white matter, with the feature of bilateral white matter lesions connected by the corpus callosum, which looks like a butterfly. CT reveals low attenuation. MRI demonstrates marked hypointense on T1-weighted imaging, corresponding to hyperintensity on T2-weighted imaging and FLAIR imaging. It shows a rim of enhancement surrounding the area of affected white matter after gadolinium administration. Proton MRS shows high choline, low creatine, and low NAA in the affected regions, whereas this appearance may also be seen in relatively normal white matter suggesting a progressive injury course [8, 11, 14].

Case 3.2.2 Tuberculosis Infection
Patient 1

Clinical Presentation

A 2-year-old boy presented with fever for 9 days with occasional headaches and vomiting. He had a history of contacting with tuberculosis. Examination of the CSF reveals a predominantly monocyte pleocytosis. The PPD skin test was strongly positive.

Imaging Findings

A. Axial T2-weighted image shows high signal intensity in the left basal ganglia region (arrow) (Fig. 3.3a).
B. The DWI demonstrates restricted diffusion of the lesion (arrow) (Fig. 3.3b).
C. CE T2WI-FLAIR image show extensive abnormal enhancement of leptomeninges of bilateral frontal and temporal lobe with the lateral fissure cistern involved (arrowhead) (Fig. 3.3c).
D. CE T2WI-FLAIR image proximal to the level of Fig.3.3c demonstrates abnormal enhancement in the left basal ganglia (arrow) (Fig. 3.3d).

Patient 2

Clinical Presentation

A 4-year-old boy presented with fever and headache for several days. He had contact with a tuberculosis patient several months ago. The PPD skin test was strongly positive.

Imaging Findings

A. Axial T2-weighted image shows multiple high signal intensity lesions in the bilateral thalamus and occipital lobe (arrows and arrowheads) (Fig. 3.4a).
B. T2WI-FLAIR image at the same level of Fig.3.4a shows the lesions, part of them with peripheral edema (arrows) (Fig. 3.4b).
C. Axial CE-T1WI shows multiple spotty, nodular, and ring enhancement lesions in the brain parenchyma (arrowheads) (Fig. 3.4c).
D. Axial CE-T1WI distal to the Fig.3.4c in the same patient shows more extensive dissemination (arrowheads) (Fig. 3.4d).

Discussion

Mycobacterium tuberculosis is one of the common pathogens in children and causes tuberculosis. Central nervous system (CNS) tuberculosis accounts for approximately 10% of all forms of TB and carries the highest mortality [15].

CNS TB may involve the meninges, brain, calvarium, spinal cord, or bony spine. Intracranial tuberculous infection mainly involves meninges, parenchyma. In rare cases, TB may also involve calvarium, orbit, temporal bone, pituitary gland, etc. Tuberculous meningitis (TBM) is the most common and severe form of CNS TB, composing 9 ~ 16% of extrapulmonary tuberculosis in children [16]. Parenchymal TB may occur in isolation or in association with TBM, of which tuberculoma is the most common form. TBM is often combined with vasculitis, infarction (about 20–40%), progressive hydrocephalus, and cranial neuropathies [15, 17].

Central nervous system involvement has a clinical appearance within 6 months of the primary infection, and almost always accompanies acute miliary tuberculosis. Early onset of TBM in children includes headache, vomiting, irritability or lethargy, and sometimes fever [18]. If untreated, affected patients may develop cranial nerve palsies, focal deficits, or signs of increased intracranial pressure. PCR detection of mycobacterium in cerebrospinal fluid and positive tuberculin skin test are helpful for diagnosis of TB infection [17, 19].

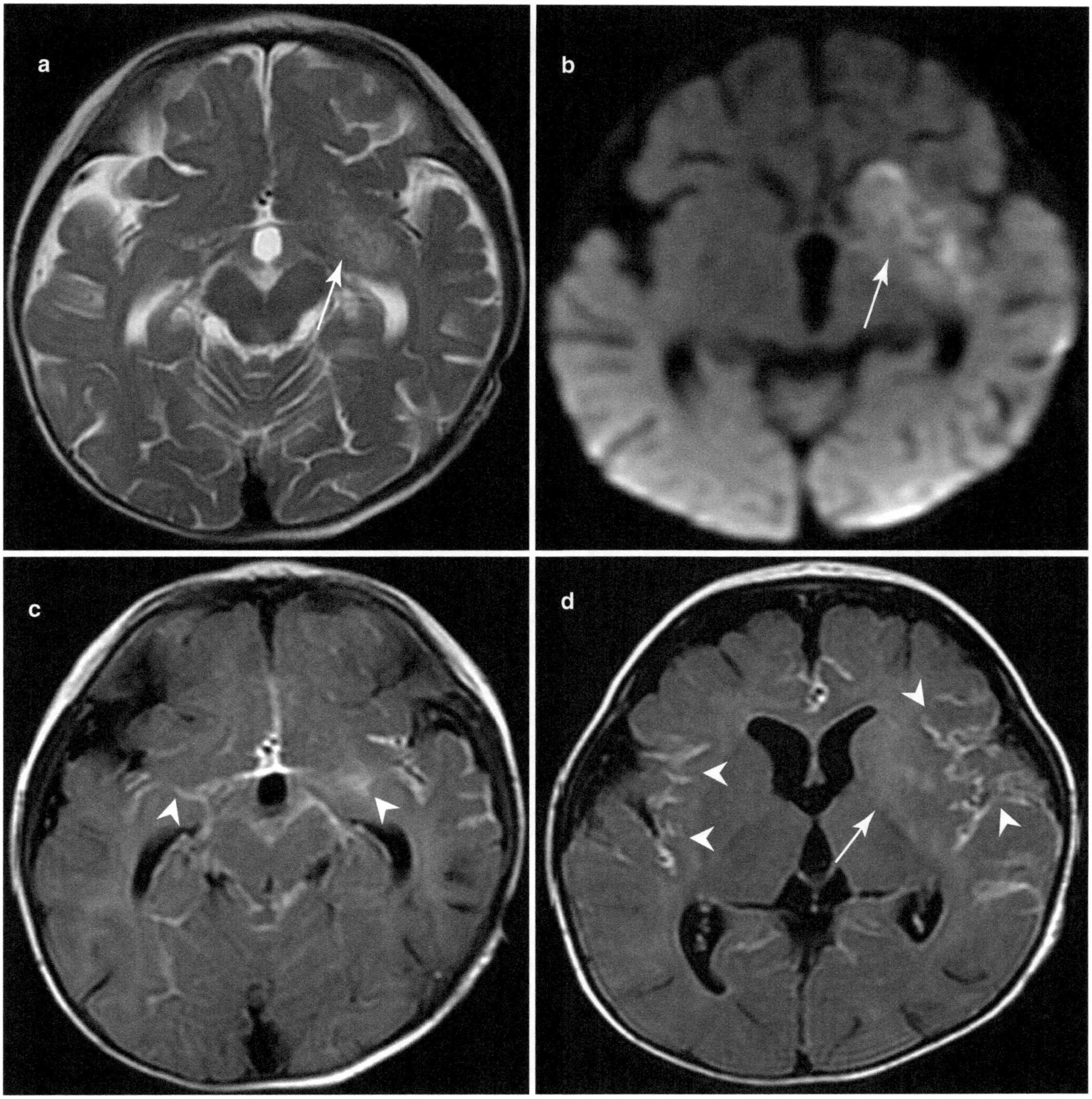

Fig. 3.3 Tuberculosis infection

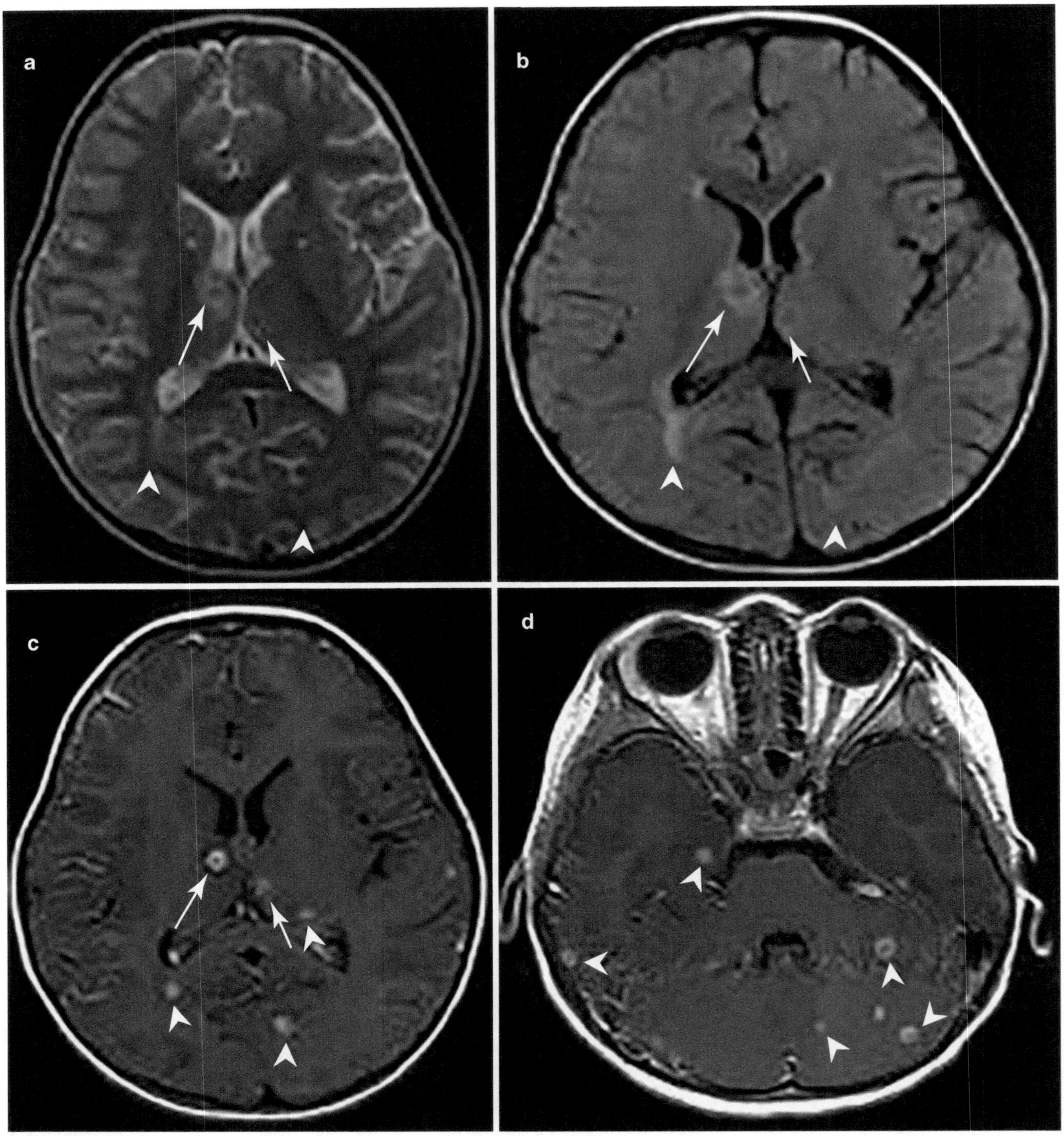

Fig. 3.4 Tuberculosis infection

The cranial routine CT shows the narrowed and density increased cisterns, which are more common in the basal cistern and the lateral fissure cistern. After enhancement, the involved cisterns are significantly enhanced. Often accompanied by hydrocephalus. Part of cases can be complicated with cerebral infarction, found in the brain parenchyma slightly lower density lesions, often involved basal ganglia and internal capsule. Magnetic resonance imaging (MRI) is more sensitive than CT in depicting meningeal abnormalities. The affected cisterns show high signal intensity on T2WI-FLAIR images and variably enhancement after contrast administration, typically as thicken or nodular enhancement of leptomeningeal. Diffusion-weighted images (DWI) help in the early detection of infarct [19, 20].

Tuberculomas are parenchymal tuberculosis typically located at the junction of the gray matter and white matter in cerebrum and cerebellum. They can present isodense to slightly higher attenuation with less surrounding vasogenic edema on CT. The lesions less than 2 mm in size usually show solid enhancement, and ring-like enhancement for larger ones. Tuberculomas are not commonly present calcification [5, 21]. Liquefying of caseous component in granuloma may form tuberculous abscesses that the central portion showing hyperintense on T2WI. The manifestation of the tuberculomas on diffusion-weighted images is varied [19, 20, 22, 23].

Tuberculous meningitis should be differentiated from other kinds of diseases which can also cause abnormal meningeal enhancement, such as tumors, purulent meningitis, Sturge–Weber syndrome. It is not difficult to identify on the basis of history, clinical symptoms, laboratory examination, and typical radiographic findings. In addition, pre- and postcontrast magnetization transfer imaging ratio (MTR) quantification can help in differentiating TBM from nontuberculous meningeal inflammation. Low MTR indicates TBM. Tuberculomas should be differentiated from neurocysticercosis, pyogenic brain abscess, glioma, and metastases. Neurocysticercosis can be distinguished from tuberculomas on the basis of history, laboratory examination, and multiple calcified plaques on CT images. Proton MR spectroscopy (MRS) differentiates tuberculomas from pyogenic abscess and neoplasms such as high-grade gliomas and metastases. Tuberculomas have a specific lipid peak.

Case 3.2.3 Bacterial Infection

Clinical Presentation

A 9-year-old girl presented with headache and intermitted fever for 2 weeks with seizures for 2 times. The peripheral leukocyte count was 11 × 10^9/L. The CSF examination displayed increased WBC with neutrophils as the main part and protein 1.5 g/L. The patient had a history of right otitis media.

Imaging Findings

A. Axial T1-weighted image demonstrates a round like abnormal signal lesion with peripheral edema and mild mass effect in the temporal lobe with central hypointense (Fig. 3.5a).
B. Axial T2-weighted image shows abnormal hyperintense in central part of the lesion with a relatively visible isointense cyst wall (Fig. 3.5b).
C. DWI image shows heterogeneous hyperintense (Fig. 3.5c).
D. CE-T1WI image shows uniform ring-like enhancement of the cystic wall and no enhancement of the interior cystic portion (Fig. 3.5d).

Discussion

Brain abscess caused by bacteria is not rare in pediatrics, include the staphylococcal species and several Gram-negative bacteria. The clinical manifestations usually include headache, vomiting, malaise, and certain focal neurological symptoms. Hematogenous dissemination and contiguous infection extension are the main routes. The former way is common in patients with congenital heart disease [24]. The subcortical regions of parietal lobes are the typically affected areas and the lesions are often multiple. The latter way is common in patients with adjacent infections such as sinusitis and otomastoiditis. This kind of cerebritis lesion typically near the primary infectious lesions, as otogenic brain cerebritis or abscess typically occurs in the temporal lobe or cerebellum. Other risk factors contain central nervous system trauma, immunosuppressive therapy, and underlying immunodeficiency disorder, such as HIV [20, 25].

The formation of brain abscess is composed of four stages: early cerebritis, late cerebritis, early capsule formation, and late capsule formation [21]. Bacterial cerebritis is the earliest stage of purulent brain infection. The affected region liquefies and forms a surrounding capsule of granulation tissue and collagen forms, resulting in abscess formation [25].

In the early two stages, the affected region shows increased water content as an ill-circumstance area of low attenuation on CT consistent with prolonged T1 and T2 signal intensity on MRI. Mass effect can usually be seen. In the late two stages, increasing collagen and reticulin surround the necrotic center of the abscess and form the wall of abscess, meanwhile the edema and consequent mass effect regress. The characteristic imaging finding in these stages is well-defined abscesses with a ring-like enhancement pattern representing the abscess wall. The abscess wall shows isointense on T1-weighted images and markedly hypointense on T2-weighted images. The abscess center is isointense to slightly hypointense on T1-weighted images and hyperintense on T2-weighted images. The lesions are commonly located near the junction of gray matter and white matter. The wall is often thicker on the cortical side than the ventricular side. The whole evolution takes about 1–2 weeks [11, 24, 26].

Central nervous system bacterial infection may also present as meningitis. The organisms spread into the ventricles and subarachnoid space causing ventriculitis, hydrocephalus, and empyema. The characteristic imaging manifestation is the enhancement of the meninges on postcontrast CT and MRI. MRI is also superior in revealing dilatation of the sulci

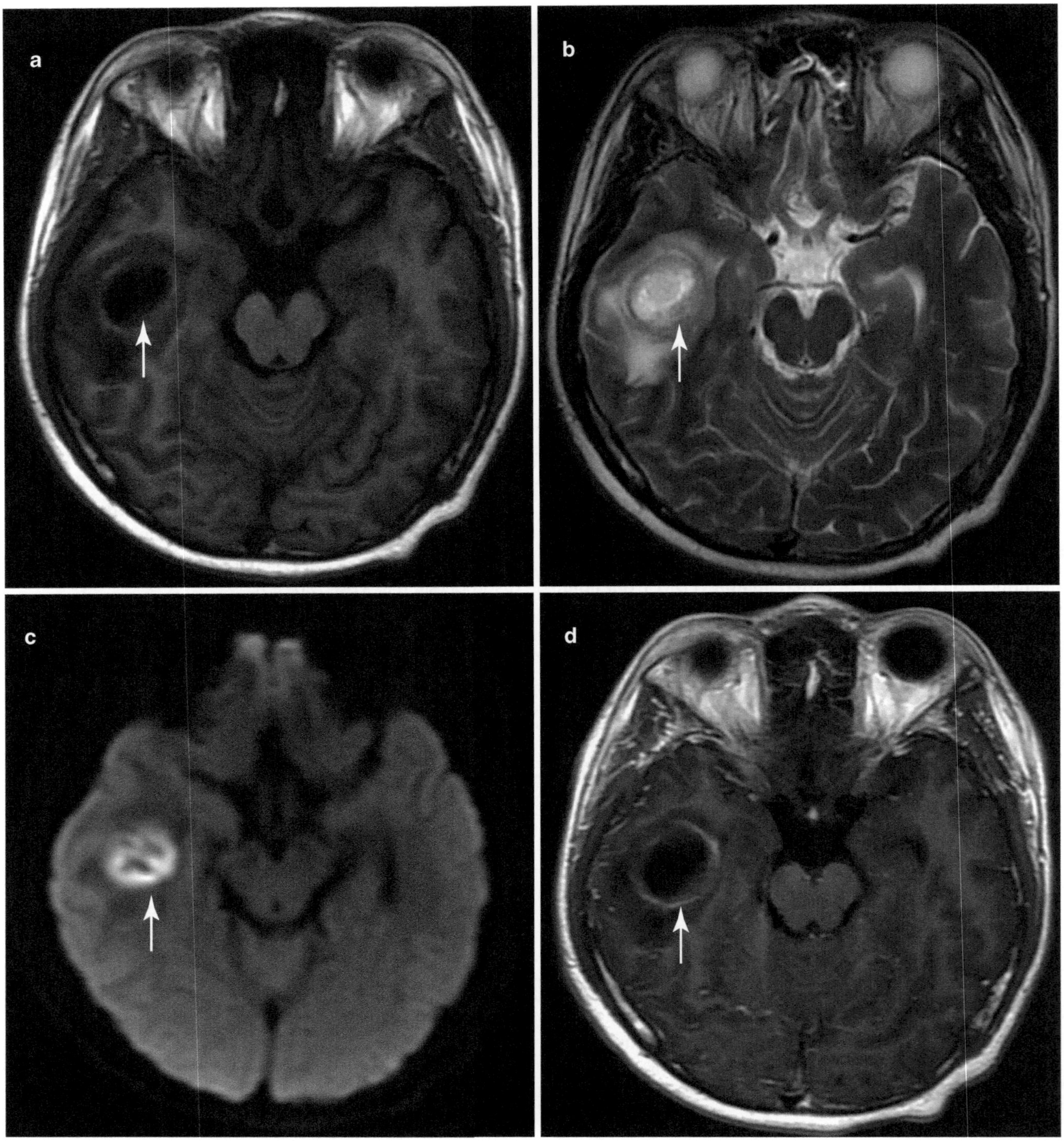

Fig. 3.5 Bacterial infection

and cisterns [21]. Purulent meningitis usually causes subdural effusion. The presence of intraventricular debris in the occipital horns of the lateral ventricle and dilation of ventricles are the best imaging signs of ventriculitis as enhancement of the inflamed ependyma on postcontrast CT and MRI [11].

Case 3.2.4 Brain Parasite Infection
Patient 1

Clinical Presentation
A 14-year-old boy presented with a headache. His past medical, surgical, and family histories were negative. He had a history of unclean drinking water. Serum cysticercosis antibody was detected by ELISA.

Imaging Findings

A. T2WI-FLAIR image demonstrates multiple round, nodular and patchy abnormal signal intensity lesions mainly distributed in the cortex and medulla junction area and para-ventricular parenchyma, most of the lesions presented with central hypointense accompanied by peri-hyperintensity (arrow), patchy hyperintense lesions can be seen around the lateral ventricles (arrowhead) (Fig. 3.6a).
B. Axial CE-T1WI shows obvious ring-like or nodular enhancement (arrow) of the lesions (Fig. 3.6b).

Patient 2

Clinical Presentation
An 18-year-old girl presented with a long-term history of headache. Her past medical, surgical, and family histories were negative. He had no trauma or traveling in the epidemic area recently. She had a suspicious history of raw meat consumption. Serum cysticercosis antibody was detected by ELISA.

Imaging Findings

A. Axial non-contrast CT image shows nodular calcification in the left cerebral parenchyma bilateral periventricular hypoattenuating lesions (arrow head) and multiple subependymal calcifications (arrow) (Fig. 3.7a).

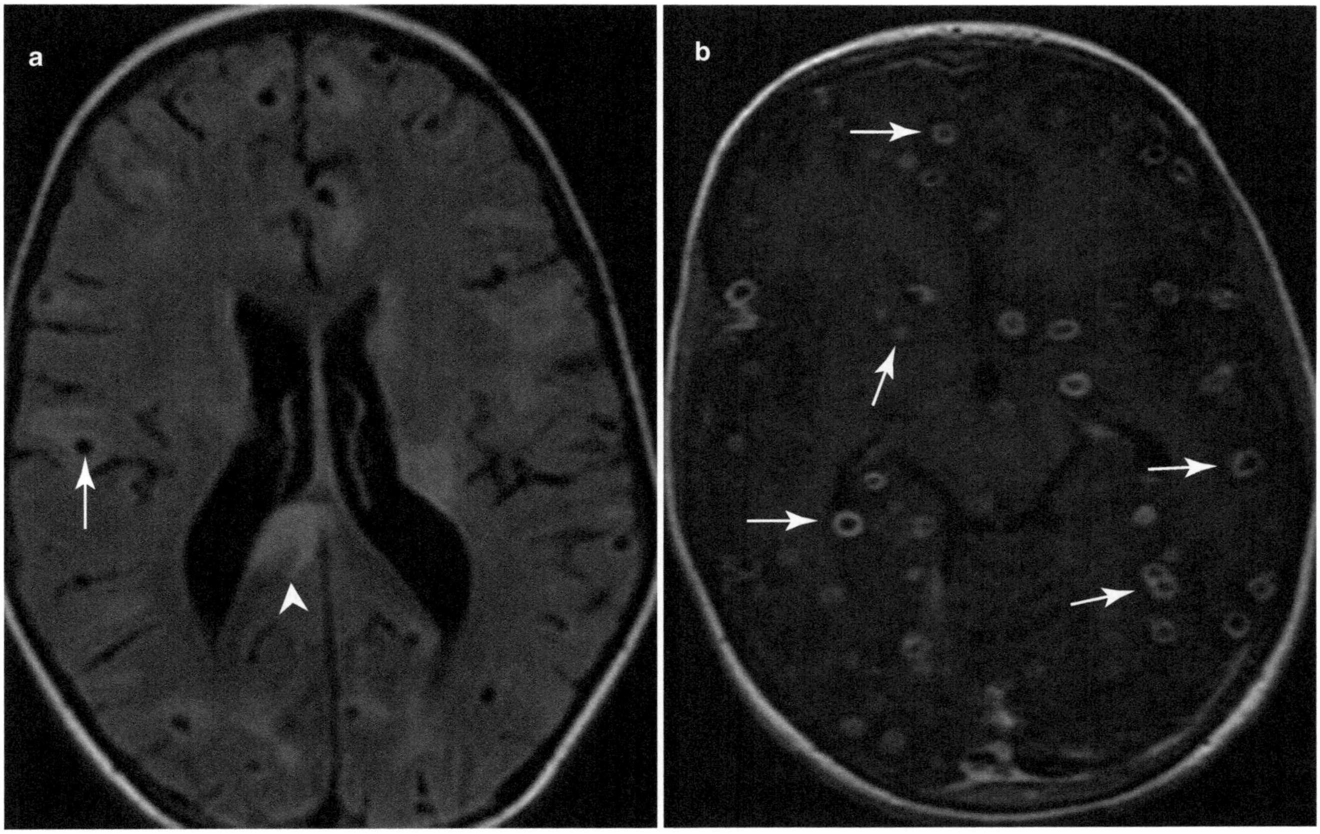

Fig. 3.6 Neurocysticercosis (NCC), colloidal vesicular stage

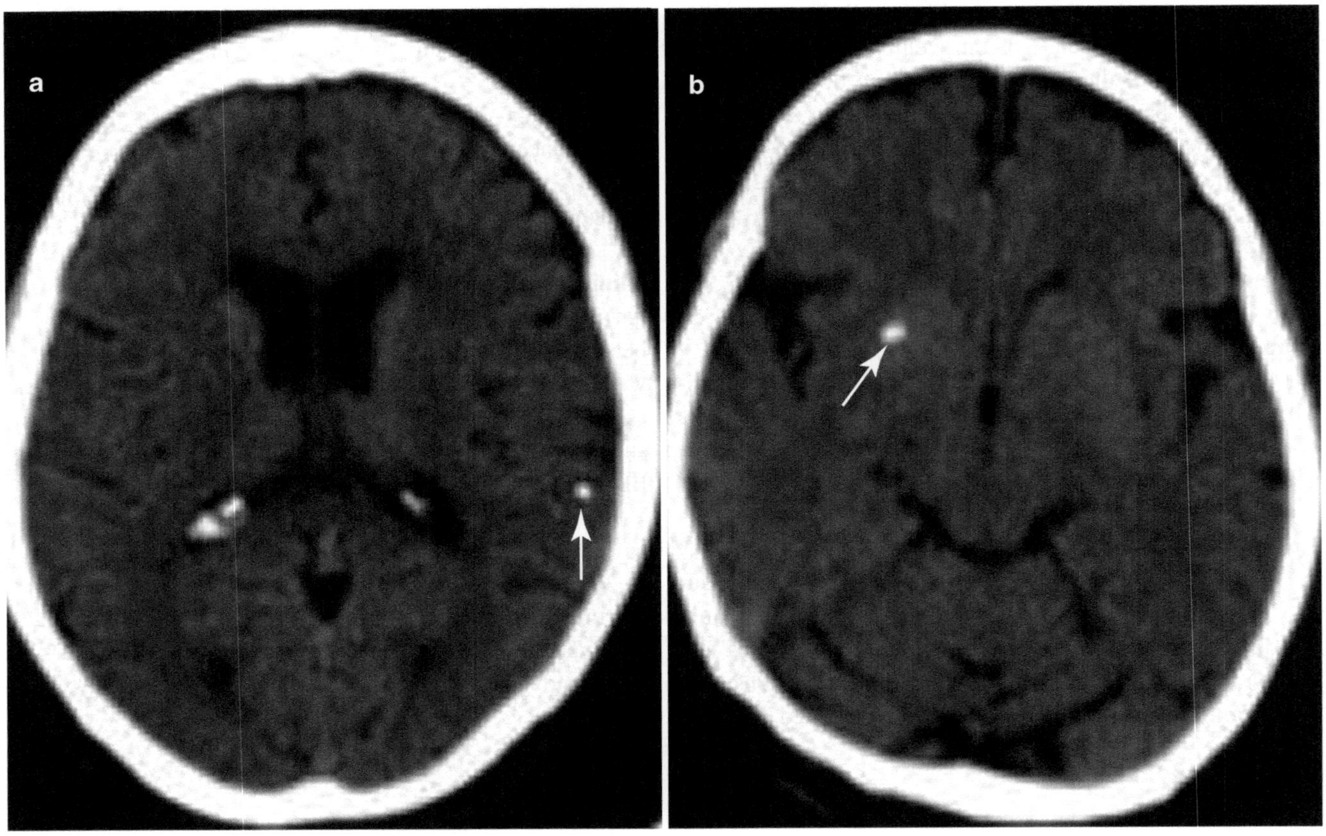

Fig. 3.7 Neurocysticercosis (NCC), nodular calcified stage

B. The proximal level of the Fig.3.7a in the same patient shows nodular calcification in the right basal ganglia (arrow) (Fig. 3.7b).

Discussion

Brain parasite infection includes various diseases, such as cerebral cysticercosis, hydatid disease of brain, cerebral paragonimiasis, cerebral malaria, and so on. This section focuses on neurocysticercosis (NCC). It is not rare in children and has the highest incidence in Latin America [27].

NCC is caused by Taenia solium, a parasitic helminth worm. The initial infection of Taenia solium occurs from the ingestion of its eggs or undercooked pork containing the larval cysts (cysticerci). Once ingested and in the intestines, the eggs hatch into oncospheres (embryos) that cross the intestinal wall where they are transported by blood to various body tissues in which they form the larval cysts. Brain is the most common site of cysticercosis. At first, they stimulate an immune response that will induce both granuloma formation as well as perilesional edema around the granuloma. Later on, after the cyst degenerates, the lesion undergoes a further immunologic process in which there is a deposition of fibrotic material and the cyst eventually hardens and turns into a calcific nodule [28, 29].

Late-onset epilepsy and intracranial hypertension are the most common clinical manifestations. The diagnosis of NCC is mainly based on neuroimaging and serological assessment. According to the position of lesions on CT or MRI, NCC can be classified into four types: brain parenchyma type, ventricle type, subarachnoid type, and the mixed type [29, 30].

CT and MRI are the best methods for detecting neurocysticercosis. CT is more sensitive to reveal calcification, while MRI is more sensitive in distinguishing edema, scolex, and small lesions. There are four stages of NCC: (1) Vesicular: Viable larva; smooth-walled cyst with central scolex. (2) Colloidal vesicular: Degenerating larva; rim-enhancing cyst and marked surrounding edema. (3) Granular nodular: Healing stage; mild edema and rim enhancement. (4) Nodular calcified: Healed stage; small, involuted cyst with or without calcifications. Depending on the stage of infection and location of lesions, neuroimaging performs are different. On CT, viable cysts appear as hypodense, rounded, cystic lesions. Some may be enhanced on postcontrast images. The scolex can be occasionally seen as a hyperintense dot within the cyst. On MRI, the cysts show hypointense on T1WI and FLAIR images, hyperintense on T2WI images. Degenerating cysts appear as ring-like or nodular enhancement surrounded by edema. Calcified cysts appear as punctate hyperdense dots on CT, while areas of subtracted signal intensity on MRI of all sequences [29–31].

NCC should be differentiated from other infections according to medical history and skin test. Large and complex cysts with edema may be confused with intracranial neoplasms. FLAIR or diffusion-weighted MRI can show the cephalic segment of some degenerative cysts, helping to make the correct diagnosis of these cases. One of the most important and difficult differential diagnoses of a single degenerating cysticercosis is tuberculoma. Magnetic resonance spectroscopy seems to detect a peak of lipids in tuberculomas not present in degenerating cysticercosis [29].

3.3 Immune-Associated Encephalitis

Case 3.3.1 Multiple Sclerosis

Clinical Presentation

A 10-year-old boy presented with headache and paresthesia for 2 weeks and subsequently developed nystagmus and dysarthria. His past medical, surgical, and family histories were negative. He had no recent trauma or traveling in the epidemic area. After many follow-up visits, she was diagnosed as MS.

Imaging Findings

A. Axial T1-weighted image demonstrates multiple oval shape low signal intensity lesions around bilateral ventricles (arrow) (Fig. 3.8a).
B. Axial T2-weighted image demonstrates multiple oval shape high signal intensity lesions around bilateral ventricles (arrow) (Fig. 3.8b).
C. T2WI-FLAIR image shows all of the lesions high signal intensity (arrow) (Fig. 3.8c).
D. Sagittal CE-T1WI shows marginal or patchy enhancement of the lesions, which are distributed perpendicular to the body of the lateral ventricles (arrow) (Fig. 3.8d).

Discussion

Multiple sclerosis (MS) is an inflammatory autoimmune disease of the central nervous system. It is more common in young and middle-aged females characterized by demyelination and degeneration. Pediatric-onset multiple sclerosis (POMS) usually refers to children and adolescents under the age of 18. POMS is rare and accounts for less than 5% of all MS patients with a median age of 11 ~ 13 years [32]. Although POMS have an equal gender distribution before the age of puberty, with a female predominance afterwards [32].

The pathogenesis of MS is complex and elusive. Risk factors include genetic and environmental factors such as specific viral infections, smoking, obesity, and low serum 25-hydroxyvitamin D [33].

The clinical course of MS can be broadly classified into three patterns: relapsing-remitting (RRMS), secondary progressive (SPMS), and primary progressive MS (PPMS). More than 98% of POMS patients demonstrate an RRMS course [34]. The clinical manifestations are different. POMS usually manifests with focal deficits such as unilateral weakness, numbness, or paresthesia. Visual loss (optic neuritis), ataxia, and transverse myelitis are also common. Specifically, the presence of intrathecal oligoclonal bands (OCB) is supportive of POMS. POMS patients are more likely to develop early physical disabilities and early cognitive impairment due to their younger age of onset, high-level of inflammatory activity, and higher relapse [34].

MRI is helpful to identify and monitor demyelinating activity of MS. POMS lesions are located in periventricular and subcortical regions, and can also arise in the brainstem and spinal cord, with mostly multiple. White matter is mainly involved. The size and shape of lesions are variable. Lesions appear equal or low signal intensity on T1-weighted images and high signal intensity on T2-weighted images, the lesions which are at active stage show "ring open," annular or nodular enhancement on postcontrast T1-weighted images. Specifically, periventricular lesions expand perpendicular to the ventricles, especially on sagittal or coronal T2 FLAIR. The central vein sign and "Dawson's Finger" appearance are imaging features that are suggestive of MS. DTI can show the damage of white matter [34–37].

Acute disseminated encephalomyelitis (ADEM) is an important differential diagnosis of POMS. Two or more periventricular lesions, absence of a diffuse bilateral lesion pattern, and enhancement of active lesions are usually seen in POMS patients compared to those with ADEM. The appearance of new lesions in different locations on follow-up MRI strongly suggests POMS. Clinical, imaging, and serological detection should be considered in the diagnosis of MS [37].

Case 3.3.2 Anti-NMDAR Encephalitis

Clinical Presentation

A 7-year-old girl presented to the emergency department (ED) for altered mental status and seizure. She had been seen in the ED 3 weeks ago for fever, diarrhea, and vomiting. She had no recent trauma or traveling in the epidemic area. IgG GluN1 antibody (CSF) test was positive.

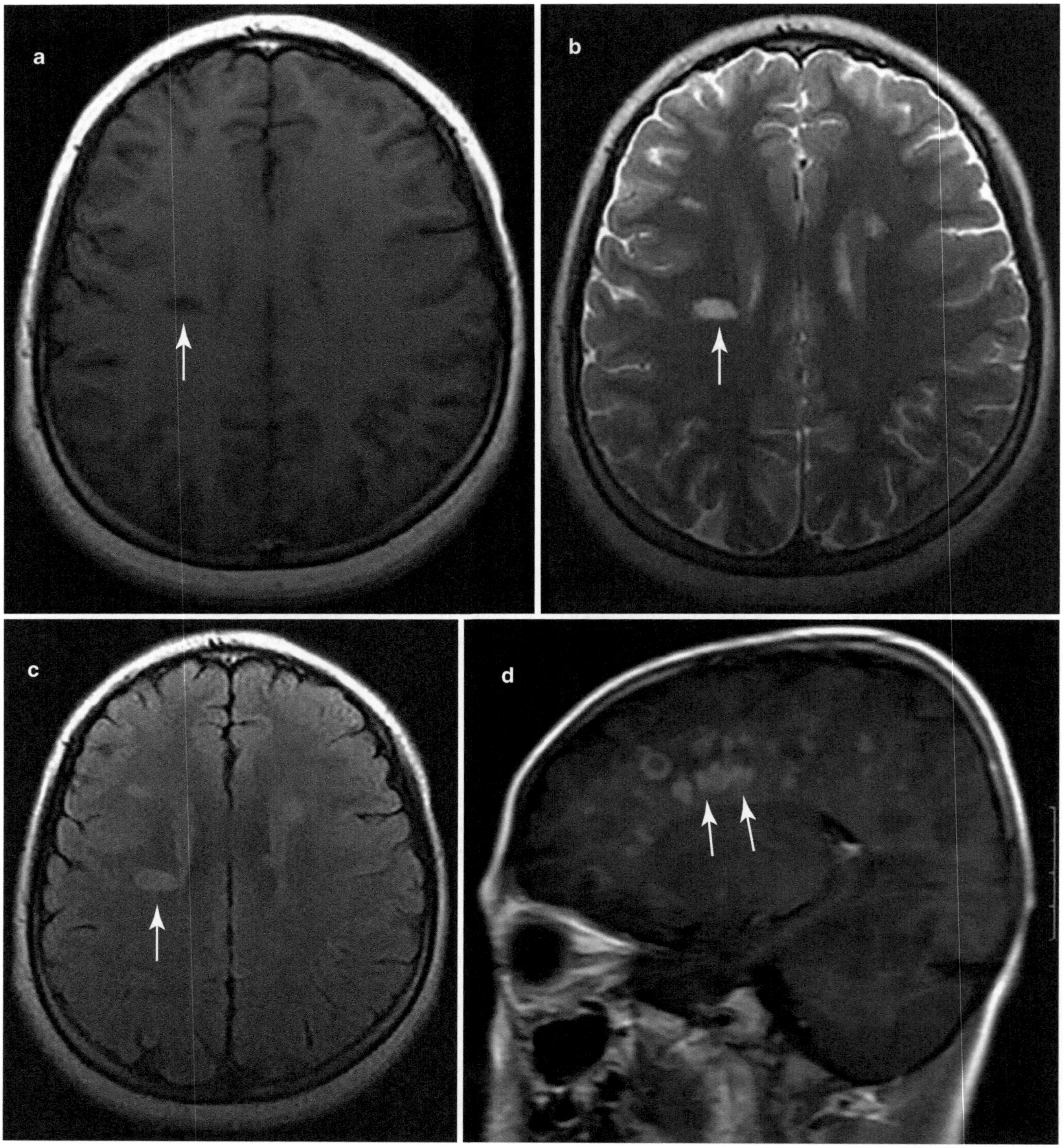

Fig. 3.8 Multiple sclerosis

Imaging Findings

A. Axial T2-weighted image shows mild swell and high signal intensity lesion in the left hippocampal area (arrow) (Fig. 3.9a).
B. Axial T1-weighted image shows slightly low signal intensity lesion in the left hippocampal area (arrow) (Fig. 3.9b).
C. T2WI-FLAIR image shows high signal intensity of the lesion (arrow) (Fig. 3.9c).
D. Axial CE-T1WI shows no enhancement of the lesion (arrow) (Fig. 3.9d).

Discussion

Anti-*N*-methyl-D-aspartate receptor (NMDAR) encephalitis is an immune-mediated disease caused by antibodies that act on the synaptic protein NMDA receptor. It is also the most common Antibody-Mediated Encephalitis in children [38]. Mental and behavioral abnormalities, seizures, movement

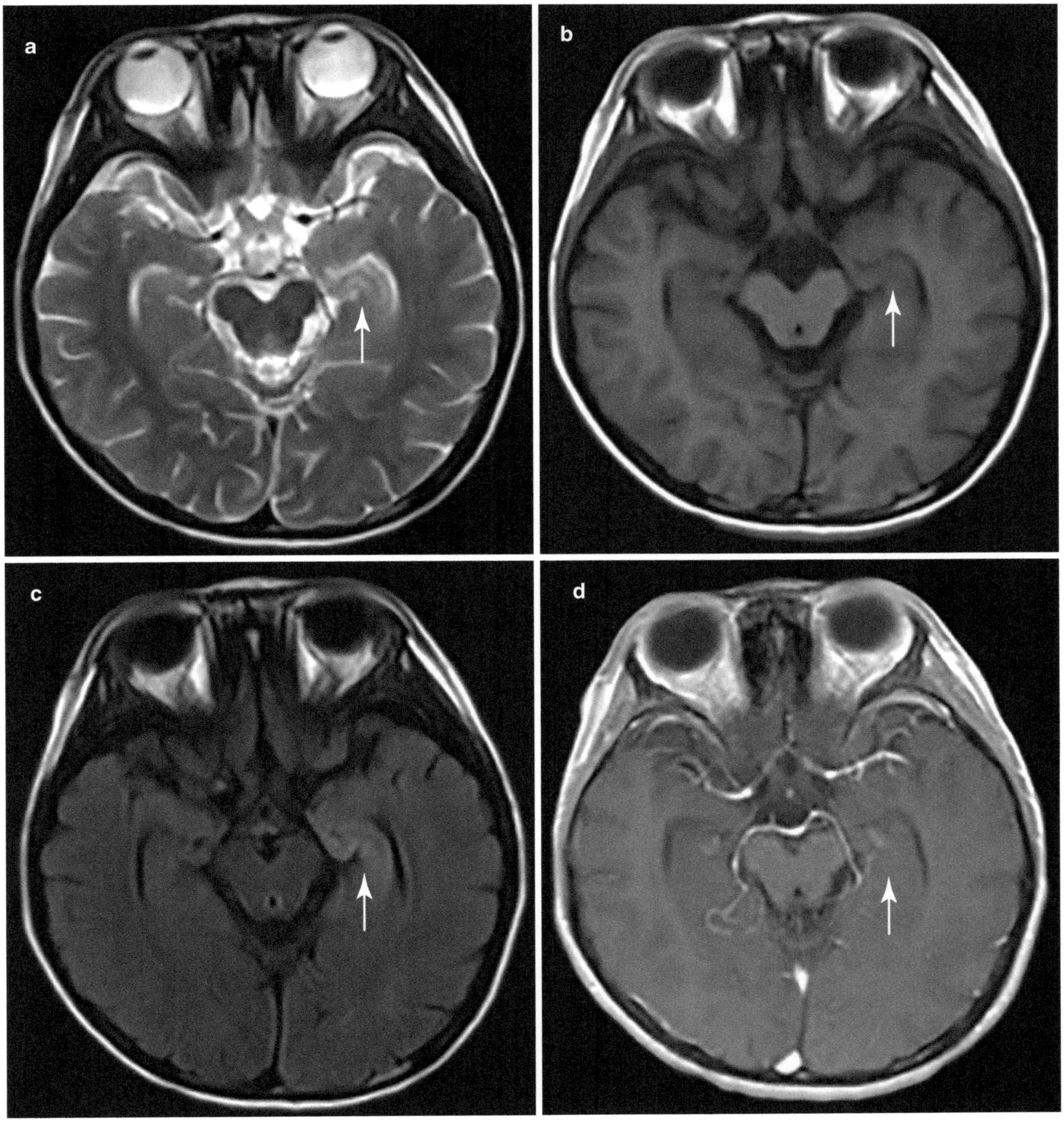

Fig. 3.9 Anti-NMDAR encephalitis

disorders, speech disorders, and autonomic dysfunction are common clinical manifestations of anti-NMDAR encephalitis in children [39]. At onset or relapse of anti-NMDAR encephalitis, about 90% of patients have psychiatric or behavioral symptoms that can be very difficult to differentiate from a primary psychiatric disease [40]. However, abnormal brain MRI findings should prompt screening for NMDAR antibodies.

Anti-NMDAR encephalitis has a significant correlation with age, gender, and associated tumors (mostly ovarian teratoma). Anti-NMDAR encephalitis is generally more common in women than men, with a male to female ratio of approximately 1:4, especially in women with ovarian teratomas. 40% of patients are younger than 18 years old. About 90% of children with anti-NMDAR encephalitis are usually not associated with tumor [41].

50–95% of patients with anti-NMDAR encephalitis were negative on conventional MRI [42, 43]. Anti-NMDAR encephalitis mainly involves cerebral cortex, and Lesions in the hippocampus were the most commonly affected site. Other affected sites currently reported include the frontal lobe, cerebellar hemisphere, basal ganglia, and so on. The lesion usually presents with mild swelling at onset, but bleeding is rare. Conventional T1WI sequence shows mild low signal intensity, T2WI and T2WI-FLAIR sequence shows high signal intensity, and postcontrast injection demonstrates no enhancement. Diffusion-weighted imaging (DWI) sequence generally showed hyperintensity in ADC, but there were a few patients with limited diffusion. In the later stages of the disease, volumetric MRI analysis showed that the whole brain (especially hippocampus and basal ganglia) of children with anti-NMDAR encephalitis decreased in volume [44].

T. Zhang etc. [43] classified brain MR imaging appearance into four types. Type 1 is normal; type 2 only had hippocampal lesion; lesions of type 3 were in other brain areas; and type 4 presented hippocampal lesion and lesions in other areas. And the presence of hippocampal lesions may be an important imaging predictor for poor prognosis in patients with anti-NMDAR encephalitis [43].

The disease needs to be differentiated from acute disseminated encephalitis and viral encephalitis. Acute disseminated encephalitis is characterized by both cortical and white matter involvement and is generally dominated by white matter involvement. The onset of viral encephalitis is relatively more urgent, and the course of disease progresses rapidly. And there are many obvious changes in the lesions such as edema, necrosis, and hemorrhage. In addition, cerebrospinal fluid pathogen detection can detect the corresponding viral DNA.

Case 3.3.3 Acute Disseminated Encephalomyelitis

Clinical Presentation

A 5-year-old boy presented with fever, poor mental status, and seizure for 1 day. A routine blood test showed a white blood cell count of 10.51 × 10^9 g/L. The erythrocyte sedimentation rate was 28 mm/h. The immunoglobulin of cerebrospinal fluid examination was 43.20 mg/L. Other routine tests were negative. ADEM was diagnosed after more than 1 year of follow-up.

Imaging Findings

A. Axial T2-weighted image shows multiple hyperintense lesions located in the cortical and subcortical areas of bilateral cerebrum at symptom onset of the patient (arrow) (Fig. 3.10a).
B. Axial T1-weighted image shows slightly low signal intensity of the lesions (arrow) (Fig. 3.10b).
C. T2WI-FLAIR image shows high signal intensity of the lesions (arrow) (Fig. 3.10c).
D. DWI shows restricted diffusion of the lesions (arrow) (Fig. 3.10d).

Discussion

Acute disseminated encephalomyelitis (ADEM) is a rare autoimmune inflammatory and demyelinating disorder of the central nervous system. ADEM may occur at any age, usually within 15 years old, with an average onset age of 5–8 years [45, 46]. The prevalence is more common in males than females (1.3:1 male to female) and tends to occur in colder seasons, such as winter and spring [47]. The incidence of ADEM is reported to be 0.4 per 100,000 person-years [45]. Although ADEM is a typically monophasic illness, relapses may occur within the first 3 months. Anti-myelin oligodendrocyte glycoprotein (MOG) immunoglobulin G antibodies are present in one-half of patients with ADEM, and cerebrospinal fluid pleocytosis is frequently present. ADEM usually has a favorable prognosis, but mortality in the initial phase can be as high as 10–20% [45].

ADEM typically follows a rapidly progressive course, with prodromal symptoms including headache, fever, nausea, vomiting, and even coma. In approximately 50–75% of cases, maximum symptoms arise 4–15 days after an upper respiratory tract infection or after vaccination [2]. Multifocal neurologic deficits are the most common clinical presentations and are dependent on the location of the lesions including hemiplegia, epilepsy, ataxia, visual changes, and speech disorders [47, 48].

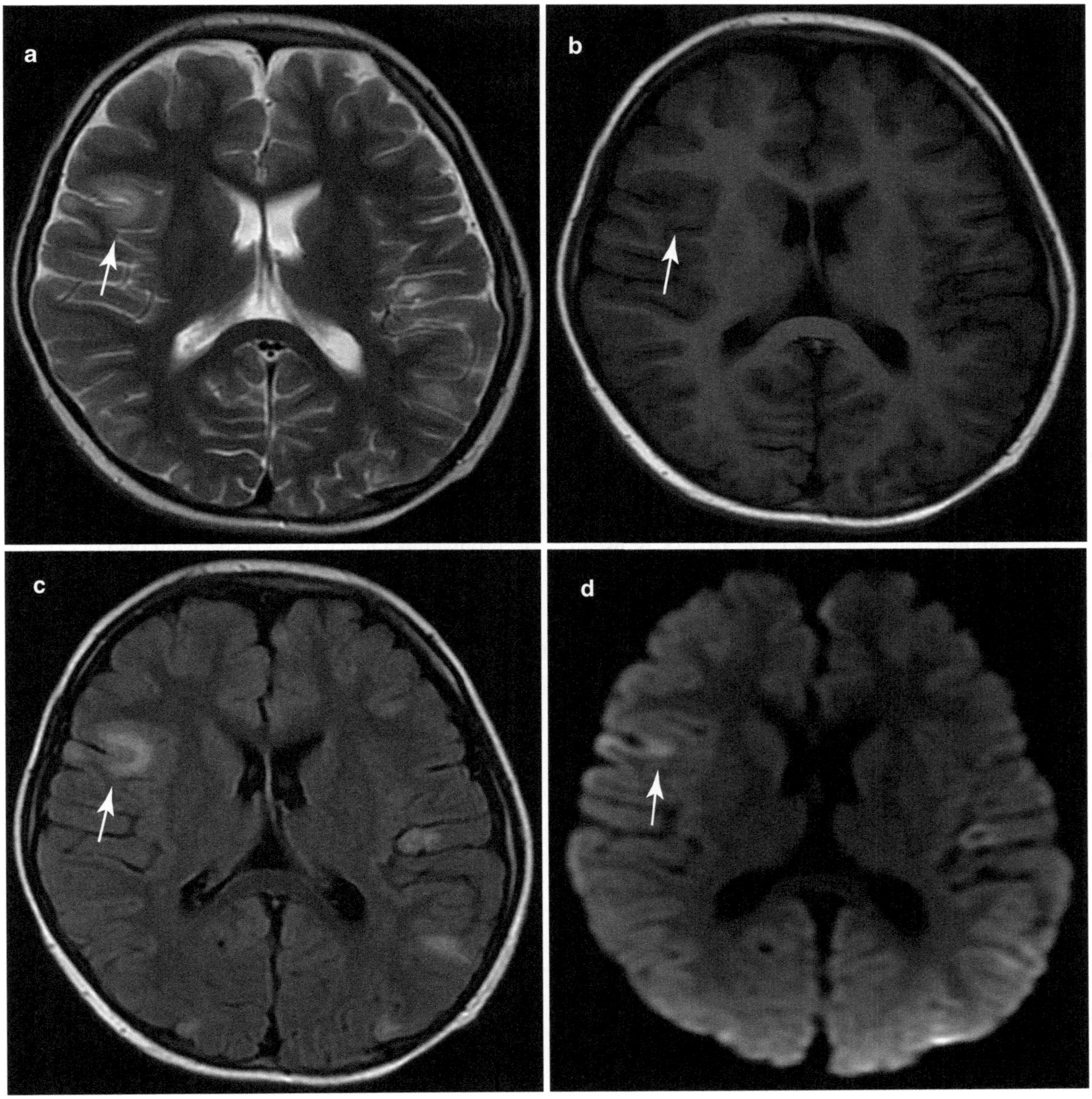

Fig. 3.10 Acute disseminated encephalomyelitis

The pathogenesis and pathophysiology of ADEM are not fully understood. Most studies proposed that it may be disseminated multifocal inflammation and patchy demyelination associated with a transient autoimmune response toward myelin oligodendrocyte glycoprotein or other self-antigens. It is believed that the autoimmune response is the result of either molecular mimicry or direct infection of the central nervous system, which leads to T-cells activation and elicits a central nervous system-specific autoimmune response [45–49].

ADEM may appear as normal MRI. MRI lesions may also appear several weeks after the onset of symptoms and require multiple repetitions, especially in the early stage. Most MRI lesions disappear within 18 months [48]. Typical lesions are multiple, bilateral, asymmetric, large (>2 cm), and ill-defined, with involvement of white matter and gray matter [50]. Deep cerebral hemispheric and subcortical white matter are the most common, as well as lesions in the deep gray matter nuclei, thalamus, brainstem, corpus callosum, and spinal cord can also be been. Brainstem lesions in ADEM more frequently involve the ventral midbrain and are usually bilateral and symmetric with poorly defined margins. ADEM lesions show hyperintensity on T2-weighted and FLAIR images and are not obvious on T1-weighted images. Active lesions may enhance at the same time appearing as peripheral rim of enhancement. DWI sequence shows high signal intensity indicating restricted diffusion. Petechial hemorrhages may be present within the lesions which can be demonstrated by susceptibility-weighted images. Besides, elevated choline and lactate levels can be observed at MR spectroscopy [45–54].

The main differential diagnosis is multiple sclerosis (MS), which is usually misdiagnosed as ADEM at the first attack. MS has predilection of females whereas ADEM has no definite gender predilection. The onset age of MS is usually between the ages of 20–40 years with a peak at 30 years, which is older than ADEM. In addition, MS is a kind of multiphasic disease, often with a course of relapsing-remitting. ADEM is a monophasic illness, relapses are rare. Compared with imaging manifestations of MS lesions, ADEM lesions can be more rounded and larger with ill-defined margins and more prominent involvement of the deep gray matter nuclei, thalamus, and brainstem. Corpus callosum involved lesions arise from the callososeptal interface, which may help to prompt the diagnosis of MS. In addition, the presence of lesions with ovoid and perpendicular to the ventricle is more indicative of MS which is a characteristic feature of Dawson fingers. The appearance of new lesions suggests the diagnosis of MS, which is rare in ADEM unless a clinical relapse has occurred. MS lesions have lower signal intensity on T1-weighted images ("black holes") than ADEM lesions. Both contrast-enhancing and non-enhancing lesions can be seen in a single MR imaging examination for MS. However, ADEM lesions often enhance at the same time [52, 53].

Case 3.3.4 Neuromyelitis Optica Spectrum Disorders

Clinical Presentation

A 14-year-old girl presented with dyspraxia for 3 months and vision loss of the left eye for 8 days. Serum AQP4-IgG was positive.

Imaging Findings

A. T2WI-FLAIR shows the left optic nerve thickening (arrow) at symptom onset of the patient (Fig. 3.11a).
B. Coronal T2-weighted image shows the hyperintense of the left optic nerve (arrow) (Fig. 3.11b).
C. T2WI-FLAIR shows patchy hyperintense lesions located in the bilateral ventricle posterior horn (arrow) (Fig. 3.11c).
D. The distal level of the Fig.3.11c in the same patient shows patchy hyperintense lesions located in hypothalamus (arrow) (Fig. 3.11d).
E. Sagittal T1-weighted image shows no significant abnormality which showed in Sagittal T2-weighted (Fig. 3.11e).
F. Sagittal T2-weighted image shows strip lesion in the thoracic medulla with hyperintense (arrow) (Fig. 3.11f).

Discussion

Neuromyelitis Optica (NMO) spectrum disorder (NMOSD) is a severe autoimmune inflammatory demyelinating disease of the central nervous system characterized by severe optic neuritis (ON) and longitudinally extensive transverse myelitis (LETM) with encephalitis manifestations. The prevalence ranges from 0.5 to 4.4 per 100,000, being more common in non-white populations (Asian, Indian, and African) [45]. Pediatric NMOSD accounts for about 3 ~ 5% of all NMOSD cases [54]. The median age of the first onset is typically around 10 ~ 12 years [54]. Women are more commonly affected, with a ratio of 6.5:1 [45].

Anti-aquaporin-4 antibodies (AQP4-Abs) are present in the serum of approximately 75–90% of patients with NMOSD [50]. The AQP4 channel is the most abundant water channel in the central nervous system which is concentrated expressed in the circumventricular organs that contain extensive vasculature and fenestrated capillaries without a restrictive blood–brain barrier and is linear in astrocyte foot processes. The antibody–antigen complex leads to demyelinating disorders by disrupting water homeostasis, activating astrocytes to produce complement, and disrupting the blood–brain barrier. Anti-myelin-oligodendrocyte glycoprotein antibodies (MOG-Abs) may be related to the pathogenesis of AQP4-Ab-seronegative NMOSD [45, 50, 54, 55].

The core characteristics symptoms of NMOSD include unilateral or bilateral optic neuritis, acute myelitis, area pos-

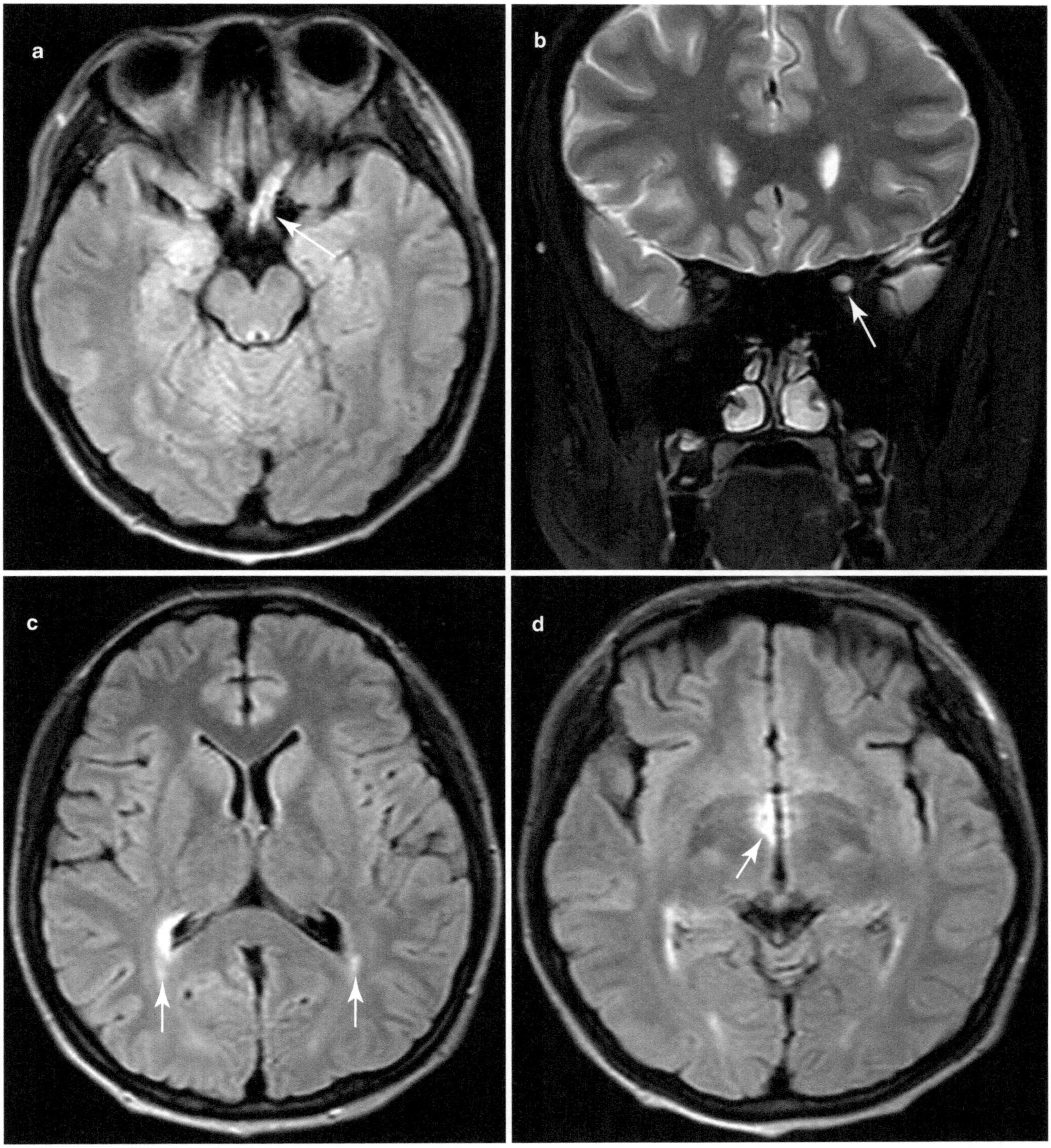

Fig. 3.11 Neuromyelitis optica spectrum disorders

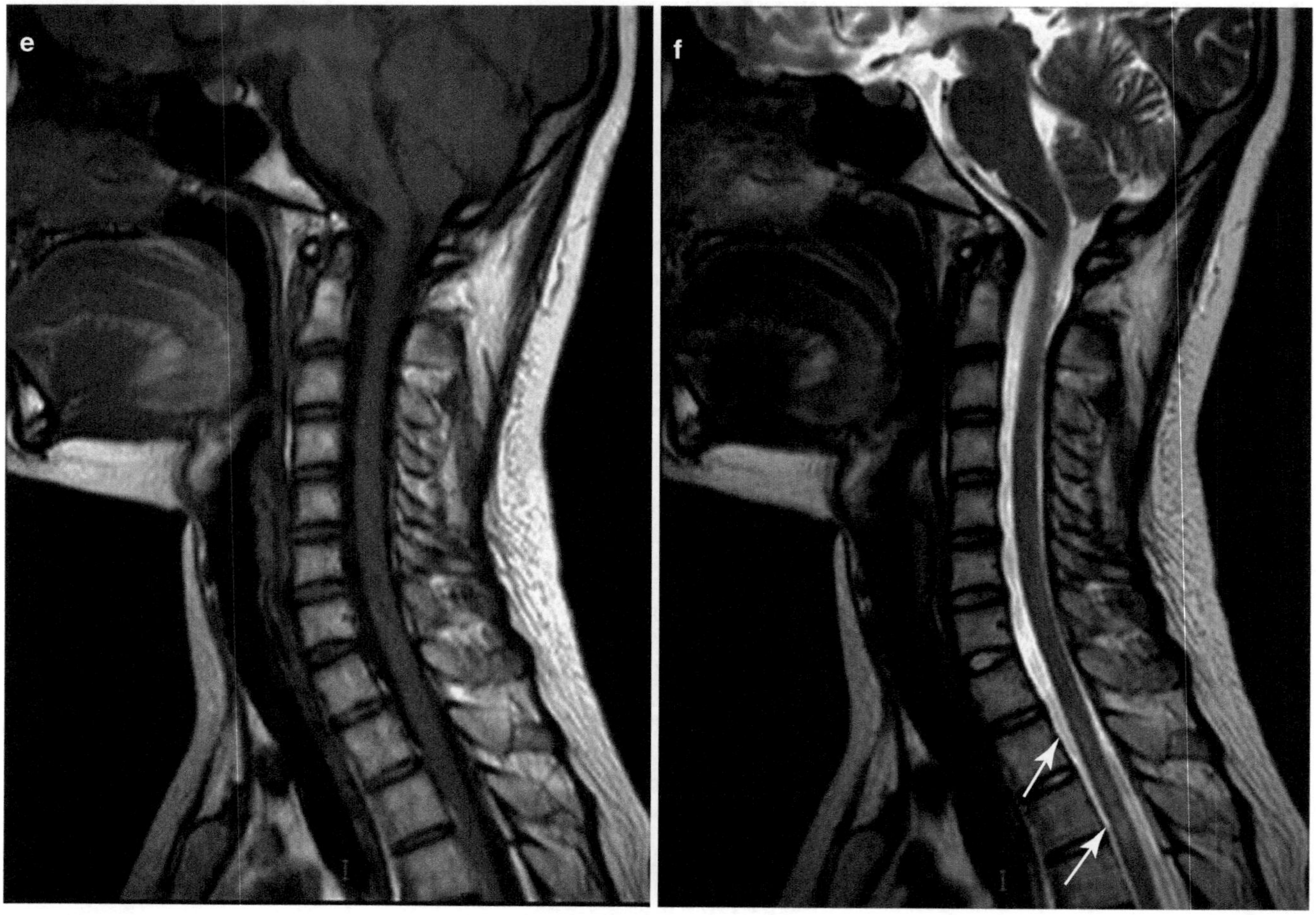

Fig. 3.11 (continued)

trema syndrome, acute brainstem syndrome, acute diencephalic syndrome, and cerebrum syndrome. Optic nerve involvement typically manifests as severe vision loss. Acute spinal cord syndrome manifests as limb movement weakness and sensory disturbance. Area postrema syndrome manifests as intractable nausea, hiccups, and vomiting. Patients with diencephalic involvement may have anorexia, hypothermia, and hypersomnia. In the brainstem involvement, oculomotor dysfunctions, long tract signs, and ataxia can be seen. AQP4-Ab-seropositive patients usually have more severe clinical attacks, worse outcome, and more relapses (81 ~ 91%) compared with AQP4-Ab-seronegative patients [5]. Children usually have a better outcome in terms of disability than adults [50, 54–56].

Optic neuritis is typically characterized as extensive thickening of bilateral and longitudinally optic nerve with hyperintensity on T2-weighted images and enhancement on gadolinium-enhanced T1-weighted images. LETM usually involves three or more vertebral segments of the central gray matter of the spinal cord. Bright spotty lesions on T2-weighted images and corresponding dark lesions on T1-weighted images are the most typical MR imaging features of LETM. Typical brain imaging findings on MRI are added to the classic spinal cord and optic nerve involvement, most of which share the same AQP4 distribution of periventricular areas, hypothalamus, and subpial regions, as well as the brainstem and area postrema. Intracerebral lesions are usually asymmetrically and large with partial enhancement. The corpus callosum is typically involved at its ependymal surface with edematous and heterogeneous hyperintensity on T2-weighted and FLAIR sequence images, assuming a typical marbled or "arch bridge" appearance. The lesions in the posterior polar region and nucleus solitarius are one of the most specific head MRI manifestations of NMOSD, which can be seen in 7 ~ 46% of NMOSD patients [6]. These medullary lesions commonly extend to the upper ependymal region in the central canal of the cervical spinal cord, usually assuming a linear shape with variable hyperintensity on FLAIR/T2-weighted images and variable enhancement on T1-weighted images [56, 57].

There are many differential diagnoses based on NMOSD imaging features (multiple sclerosis, acute disseminated encephalomyelitis, primary angiitis of the central nervous system, et al). However, multiple sclerosis (MS) remains the main differential entity. MS usually involves the optic nerve in the unilateral and short-segment, rarely involves the optic chiasm. MS has a smaller longitudinal extension than LETM and less than 50% of the cross-sectional area of the spinal cord in the axial plane, often affecting the peripheral white matter [56]. Besides, the classic "Dawson finger" perpendicular to the ventricle of MS helps to distinguish it from the NOMSD intracranial lesions. Corpus callosum lesions of MS mostly arise from the callososeptal interface, with "dot-dash" appearance, which is helpful for identification [56–58].

Case 3.3.5 Primary Central Nervous System Vasculitis

Clinical Presentation

A 6-year-old boy was admitted to the hospital with recurrent fever, cough for more than 20 days, convulsions once, accompanied by vomiting. The CSF examination: WBC: 114×10^9/L, N%:47%, lymphocyte: 29%. He was improved after treatment with hormone after admission.

Imaging Findings

A. Axial T1-weighted image shows slightly low signal intensity of bilateral thalamus (arrowhead) (Fig. 3.12a).
B. Axial T2-weighted image shows high signal intensity of bilateral thalamus (arrowhead) (Fig. 3.12b).
C. T2WI-FLAIR shows multiple lesions in the intracranial parenchyma involving bilateral thalamus, the cortical and subcortical areas (arrowhead) (Fig. 3.12c).
D. The distal level of the Fig. 3.12c in the same patient (Fig. 3.12d).
E. Axial CE-T1WI shows the lesions mentioned above with obvious enhancement (arrow) (Fig. 3.12e).
F. Coronal CE-T1WI shows multiple patchy enhanced lesions (arrow) (Fig. 3.12f).
G. T2WI-FLAIR shows that the range of lesions decreased and some lesions disappeared after half a month (comparison with Fig. 3.12c) (Fig. 3.12g).
H. Coronal CE-T1WI shows no abnormality enhancement after half a month (comparison with Fig. 3.12f) (Fig. 3.12h).

Discussion

Primary angiitis of the central nervous system (PACNS) also known as primary cerebral vasculitis, is a rare idiopathic vasculitis and restricted to the vessels of CNS, frequently involving the leptomeningeal and cortical vessels [59]. PACNS is also a rare cause of stroke in children [60]. At present, PACNS in childhood (cPACNS) can be classified into angiography-positive (AP-cPACNS) and angiography-negative small vessel PACNS (AN-cPACNS) according to the affected cerebral vessel size (large-, medium-, and small-sized vessel) [61].

PACNS showed an estimated incidence of 2.4 cases per 100,000 person-years, with similar frequency in both sexes. All age groups may be affected, with the majority occurring between 37 and 59 years of age, and it is rare in children [62]. No incidence rates on cPACNS are available. Fullerton et al. [63] found that cPACNS accounted for 24% of arterial ischemic stroke (AIS) cases in children, and this was probably an underestimate.

Pathologically, PACNS consists of inflammation, intimal proliferation, and occlusion and necrosis of the small and medium-sized arteries [45]. The presumed mechanism of cPACNS involves an immune-mediated inflammatory process that leads to endothelial injury, activates the coagulation cascade, and leads to acute thromboembolism and varying degrees of arterial stenosis and occlusion [60].

Clinical symptoms of PACNS are rather diverse, ranging from psychiatric and behavioral problems, transient focal deficits, to persistent neurological symptoms. Headache and focal neurological dysfunction are common manifestations, while stroke, hemorrhage, and transient ischemic attack can occasionally be seen, but cranial nerve damage, myelitis, or epilepsy are relatively rare. In 60%, patients with progressive forms AP-cPACNS develop permanent neurological deficits [61].

The imaging manifestations of PACNS are varied and non-specific, but MR imaging is almost always abnormal, which means that normal MR imaging can help rule out PACNS. The lesions of PACNS mostly present as patchy and gyri abnormal signals of different sizes located in the cortical and subcortical white matter. Most of the lesions are unclear. Bilateral lesions are more common than unilateral lesions. The distribution of the lesions is not consistent with certain vascular areas. The frontal lobe is the most common involved region, followed by the partial and occipital lobes. Lesions showed different signal characteristics in different sequences and different periods. Conventional T1WI sequence shows mild low signal intensity, T2WI and T2WI-FLAIR sequence shows high signal intensity. After contrast enhancement, the lesions showed different enhancement performances at different periods. Meninges can be enhanced. Other changes include parenchymal hemorrhage and microbleeds, cerebral infarction, which can be detected on susceptibility-weighted imaging (SWI) and diffusion-weighted imaging (DWI) sequences. Tumor-like mass lesions have also been reported that appear to resemble abscesses or neoplasms, with clump or garland-like enhancement. MRA is helpful in confirming the presence of cerebrovascular disease, which is typically manifested by intracranial artery stenosis, beaded changes, or occlusion [59, 62, 64, 65].

The imaging findings of PACNS lack specificity and need to be differentiated from a variety of diseases, such as viral

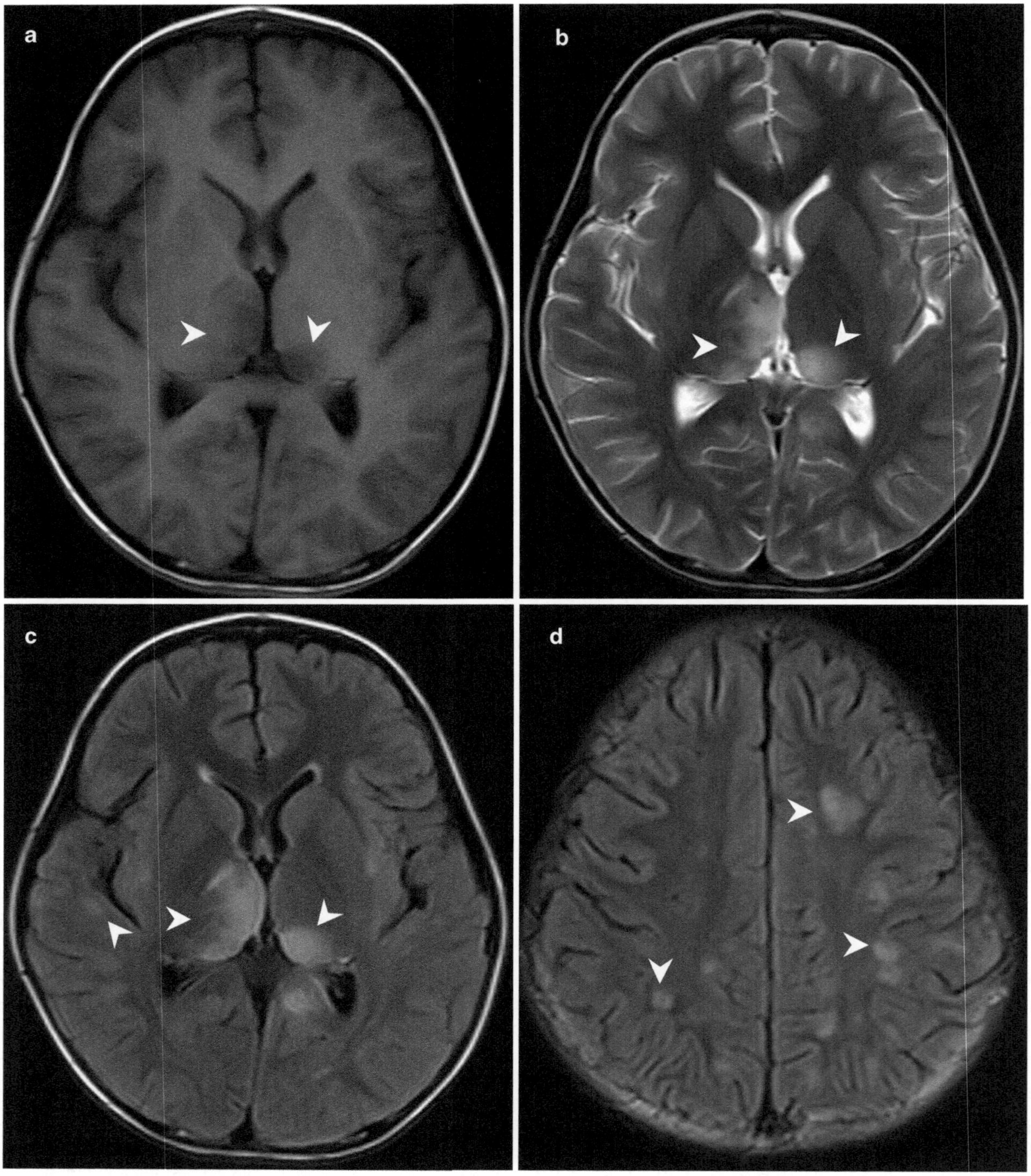

Fig. 3.12 Primary central nervous system vasculitis

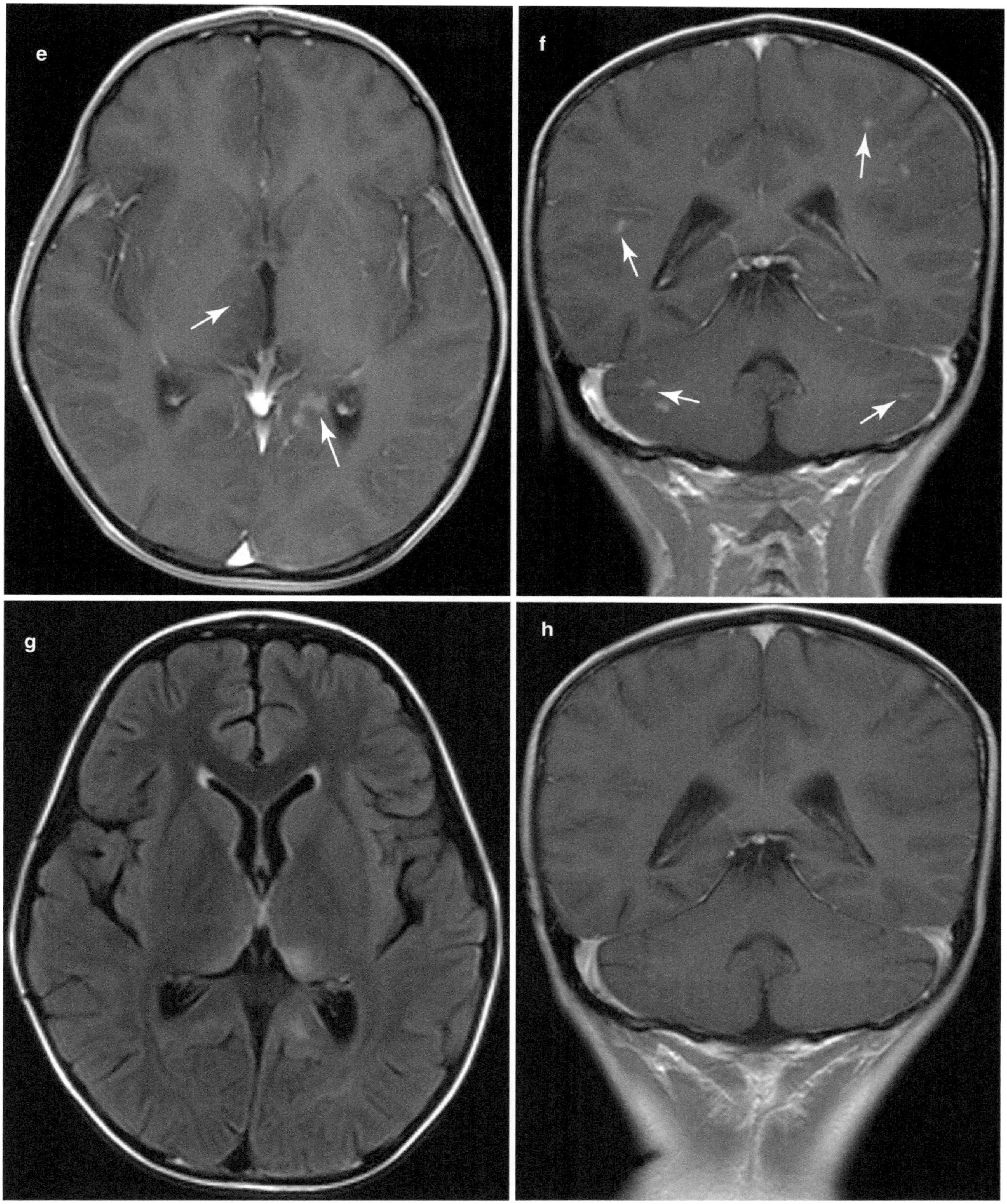

Fig. 3.12 (continued)

encephalitis, mitochondrial encephalopathy, multiple sclerosis, and neuromyelitis optica spectrum diseases. Viral encephalitis can be distinguished by clinical history, laboratory examination. The lesions of mitochondrial encephalopathy are migratory. The enhancement of the meninges can help to differentiate PACNS from multiple sclerosis and neuromyelitis optica spectrum diseases. Microbleeds within the lesions and positive MRA examination are helpful in differentiating PACNS from other diseases. In addition, tumor-like mass lesions of PACNS should be differentiated from tumors and abscesses, MRA and MRS examinations may be helpful in diagnosis [64, 65].

Case 3.3.6 Rasmussen's Encephalitis

Clinical Presentation

An 8-year-old girl was admitted to the hospital with no apparent cause for convulsions. She had no fever. Five months ago, she had a sudden seizure of left limb rigidity, accompanied by binocular staring. She was conscious during the seizure and relieved after 4 ~ 5 min. She was admitted to a local hospital and received symptomatic treatment.

Imaging Findings

A. Axial T1-weighted image shows the right hemisphere atrophy with the right caudate head is involved (arrow) and slightly low signal intensity in the right frontal subcortical white matter (arrowhead) (Fig. 3.13a).
B. Axial T2-weighted image shows high signal intensity in the right frontal subcortical white matter (arrowhead) and atrophy of the right caudate head (arrow) (Fig. 3.13b).
C. T2WI-FLAIR shows high signal intensity in the right frontal subcortical white matter (arrowhead) and atrophy of the right caudate head (arrow) (Fig. 3.13c).
D. Axial CE-T1WI shows no enhancement of the lesions (arrow head) (Fig. 3.13d).

Discussion

Rasmussen's encephalitis (RE) is a rare neurological disease first described in 1958 that is characterized as medico-refractory seizures, focal unilateral cerebral inflammation, and deficits such as hemiparesis [66].

Epidemiological research in Germany showed an estimated incidence rate of RE of about 2.4 patients per 10 million persons under 18 years old [67]. The mean age of onset is 6 years, thus the disease occurs mainly in childhood or school-age children, with no gender, geography, or ethnicity difference [68].

The primary etiology of RE remains elusive, and the possible pathogenesis is currently considered to include: virus infection, antibody-mediated, cell-mediated (cytotoxic T cells), and microglia-activation-mediated neurodegeneration. In recent years, studies have suggested the possibility of dual pathology in RE [67].

Patients are typically normal until the onset of seizures, the most common pattern of which is partial motor epilepsy, followed by epilepsia partialis continua, usually localized to the face or upper extremities. Other types of RE seizures include generalized tonic clonic seizures, partial complex seizures, and somatosensory or postural seizures. Ultimately, all patients develop hemiplegia. Electroencephalography (EEG) shows the slow activity of unilateral hemisphere with or without epileptiform activity and unilateral seizure onset. Cognitive impairment is another distinguishing feature of RE that is related to the severity of seizure. Other symptoms include dysarthria, dysphasia, in order of decreasing frequency, homonymous hemianopsia, sensory deficits, and personality changes. Patients deteriorate progressively unless the affected regions of the brain are surgically resected [67, 68].

The initial imaging findings of RE are typically normal. In time, hyperintensity develops in the cerebral cortex and subcortical white matter on T2-weighted and FLAIR images atrophy subsequently develops. The frontal and temporal lobes are most commonly affected, usually with associated atrophy in the insular. Progressive T2/FLAIR hyperintensity and atrophy in the caudate head is another important radiographic feature [69]. Other manifestations include enlargement of the lateral ventricle and the lateral fissure. The thalamus is rarely involved [70]. The reduction of NAA and creatine in Proton MRS and the dynamic changes of inter-paroxysmal cerebral hypoperfusion in SPECT of the affected hemisphere may become positive earlier than conventional MRI. In addition, automated MRI volumetric hemisphere analysis can be offered as an independent means of assessing RE progression [71–73].

Rasmussen encephalitis needs to be differentiated from bacterial or viral encephalitis, mitochondrial encephalopathy, cerebrovascular inflammation, Sturge–Weber syndrome that can cause hemispheric brain atrophy. Bacterial or viral encephalitis and Sturge–Weber syndrome are not difficult to distinguish according to clinical history, laboratory examination, and imaging characteristics. Mitochondrial encephalopathy is mostly bilateral hemispheric involvement, the lesion is transient, and rarely causes progressive unilateral hemispheric atrophy. Enhanced MR examination is helpful in differentiating cerebrovascular inflammation from RE, cerebrovascular inflammation can be excluded if lesions without enhancement [70].

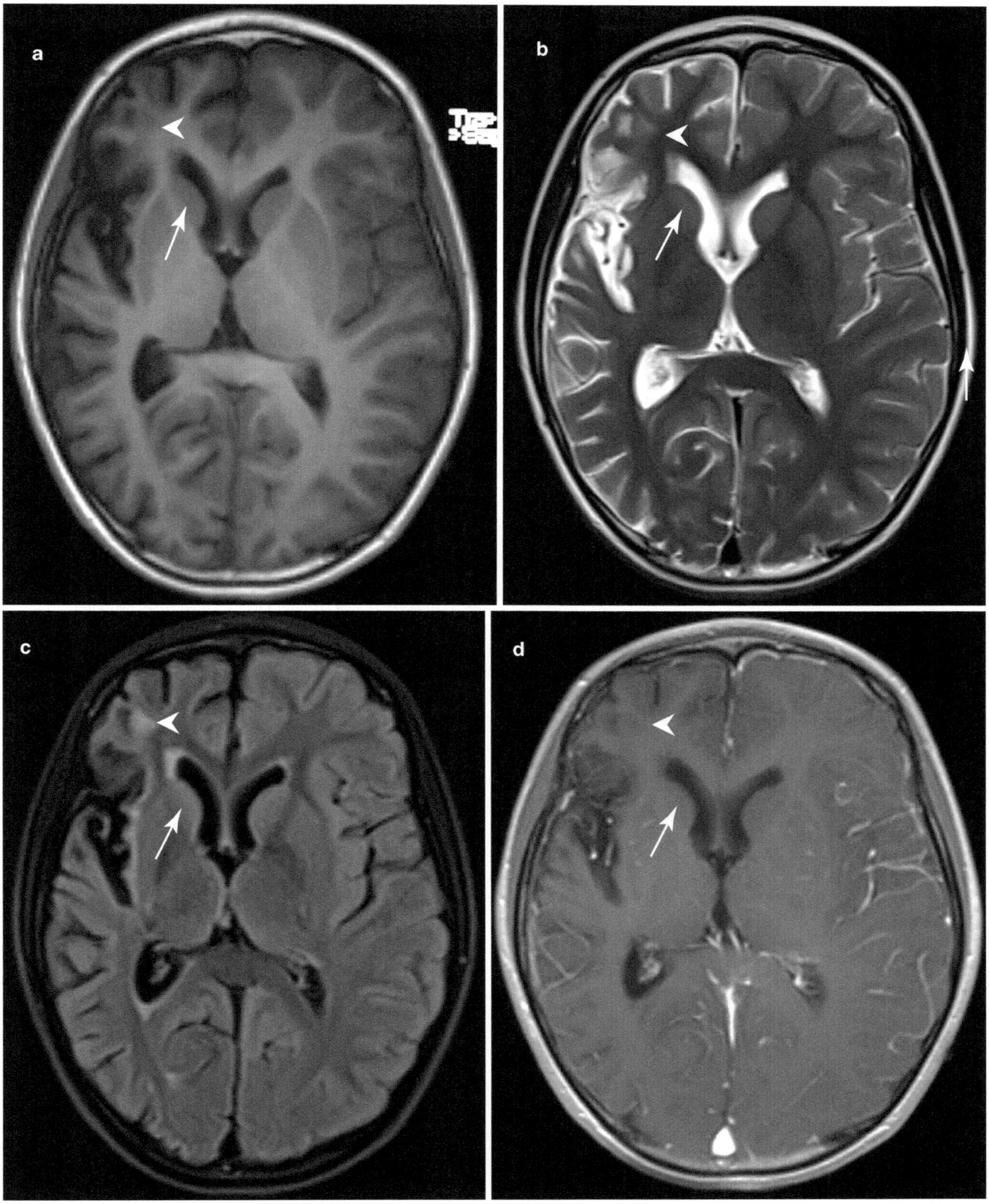

Fig. 3.13 Rasmussen's encephalitis

References

1. Neuberger I, Garcia J, Meyers ML, et al. Imaging of congenital central nervous system infections. Pediatr Radiol. 2018;48(4):513–23. https://doi.org/10.1007/s00247-018-4092-1.
2. de Vries LS. Viral infections and the neonatal brain. Semin Pediatr Neurol. 2019;32:100769. https://doi.org/10.1016/j.spen.2019.08.005.
3. Soares de Oliveira-Szejnfeld P, Levine D, Melo AS, et al. Congenital brain abnormalities and Zika virus: what the radiologist can expect to see prenatally and postnatally. Radiology. 2016;281(1):203–18. https://doi.org/10.1148/radiol.2016161584.
4. Abdel-Salam GMH, Abdel-Hamid MS, Mohammad SA, et al. Aicardi-Goutieres syndrome: unusual neuro-radiological manifestations. Metab Brain Dis. 2017;32(3):679–83. https://doi.org/10.1007/s11011-017-9993-4.
5. Goncalves FG, Caschera L, Teixeira SR, et al. Intracranial calcifications in childhood: part 1. Pediatr Radiol. 2020;50(10):1424–47. https://doi.org/10.1007/s00247-020-04721-1.
6. Goncalves FG, Caschera L, Teixeira SR, et al. Intracranial calcifications in childhood: part 2. Pediatr Radiol. 2020;50(10):1448–75. https://doi.org/10.1007/s00247-020-04716-y.
7. Bale JF. Fetal infections and brain development. Clin Perinatol. 2009;36(3):639–53. https://doi.org/10.1016/j.clp.2009.06.005.
8. Nickerson JP, Richner B, Santy K, et al. Neuroimaging of pediatric intracranial infection—part 2: TORCH, viral, fungal, and parasitic infections. J Neuroimaging. 2012;22(2):e52–63. https://doi.org/10.1111/j.1552-6569.2011.00699.x.
9. Ai J, Xie Z, Liu G, et al. Etiology and prognosis of acute viral encephalitis and meningitis in Chinese children: a multicentre prospective study. BMC Infect Dis. 2017;17(1):494. https://doi.org/10.1186/s12879-017-2572-9.
10. Shah G. Neuroimaging clinics of North America. Central nervous system infections. Preface. Neuroimaging Clin N Am. 2012;22(4):xiii. https://doi.org/10.1016/j.nic.2012.08.001.
11. Rath TJ, Hughes M, Arabi M, et al. Imaging of cerebritis, encephalitis, and brain abscess. Neuroimaging Clin N Am. 2012;22(4):585–607. https://doi.org/10.1016/j.nic.2012.04.002.
12. Misra UK, Kalita J, Phadke RV, et al. Usefulness of various MRI sequences in the diagnosis of viral encephalitis. Acta Trop. 2010;116(3):206–11. https://doi.org/10.1016/j.actatropica.2010.08.007.
13. Sarma A, Heck JM, Bhatia A, et al. Magnetic resonance imaging of the brainstem in children, part 2: acquired pathology of the pediatric brainstem. Pediatr Radiol. 2021;51(2):189–204. https://doi.org/10.1007/s00247-020-04954-0.
14. Quattrocchi CC, Longo D, Delfino LN, et al. MR differential diagnosis of acute deep grey matter pathology in paediatric patients. Pediatr Radiol. 2013;43(6):743–61. https://doi.org/10.1007/s00247-012-2491-2.
15. World Health Organization. Global tuberculosis report 2020. 2020.
16. Kritsaneepaiboon S, Andres MM, Tatco VR, et al. Extrapulmonary involvement in pediatric tuberculosis. Pediatr Radiol. 2017;47(10):1249–59. https://doi.org/10.1007/s00247-017-3867-0.
17. Holmberg PJ, Temesgen Z, Banerjee R. Tuberculosis in children. Pediatr Rev. 2019;40(4):168–78. https://doi.org/10.1542/pir.2018-0093.
18. Wang DM, Li QF, Zhu M, et al. Epidemiological, clinical characteristics and drug resistance situation of culture-confirmed children TBM in southwest of China: a 6-year retrospective study. BMC Infect Dis. 2020;20(1):318. https://doi.org/10.1186/s12879-020-05041-3.
19. Chaudhary V, Bano S, Garga UC. Central nervous system tuberculosis: an imaging perspective. Can Assoc Radiol J. 2017;68(2):161–70. https://doi.org/10.1016/j.carj.2016.10.007.
20. Nickerson JP, Richner B, Santy K, et al. Neuroimaging of pediatric intracranial infection—part 1: techniques and bacterial infections. J Neuroimaging. 2012;22(2):e42–51. https://doi.org/10.1111/j.1552-6569.2011.00700.x.
21. Swinburne NC, Bansal AG, Aggarwal A, et al. Neuroimaging in central nervous system infections. Curr Neurol Neurosci Rep. 2017;17(6):49. https://doi.org/10.1007/s11910-017-0756-8.
22. Azeemuddin M, Alvi A, Sayani R, et al. Neuroimaging findings in tuberculosis: a single-center experience in 559 cases. J Neuroimaging. 2019;29(5):657–68. https://doi.org/10.1111/jon.12627.
23. Schaller MA, Wicke F, Foerch C, et al. Central nervous system tuberculosis : etiology, clinical manifestations and Neuroradiological features. Clin Neuroradiol. 2019;29(1):3–18. https://doi.org/10.1007/s00062-018-0726-9.
24. Parmar H, Ibrahim M. Pediatric intracranial infections. Neuroimaging Clin N Am. 2012;22(4):707–25. https://doi.org/10.1016/j.nic.2012.05.016.
25. Shih RY, Koeller KK. Bacterial, fungal, and parasitic infections of the central nervous system: radiologic-pathologic correlation and historical perspectives. Radiographics. 2015;35(4):1141–69. https://doi.org/10.1148/rg.2015140317.
26. Muccio CF, Caranci F, D'Arco F, et al. Magnetic resonance features of pyogenic brain abscesses and differential diagnosis using morphological and functional imaging studies: a pictorial essay. J Neuroradiol. 2014;41(3):153–67. https://doi.org/10.1016/j.neurad.2014.05.004.
27. Reddy DS, Volkmer R 2nd. Neurocysticercosis as an infectious acquired epilepsy worldwide. Seizure. 2017;52:176–81. https://doi.org/10.1016/j.seizure.2017.10.004.
28. Garcia HH, Del Brutto OH. Cysticercosis working group in P. Neurocysticercosis: updated concepts about an old disease. Lancet Neurol. 2005;4(10):653–61. https://doi.org/10.1016/S1474-4422(05)70194-0.
29. Siddiqua T, Habeeb A. Neurocysticercosis. Saudi J Kidney Dis Transpl. 2020;31(1):254–8. https://doi.org/10.4103/1319-2442.279948.
30. Gupta MM, Chaudhary N, Pathak S, et al. Neurocysticercosis in children with seizures: a cross-sectional study. Int J Pediatr. 2018;2018:1030878. https://doi.org/10.1155/2018/1030878.
31. Kufel J. Pathological structural changes in the brain in the course of neurocysticercosis—pathogenesis, serological diagnostics and imaging: a literature review. Ann Parasitol. 2020;66(4):441–6. https://doi.org/10.17420/ap6604.284.
32. Chou IJ, Wang HS, Whitehouse WP, et al. Paediatric multiple sclerosis: update on diagnostic criteria, imaging, histopathology and treatment choices. Curr Neurol Neurosci Rep. 2016;16(7):68. https://doi.org/10.1007/s11910-016-0663-4.
33. Otallah S, Banwell B. Pediatric multiple sclerosis: an update. Curr Neurol Neurosci Rep. 2018;18(11):76. https://doi.org/10.1007/s11910-018-0886-7.
34. Ruet A. Update on pediatric-onset multiple sclerosis. Rev Neurol (Paris). 2018;174(6):398–407. https://doi.org/10.1016/j.neurol.2018.04.003.
35. McGinley MP, Goldschmidt CH, Rae-Grant AD. Diagnosis and treatment of multiple sclerosis: a review. JAMA. 2021;325(8):765–79. https://doi.org/10.1001/jama.2020.26858.
36. Fadda G, Armangue T, Hacohen Y, et al. Paediatric multiple sclerosis and antibody-associated demyelination: clinical, imaging, and biological considerations for diagnosis and care. Lancet Neurol. 2021;20(2):136–49. https://doi.org/10.1016/S1474-4422(20)30432-4.
37. Alroughani R, Boyko A. Pediatric multiple sclerosis: a review. BMC Neurol. 2018;18(1):27. https://doi.org/10.1186/s12883-018-1026-3.

38. Dalmau J, Armangue T, Planaguma J, et al. An update on anti-NMDA receptor encephalitis for neurologists and psychiatrists: mechanisms and models. Lancet Neurol. 2019;18(11):1045–57. https://doi.org/10.1016/S1474-4422(19)30244-3.
39. Scheer S, John RM. Anti-N-methyl-D-aspartate receptor encephalitis in children and adolescents. J Pediatr Health Care. 2016;30(4):347–58. https://doi.org/10.1016/j.pedhc.2015.09.004.
40. Kayser MS, Titulaer MJ, Gresa-Arribas N, et al. Frequency and characteristics of isolated psychiatric episodes in anti-N-methyl-d-aspartate receptor encephalitis. JAMA Neurol. 2013;70(9):1133–9. https://doi.org/10.1001/jamaneurol.2013.3216.
41. Dalmau J, Graus F. Antibody-mediated encephalitis. N Engl J Med. 2018;378(9):840–51. https://doi.org/10.1056/NEJMra1708712.
42. Titulaer MJ, Hoftberger R, Iizuka T, et al. Overlapping demyelinating syndromes and anti-N-methyl-D-aspartate receptor encephalitis. Ann Neurol. 2014;75(3):411–28. https://doi.org/10.1002/ana.24117.
43. Zhang T, Duan Y, Ye J, et al. Brain MRI characteristics of patients with anti-N-methyl-D-aspartate receptor encephalitis and their associations with 2-year clinical outcome. AJNR Am J Neuroradiol. 2018;39(5):824–9. https://doi.org/10.3174/ajnr.A5593.
44. Bartels F, Krohn S, Nikolaus M, et al. Clinical and magnetic resonance imaging outcome predictors in pediatric anti-N-methyl-D-aspartate receptor encephalitis. Ann Neurol. 2020;88(1):148–59. https://doi.org/10.1002/ana.25754.
45. Sarbu N, Shih RY, Jones RV, et al. White matter diseases with radiologic-pathologic correlation. Radiographics. 2016;36(5):1426–47. https://doi.org/10.1148/rg.2016160031.
46. Gray MP, Gorelick MH. Acute disseminated encephalomyelitis. Pediatr Emerg Care. 2016;32(6):395–400. https://doi.org/10.1097/PEC.0000000000000825.
47. Nishiyama M, Nagase H, Tomioka K, et al. Clinical time course of pediatric acute disseminated encephalomyelitis. Brain and Development. 2019;41(6):531–7. https://doi.org/10.1016/j.braindev.2019.02.011.
48. Anilkumar AC, Foris LA, Tadi P. Acute disseminated encephalomyelitis. Treasure Island, FL: StatPearls; 2021.
49. Pohl D, Alper G, Van Haren K, et al. Acute disseminated encephalomyelitis: updates on an inflammatory CNS syndrome. Neurology. 2016;87(9 Suppl 2):S38–45. https://doi.org/10.1212/WNL.0000000000002825.
50. Frampton JE. Eculizumab: a review in neuromyelitis optica spectrum disorder. Drugs. 2020;80(7):719–27. https://doi.org/10.1007/s40265-020-01297-w.
51. Paolilo RB, Deiva K, Neuteboom R, et al. Acute disseminated encephalomyelitis: current perspectives. Children (Basel). 2020;7(11) https://doi.org/10.3390/children7110210.
52. Malagon VJ. [Demyelinizing diseases in children. Acute disseminated encephalomyelitis and multiple sclerosis]. Medicina (B Aires). 2019;79(Suppl 3): 66–70.
53. Santoro JD, Chitnis T. Diagnostic considerations in acute disseminated encephalomyelitis and the interface with MOG antibody. Neuropediatrics. 2019;50(5):273–9. https://doi.org/10.1055/s-0039-1693152.
54. Gombolay GY, Chitnis T. Pediatric neuromyelitis optica spectrum disorders. Curr Treat Options Neurol. 2018;20(6):19. https://doi.org/10.1007/s11940-018-0502-9.
55. Ungureanu A, de Seze J, Ahle G, et al. Myelin oligodendrocyte glycoprotein antibodies in neuromyelitis optica spectrum disorder. Rev Neurol (Paris). 2018;174(10):675–9. https://doi.org/10.1016/j.neurol.2018.01.378.
56. Dutra BG, da Rocha AJ, Nunes RH, et al. Neuromyelitis optica spectrum disorders: spectrum of MR imaging findings and their differential diagnosis. Radiographics. 2018;38(1):169–93. https://doi.org/10.1148/rg.2018170141.
57. Kim HJ, Paul F, Lana-Peixoto MA, et al. MRI characteristics of neuromyelitis optica spectrum disorder: an international update. Neurology. 2015;84(11):1165–73. https://doi.org/10.1212/WNL.0000000000001367.
58. Kim SM, Kim SJ, Lee HJ, et al. Differential diagnosis of neuromyelitis optica spectrum disorders. Ther Adv Neurol Disord. 2017;10(7):265–89. https://doi.org/10.1177/1756285617709723.
59. Wang LJ, Kong DZ, Guo ZN, et al. Study on the clinical, imaging, and pathological characteristics of 18 cases with primary central nervous system vasculitis. J Stroke Cerebrovasc Dis. 2019;28(4):920–8. https://doi.org/10.1016/j.jstrokecerebrovasdis.2018.12.007.
60. Elbers J, Armstrong D, Yau I, et al. Vascular imaging outcomes of childhood primary angiitis of the central nervous system. Pediatr Neurol. 2016;63:53–9. https://doi.org/10.1016/j.pediatrneurol.2016.06.009.
61. Smitka M, Bruck N, Engellandt K, et al. Clinical perspective on primary angiitis of the central nervous system in childhood (cPACNS). Front Pediatr. 2020;3(8):281. https://doi.org/10.3389/fped.2020.00281.
62. Deb-Chatterji M, Schuster S, Haeussler V, et al. Primary angiitis of the central nervous system: new potential imaging techniques and biomarkers in blood and cerebrospinal fluid. Front Neurol. 2019;6(10):568. https://doi.org/10.3389/fneur.2019.00568.
63. Fullerton HJ, Wu YW, Sidney S, et al. Risk of recurrent childhood arterial ischemic stroke in a population based cohort: the importance of cerebrovascular imaging. Pediatrics. 2007;119:495–501. https://doi.org/10.1542/peds.2006-2791.
64. Wangchun D, Hongsheng L, Jianming L, et al. Imaging findings of childhood primary angiitis of the central nervous system. Chin J Radiol. 2020;54(7):713–5. https://doi.org/10.3760/cma.j.cn112149-20190627-00531.
65. Kumar RS, Singh A, Rathore C, et al. Primary angiitis of central nervous system: tumor-like lesion. Neurol India. 2010;58:147–9. https://doi.org/10.4103/0028-3886.60417.
66. Press C, Wallace A, Chapman KE. The Janus-faced nature of Rasmussen's encephalitis. Semin Pediatr Neurol. 2014;21(2):129–36. https://doi.org/10.1016/j.spen.2014.04.018.
67. Tang C, Luan G, Li T. Rasmussen's encephalitis: mechanisms update and potential therapy target. Ther Adv Chronic Dis. 2020;11:2040622320971413. https://doi.org/10.1177/2040622320971413.
68. Cay-Martinez KC, Hickman RA, McKhann Ii GM, et al. Rasmussen encephalitis: an update. Semin Neurol. 2020;40(2):201–10. https://doi.org/10.1055/s-0040-1708504.
69. David B, Prillwitz CC, Hoppe C, et al. Morphometric MRI findings challenge the concept of the "unaffected" hemisphere in Rasmussen encephalitis. Epilepsia. 2019;60(5):e40–6. https://doi.org/10.1111/epi.14702.
70. Zhao DJ, Zhu MW, Du TQ, et al. MRI diagnosis of Rasmussen encephalitis. Chinese J Radiol. 2012;4(46)
71. Wellard RM, Briellmann RS, Wilson JC, et al. Longitudinal study of MRS metabolites in Rasmussen encephalitis. Brain. 2004;127(Pt 6):1302–12. https://doi.org/10.1093/brain/awh157.
72. Tessonnier L, Thomas P, Benisvy D, et al. Perfusion SPECT findings in a suspected case of Rasmussen encephalitis. J Neuroimaging. 2009;19(4):378–80. https://doi.org/10.1111/j.1552-6569.2008.00320.x.
73. Wagner J, Schoene-Bake JC, Bien CG, et al. Automated 3D MRI volumetry reveals regional atrophy differences in Rasmussen encephalitis. Epilepsia. 2012;53(4):613–21. https://doi.org/10.1111/j.1528-1167.2011.03396.x.

4 Vascular Diseases

Honglei Shang, Xin Zhao, and Xiaoan Zhang

Cerebrovascular diseases, such as intracranial hemorrhage (ICH), Aorto-Arteritis, vein of Galen malformation, developmental venous anomaly, cavernous malformation, arteriovenous malformation (AVM), and so on, act as the major causes that lead to disability and death of children. Although the incidence of cerebrovascular diseases in children is lower than that in adults, it does great harm. Due to the young age of children, cerebrovascular diseases may directly affect the children's life if they are not diagnosed and treated on time. In recent years, the understanding of cerebrovascular diseases in children has become more and more thorough. There are obvious differences between the clinical manifestations of cerebrovascular diseases in children and adults. For example, some children have transient ischemic attacks, but the lesion of cerebral infarction is not that apparent in imaging examination. Some children with venous sinus thrombosis only present with headache or epilepsy; Children with "stroke-like episodes," on the other hand, may have migraine or metabolic disease without obvious vascular anomalies. The types of cerebrovascular diseases in children change with age, and the risk factors for stroke in children are more complex compared with adults. As adults, stroke is mainly related to atherosclerosis, hypertension, hyperlipidemia, diabetes, alcoholism, smoking, and so on, but these risk factors are relatively rare in pediatric patients. The clinical diagnosis of stroke in children is more difficult as well. Therefore, how to diagnose cerebrovascular diseases effectively and quickly in children and provide targeted treatment in time is really an important issue in clinical practice. With the development of imaging technology, especially the wide application of magnetic resonance imaging (MRI), different types of cerebrovascular diseases can be detected and distinguished accurately, and the detection rate of cerebrovascular diseases in children has been improved. The developing imaging technologies can aid in the early detection and diagnosis of cerebrovascular diseases and are beneficial to their treatments.

4.1 Cerebral Hemorrhage

Clinical Presentation

A 15-day boy sudden convulsions. Absence of fever, congenital anomalies and recent history of trauma.

Imaging Findings

A-B. Axial T1-weighted image and Sagittal T1-weighted image demonstrate the mass in the left temporal lobe showed a hyperintense rim and hypointense center (arrows) (Fig. 4.1a–b).

C. Axial T2-FLAIR image demonstrates the mass showed hyperintense rim and hypointense center (arrow) (Fig. 4.1c).

D. Axial T2-weighted image demonstrates the mass showed hyperintense center with black rim (arrow) (Fig. 4.1d).

E. DWI demonstrates the mass with hypointense and severe edema around (arrow) (Fig. 4.1e).

Discussion

Cerebral hemorrhage (CH), which is the most lethal danger to human health, refers to the primary brain parenchymal internal hemorrhage. The main causes of cerebral hemorrhage in children include arteriovenous malformation, brain trauma, coagulation dysfunction, or thrombosis, among which congenital vascular disease is the most important cause. Cerebral hemorrhage caused by arteriovenous malformation is mainly distributed in the brain parenchyma, especially in the parietal lobe, occipital lobe, basal ganglia region, and thalamus region, which is related to the predilection

H. Shang
Department of Radiology, The Third Affiliated Hospital of Zhengzhou University, Zhengzhou, Henan, China

X. Zhao · X. Zhang (✉)
Department of Radiology, The Third Affiliated Hospital of Zhengzhou University, Institute of Neuroscience, Zhengzhou University, Zhengzhou, Henan, China
e-mail: zdsfyzx@zzu.edu.cn; zxa@zzu.edu.cn

H. Liu, X. Zhang (eds.), *Pediatric Neuroimaging*, https://doi.org/10.1007/978-981-16-7928-5_4

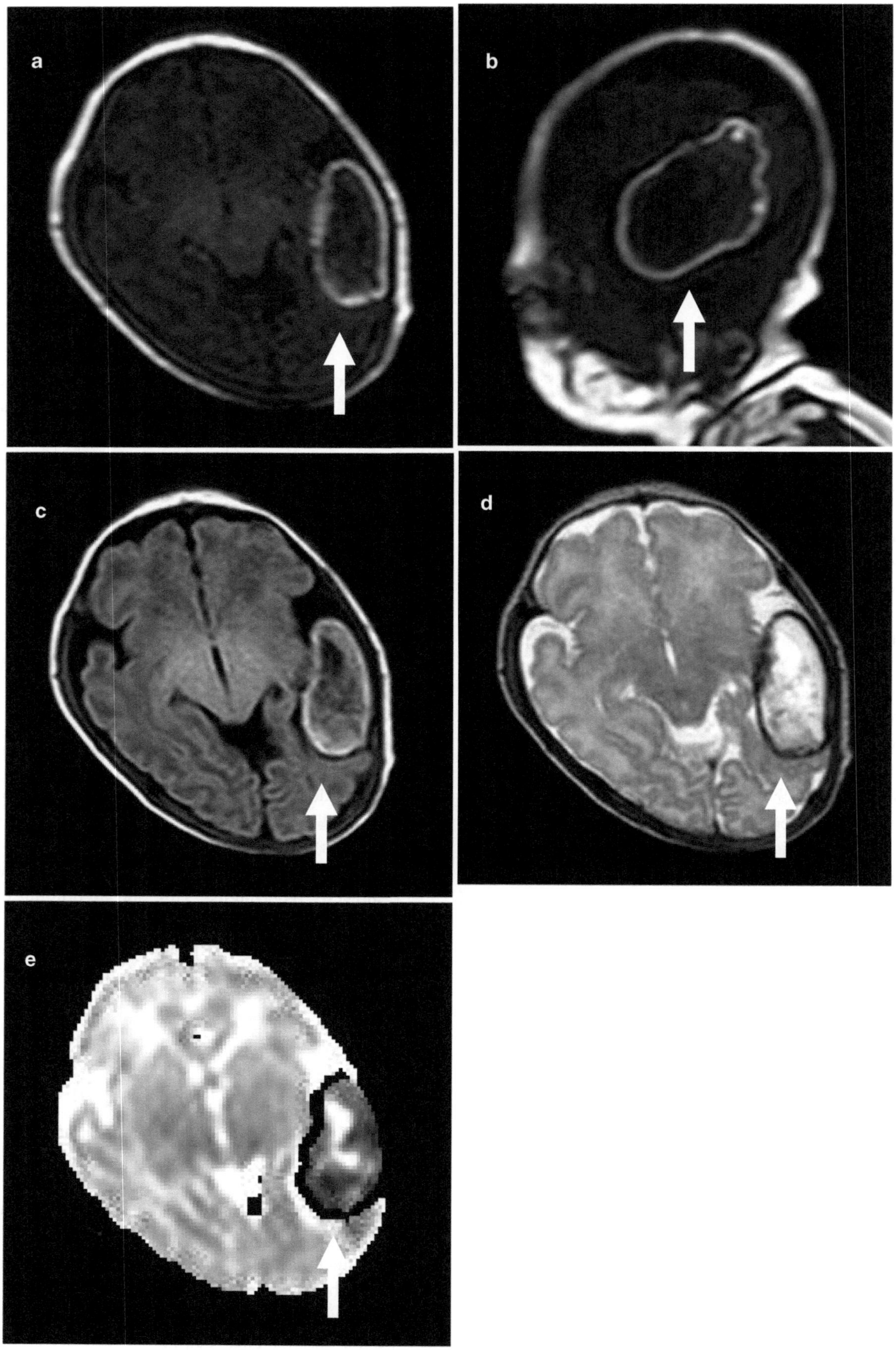

Fig. 4.1 Cardioaortic embolism

place of arteriovenous malformation. Hypertensive intracerebral hemorrhage is very rare in childhood, and the lesions are mainly distributed in the basal ganglia and thalamus, which are in the shape of kidney or oval. The pathological changes after cerebral hemorrhage include the sharp destruction of brain tissue by massive hemorrhage, the displacement of brain tissue compression caused by the occupying effect, the damage of thalamus and brain stem, and the secondary cerebral ischemia and cerebral edema around the lesion. During cerebral hemorrhage, obvious ischemic changes occur in the perifocal brain tissue, with neurocyte and glial cell degeneration. According to the pathological evolution of the lesion, cerebral hemorrhage was divided into hyperacute hemorrhage stage, acute hematoma stage, subacute hematoma stage, and chronic hematoma stage by imaging.

The clinical methods commonly used for the detection of CH include angiography, computed tomography (CT) scanning, the cerebrospinal fluid (CSF) method, and magnetic resonance imaging (MRI). Skull CT, which is the most widely used CH detection method, can clearly show the bleeding site, amount of blood released, and the shape of the hematoma. The sensitivity of CT in hyperacute stage and acute stage of cerebral hemorrhage is higher than that of MRI, and MRI is superior to CT in determining the cause of cerebral hemorrhage.

CT finding of cerebral hematoma showed a clear border and uniform density of high-density mass. Over time, the hematoma gradually liquefies from the edge to the center until all of the hematoma liquefies. The density gradually changes from high density to equal density, and becomes low density after full liquefaction. Enhanced scanning was performed after hematoma liquefaction, and the hematoma wall showed partial or complete enhancement with a circular high-density shadow, which was sometimes caused by the proliferation of granulation tissue, glial and collagen fibers at the hematoma edge. Hematoma edema and mass effect around the hematoma are also important indirect signs of cerebral hemorrhage. 7 ~ 14 days after cerebral hemorrhage, cerebral edema was the most obvious, and edema gradually reduced and subsided. According to the site, size and degree of edema of hematoma, the image showed the compression of the ventricle, cistem deformation, midline structure to the contralateral displacement. If the cerebral hemorrhage is close to the ventricle or subarachnoid space, it is easy to break into it, causing intraventricular hemorrhage and subarachnoid space hemorrhage stage, and CT examination should be the main method. MRI in the acute of hemorrhage were low T1 signal or equal signal, and T2 is obviously low signal, while in low field strength equipment T2 can be shown as equal signal, which is easily to missed diagnosis. MRI in subacute hematoma stage presents high signal at T1, but complex signal at T2, generally evolving from peripheral high signal. Chronic hematoma stage is characterized by T1 high signal, T2 high central signal with peripheral high signal, central low signal to central high signal evolution. The chronic hematoma stage is characterized by T1 high signal and T2 high central signal with peripheral low signal ring, which is caused by hemosiderosis.

4.2 Stroke

Case 4.2.1 Cardioaortic Embolism

Clinical Presentation

The 8-year-old boy received medical treatment with right limb weakness as the main complaint, accompanied by right eye blurring. Head CT examination indicated slightly high-density shadows in the right frontal lobe, and a small amount of bleeding was considered for differentiation from artifacts. Without special treatment, the limb weakness of the child gradually improved, and the mental response and limb activity recovered after 1 h.

Imaging Findings

A-B. Axial T2-weighted image and Axial T2-FLAIR image demonstrate the edema in the left occipital lobe (arrow) (Fig. 4.2a–b).

C. Axial T1-weighted image demonstrates the mass with gyrus-like hyperintensity in the right parietal lobe suggested hemorrhage (arrow) (Fig. 4.2c).

D. Enhanced image demonstrates the mass has obvious enhancement in the peripheral frontal lobe (arrow) (Fig. 4.2d).

E. Axial T1-weighted image demonstrates two weeks later, the lesion in the left occipital lobe showed a gyrus-like hyperintensity suggested hemorrhage (arrow) (Fig. 4.2e).

F-G. Axial T2-weighted image and Axial T2-FLAIR image demonstrate the mass with hyperintensity in the right parietal lobe indicated edema (arrow) (Fig. 4.2f–g).

Discussion

Cardioaortic embolism was also known as cardiogenic cerebral embolism. Cerebral embolism can be divided into cardiogenic cerebral embolism and non-cardiogenic cerebral embolism. Cardioaortic embolism is the most common cerebral embolism [1], with about 75% in the brain. Common heart diseases that cause cerebral embolism include atrial fibrillation, valvular heart disease, infective endocarditis, myocardial infarction, cardiomyopathy, heart surgery, congenital heart disease, mainly from the systemic venous system through congenital heart disease, such as atrial septum defect, patent foramen ovale, and other abnormal channels, directly into the intracranial artery caused by cerebral embolism [2]. Therefore, cardioaortic embolism can occur at any age, especially in young adults [3].

There are three mechanisms of cardioaortic embolism: local thrombosis of the left ventricle caused by abnormal blood flow or damage of cardiac structure, abnormal embolism of heart valve disease, or venous system to arterial system [2].

The clinical features of cardioaortic embolism include sudden neurological deficits (usually cortical involvement) that peak at the time of onset. In general, the initial severe functional impairment improves within hours or days, mainly due to spontaneous thrombolysis and recanalization of the embolic vessels.

In the diagnosis of acute cardioaortic embolism, the head CT takes a short time and is easy to rule out cerebral hemorrhage. MRI early shows the size and location of ischemic lesions. On CT plain scan, the thrombus of acute embolism could show the artery "High density sign." But brain MRI can reveal lesions that cannot be seen on CT, therefore the detection rate of cardioaortic embolism is increased. These two are the most important means of auxiliary examination in the diagno-

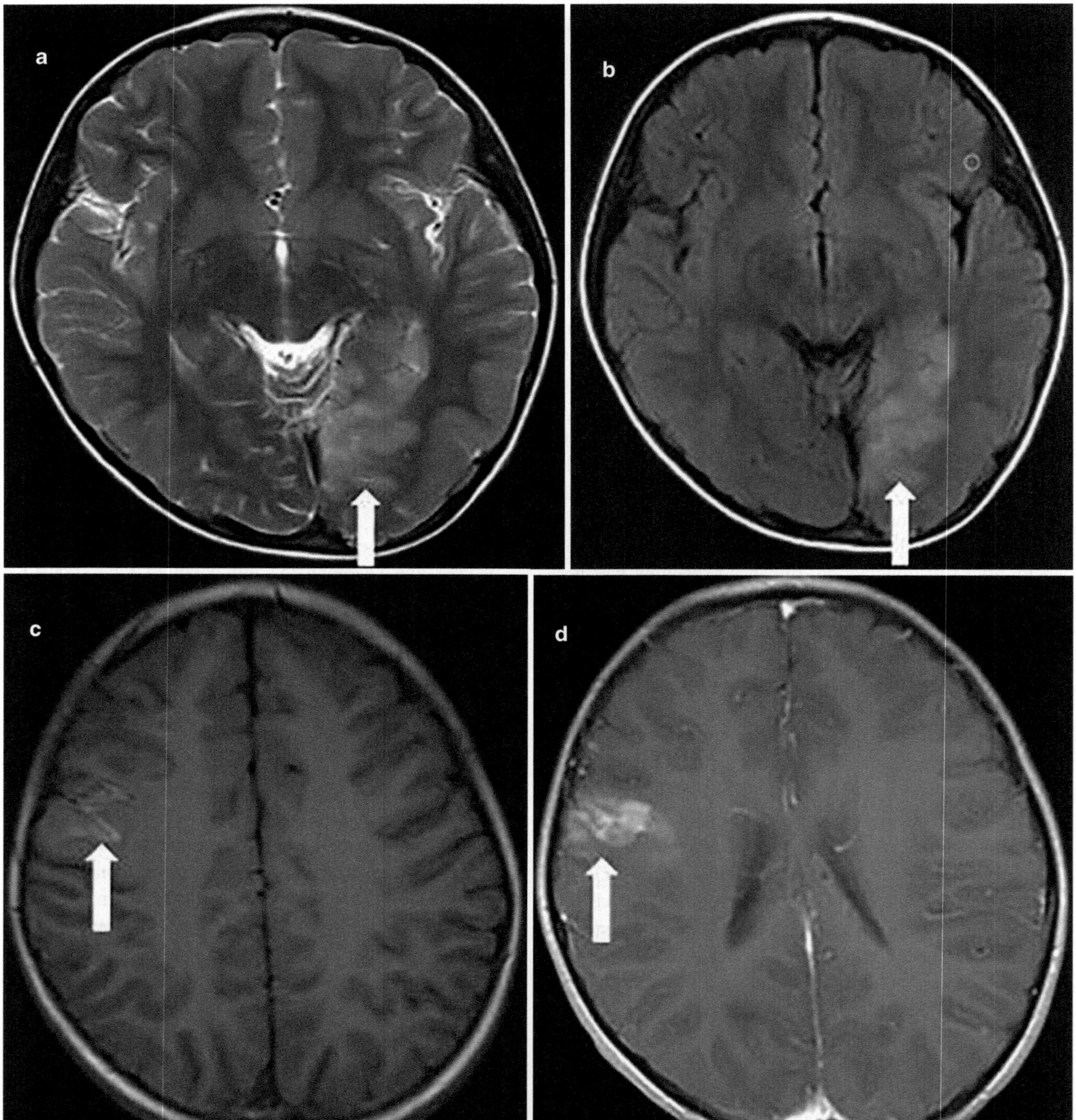

Fig. 4.2 Cardioaortic embolism

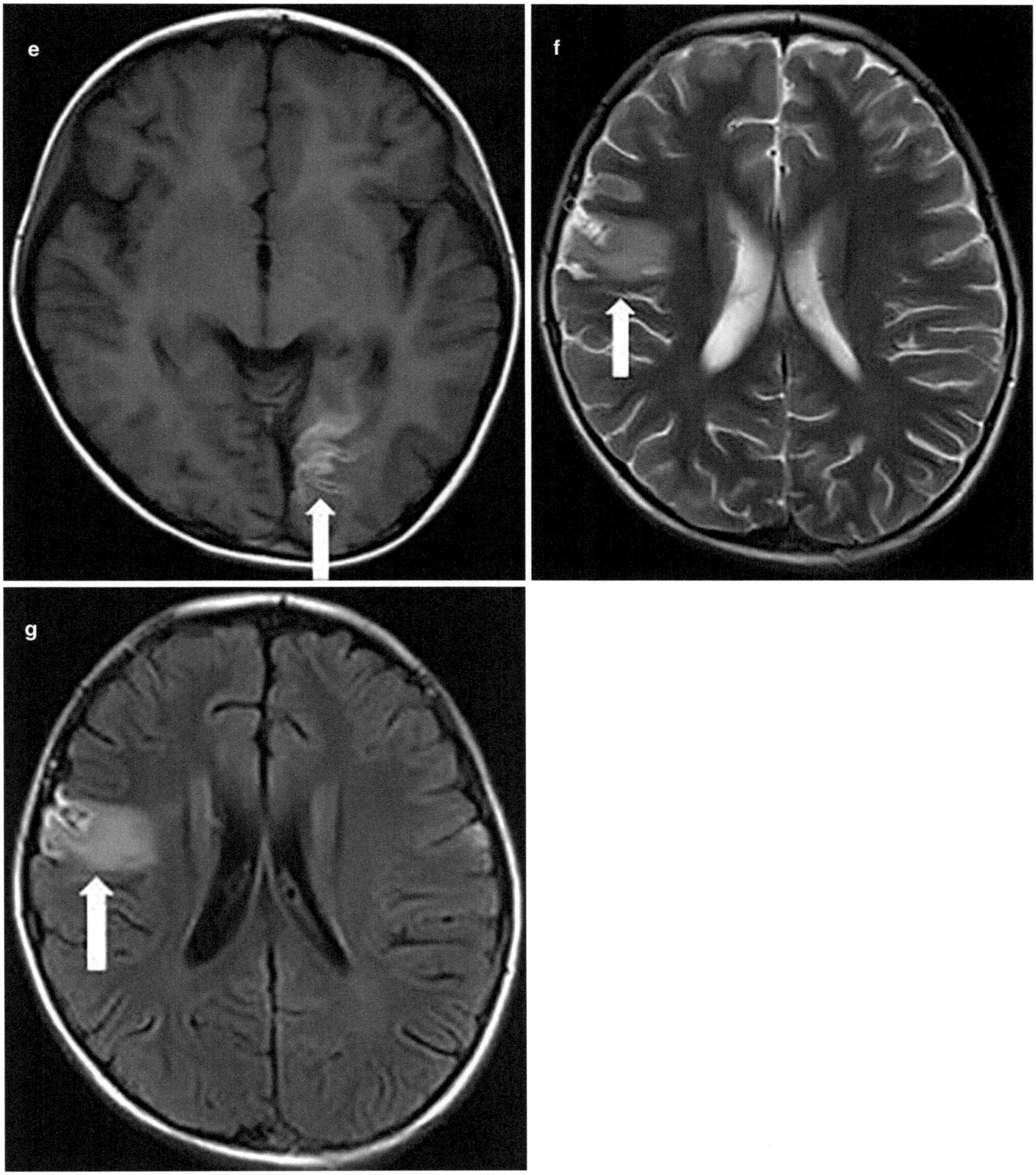

Fig. 4.2 (continued)

sis of cardioaortic embolism. Imaging findings of cardioaortic embolism have certain characteristics [4]: (1) Multiple blood supply areas are involved at the same time or the embolism occurs one after another. (2) Cortex or gray matter junction it is easy to be involved. (3) Prone to bleeding transformation.

There is no gold standard for making the diagnosis of cardioaortic embolism. The presence of a potential major cardiac source of embolism in the absence of significant arterial disease (such as atherosclerosis) remains the mainstay of clinical diagnosis. However, in many patients, history, physical examination, and routine diagnostic tests (electrocardiogram and findings on neuroimaging studies) are sufficient to easily make the differential diagnosis with non-cardioaortic embolism.

Case 4.2.2 Vascular Diseases

Clinical Presentation

A male, premature baby, gestational age of 30 W, intrauterine distress. Cesarean section was performed because of premature rupture of her mother's membranes.

Imaging Findings

A. Axial T1-FLAIR image demonstrates the lesion with hyperintensity in the posterior horn of the left lateral ventricle (arrow) (Fig. 4.3a).
B. Axial T2-weighted image demonstrates the lesion with slightly hypointensity (arrow) (Fig. 4.3b).
C. Axial T2-FLAIR image demonstrates the lesion with hyperintensity (arrow) (Fig. 4.3c).
D. DWI image demonstrates the lesion hyperintensity (arrow) (Fig. 4.3d).

Discussion

Stroke can be divided into two types: ischemic and hemorrhagic [5]. However, ischemic stroke can be divided into arterial ischemic stroke (AIS) and cerebral venous thrombosis (CSVT). Nearly, half of children with AIS suffer from cerebral artery disease [6]. AIS in childhood presents as focal defects or seizures. It locates in the ischemic area of brain injury in the known arterial region. Hemorrhagic stroke in children includes spontaneous intracerebral hemorrhage with or without intraventricular expansion, intraventricular hemorrhage (IVH), and nontraumatic subarachnoid hemorrhage.

After childhood AIS, about 75% of children develop neurological deficits and 10% die. Cervicocephalic artery dissection is an arterial lesion that accounts for 7.5–20% of AIS in children. Arterial dissection can be diagnosed by determining the appearance and location of blood vessels. Focal cerebral artery disease in children is characterized by local intracranial arterial stenosis, which accounts for approximately 25% of AIS in children. The diffusion-weighted image can clearly show the ischemic area. Three D TOF MRA maximum intensity projection (MIP) image shows a narrowing of focus in the arterial region. Moyamoya disease is characterized by chronic progressive stenosis or occlusion of the distal end of bilateral internal carotid arteries, anterior cerebral artery, and the beginning of middle cerebral artery [7]. And secondary basis cranii abnormal vascular network formation of cerebrovascular disease. Vasculitis of the central nervous system is less common in children with AIS. Fibromuscular dystrophy is a non-inflammatory arterial disease that rarely appears in childhood.

Hemorrhagic stroke refers to parenchymal hemorrhage, intraventricular hemorrhage, and subarachnoid hemorrhage. They are often manifested as mental state changes, nausea and vomiting, neck pain, seizures, and focal neurological deficits [8]. Imaging of parenchymal hemorrhage: Hyperacute phase: high-field MRI, T1WI is isosignal. Subacute stage: T1WI and T2WI showed circular hypersignal, hyposignal, or isosignal around the focal center. Chronic stage: Low-intensity ring on T1WI and T2WI with surrounding high-intensity hematoma. The softening lesions showed a high signal on T1WI and a low signal on T2WI. The most common hemorrhagic strokes in children are vascular malformation, arteriovenous malformation (AVM), cavernous vascular malformation, and aneurysm [9].

Neuroimaging is crucial for the diagnosis and differentiation of stroke. Importantly, neuroimaging is critical for the early recognition and treatment of the disease.

Case 4.2.3 Cerebral Venous Sinus Thrombosis

Clinical Presentation

A 5-year-old girl was admitted to the emergency department with intermittent fever for 6 days, intermittent vomiting, and headache for 3 days.

Imaging Findings

A. Axial T1-weighted image demonstrates the disappearance of the normal high flow void of the right sigmoid sinus (arrow) (Fig. 4.4a).
B. Axial T2-weighted image demonstrates mixed hyperintensity of the right sigmoid sinus (arrow) (Fig. 4.4b).
C. Enhanced T1-weighted image demonstrates no enhancement of the right sigmoid sinus with the adjacent transverse sinus dilatation (arrow) (Fig. 4.4c).
D. The MRV demonstrates absent flow within the right sigmoid sinus and enlargement of the right transverse sinus, superior sagittal sinus, straight sinus and sinus confluence (arrow) (Fig. 4.4d).

Discussion

Cerebral venous sinus thrombosis (CVST) is a rare and significant cause of stroke-like illness and accounts for less than 1% of all strokes. The annual incidence of CVST in the pediatric population is about 7 cases per million, with the highest incidence in newborns [10]. As with other thromboses, the causes of CVST in children and newborns are varied, such as dehydration, chronic renal failure, local infection, neonatal brain tumors, including obstetrical susceptibility conditions, such as premature rupture of membranes, infection, gestational diabetes, hypertension, and hypoxic–ischemic damage [11]. The degree of thrombosis and collateral status will determine the severity of clinical manifestations, the substantial lesions on magnetic resonance imaging, and whether the results are reasonable. The most common clinical features of CVST are headache (88–93%), epilepsy (37–71%), focal neurological deficit (20–54%), and isolated intracranial pressure increase (23%). Focal neurological deficit and sei-

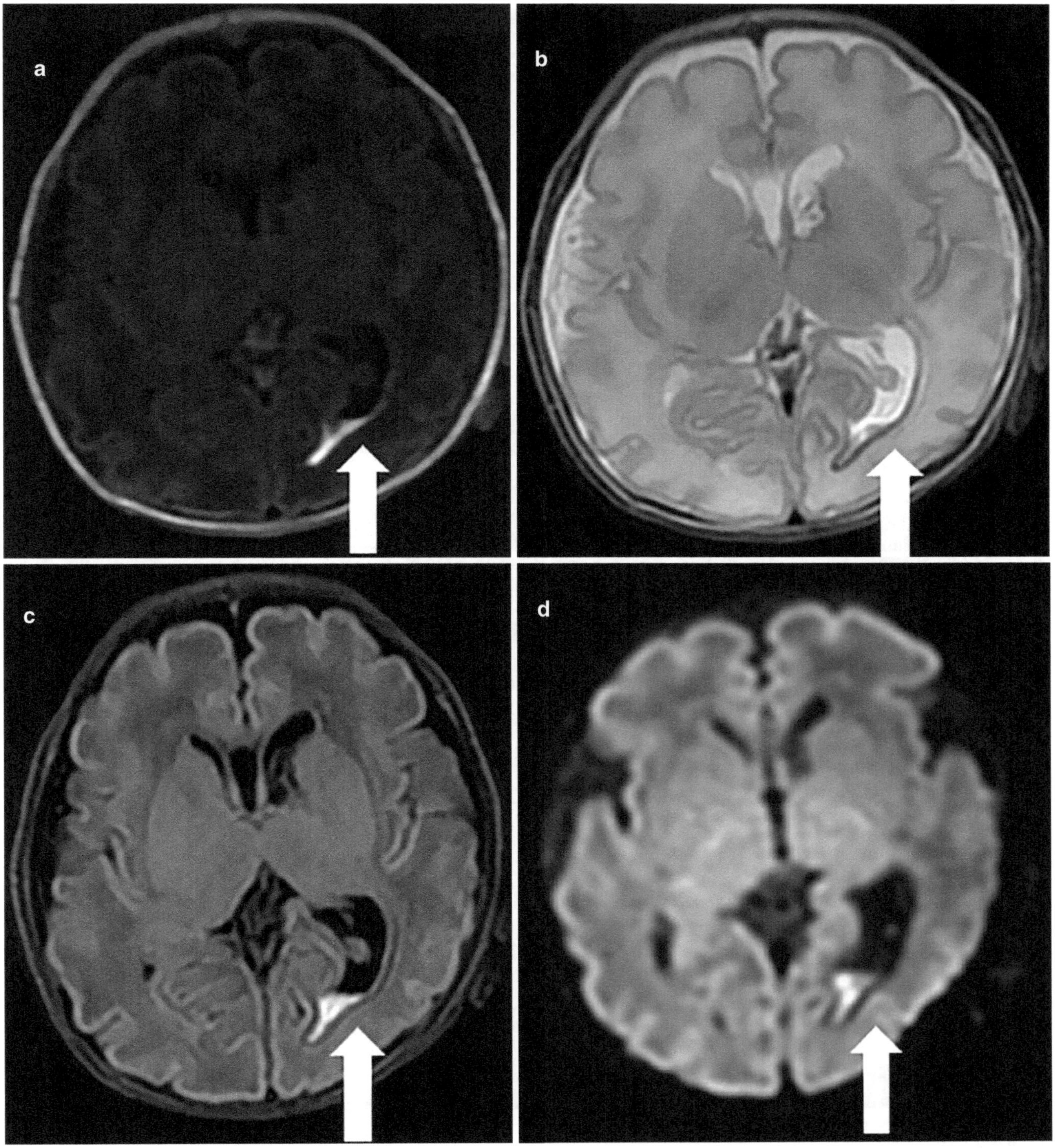

Fig. 4.3 Vascular diseases

zure may be the manifestation of potential parenchymal lesion [12]. CVST affects the superficial cerebral veins, deep cerebral veins, or dural venous sinuses. Isolated superficial cerebral vein thrombosis is rare. Most of the causes of dural venous sinus thrombosis are direct involvement of the superficial veins. The thrombosis of deep cerebral veins usually occurs in the internal cerebral vein and vein of Galen. About 60% of CVST patients involve multiple dural venous sinuses, of which the superior sagittal sinus is most commonly involved. Deep cerebral vein thrombosis mostly occurs in the internal cerebral veins and Galenic veins [13].

The imaging technology used for diagnosis in children is the same as that in adults, and transfontanine Doppler ultrasound is the first choice in neonates. It has the advantage of

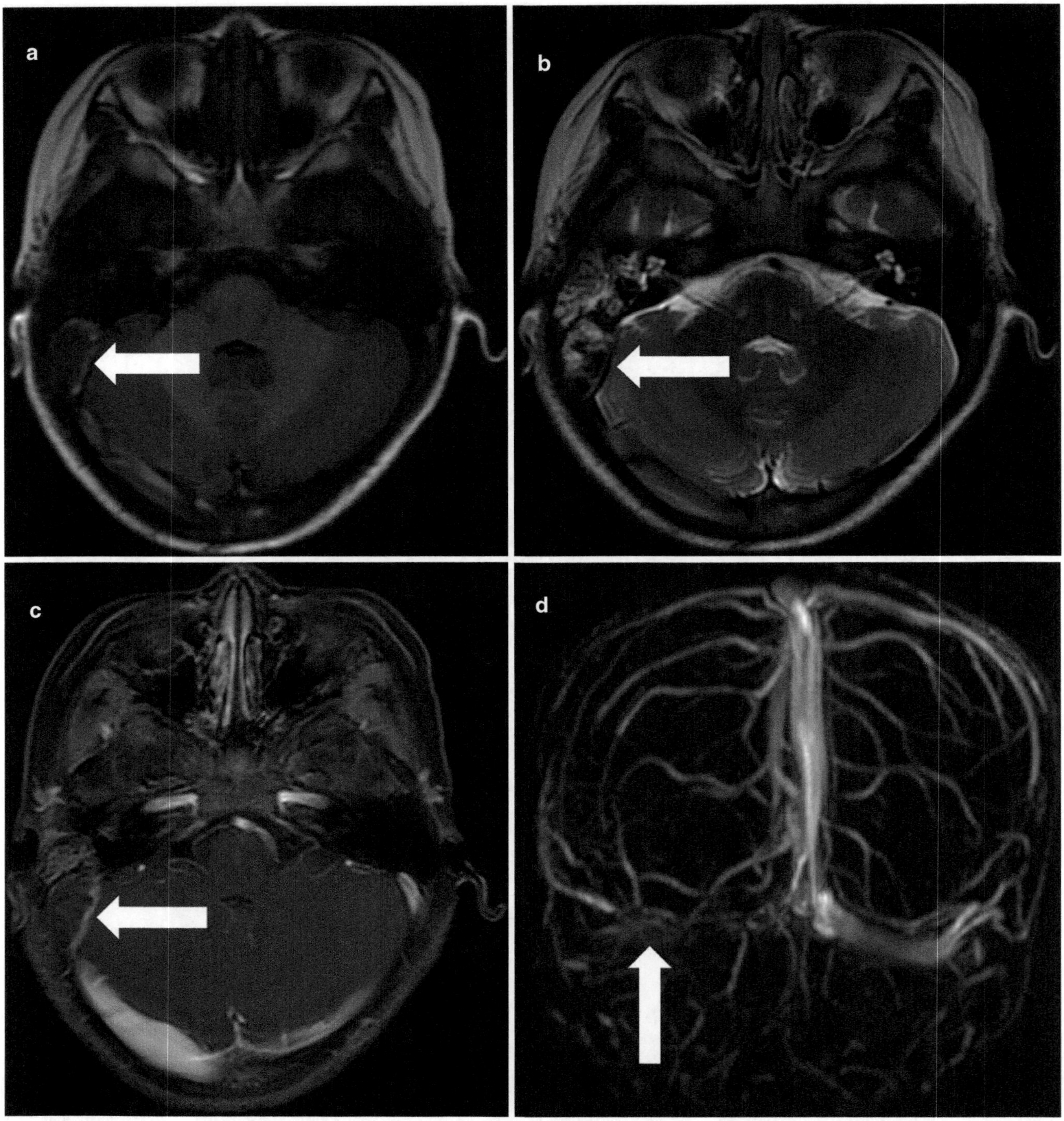

Fig. 4.4 Cerebral venous sinus thrombosis

being widely available and non-invasive, but it is strongly dependent on the operator. If there is no definite result and clinical suspicion of CVST continues, enhanced CT scan and MRI must be performed. At present, MRI is the gold standard imaging technique for diagnosing CVST.

Studies have shown that T1WI, T2WI, and FLAIR can be used to detect subacute thrombosis. Thrombus visualization and lack of signal holes in the spin echo sequence are the characteristics of thrombosis on MRI. In the acute phase, because blood products are in a state of deoxyhemoglobin, compared with brain tissue, thrombus is iso-intensity on T1WI and low-intensity on T2WI images. In the subacute phase, the thrombus signal intensity on T1WI is high. The T2WI signal intensity of thrombus in subacute phase is different. In the subacute early stage, it is low signal, and in the subacute late stage, it is high signal. This is because the blood product is in the methemoglobin state. The signal intensity of chronic thrombosis is usually isointense signal or hyperintense on T2- and T1-weighted image.

MRV uses the difference of longitudinal magnetization between flowing blood and surrounding stationary tissues to perform imaging, showing direct signs of cerebral venous sinus thrombosis, visually and vividly showing the filling of venous sinuses, occlusion, and irregular stenosis of the involved cerebral veins or venous sinuses. And filling defect is an indirect sign of cerebral venous sinus thrombosis which is different from cerebral parenchymal edema and spot-like hemorrhage. Normal cerebral veins and venous sinuses show high signals in MRV. If the cerebral venous sinus is completely blocked, MRV may demonstrate absent flow with the formation of surrounding collaterals.

The differential diagnoses of CVST are hypoplastic segment of dural sinuses, especially the transverse sinuses; a "splitting" superior sagittal sinus, which shows a high position and splitting torcular; and giant arachnoid granulations, which shows high signal on T2WI and surrounding bone remodelling may be seen. All of these are actually normal variants of the dural sinuses and typically do not present clinical manifestations as the CVST does.

Case 4.3 Moyamoya Disease

Clinical Presentation

A 6-year-old girl was examined by cranial MR imaging to investigate fever for 1 day, mouth askew for 11 h, and right limb weakness for more than 7 h.

Imaging Findings

A. Axial T2-weighted image demonstrates ischemic lesions in the left frontal lobe (arrow) (Fig. 4.5a).
B-D. MRA with TOF (time-of flight) 3D sequence, axial, sagittal, and coronal images demonstrate severe anterior and middle cerebral artery narrowed, and collateral lenticulostriate arteries enlarged with a "puff of smoke" pattern (arrow) (Fig. 4.5b–d).

Discussion

Moyamoya disease (MMD), a condition characterized primarily by angiographic findings, is a chronic, progressive vasculo-occlusive arteriopathy of uncertain etiology that typically affects the distal internal carotid arteries and proximal circle of Willis [14].

According to the diagnostic criteria of the Japanese Cooperative Research Committee, only cases with bilateral lesions are diagnosed as "definite." It has been discovered all over the world, especially in East Asian countries such as Japan, Korea, and China, with bimodal age distribution (5–10 years and second peak during fourth decade). The underlying pathological and genetic basis of MMD is still not well understood. Clinical onset of this disease includes recurrent transient ischemic strokes, epileptic attacks, or headaches, although some patients are asymptomatic [15]. MMD is the most frequent cause of stroke in Asian children. Anticoagulation therapy and surgical revascularization procedures are the main treatment methods. There are various surgical options accomplished by direct, indirect, or combined revascularization. Direct surgeries mainly include intra- and extracranial vascular reconstructions that primarily consist of superficial temporal artery-middle cerebral artery (STA-MCA) bypass; indirect surgeries include encephalo-myo-synangiosis (EMS), encephalo-duro-arterio-synangiosis (EDAS), and encephalo-duro-arterio-myo-synangiosis (EDAMS) [16].

Main imaging techniques may be used to evaluate cerebral hemodynamics in moyamoya disease. MRI has been widely used in assessing moyamoya disease because of its capacity to demonstrate anatomic vascular details. Progressive arterial stenosis results in abnormal net-like vessels that proliferate at the base of brain, forming a cloudy angiographic appearance named puff of smoke ("moyamoya" in Japanese). Perfusion MRI has been found to be effective in estimating cerebral hemodynamics in MMD and evaluating changes after bypass surgery. Similar to MR angiography (MRA), CT angiography (CTA) provides information about the anatomical state of the vessels. Though both CTA, and MRA have been shown to be quite effective, cerebral angiography is the gold standard for diagnosing MMD and assessing its progression [17].

Case 4.4 Aorto-Arteritis

Clinical Presentation

A 14-year-old girl presented with blurred vision in both eyes for more than 2 months. She was admitted to hospital with dizziness for 7 days. She had no trauma or family history.

Imaging Findings

A. Axial position of the head and neck CT angiography (CTA) demonstrates the brachiocephalic trunk, the left common carotid artery and the left subclavian artery wall thickened, and the lumen-heavy narrowed (arrow) (Fig. 4.6a).
B. Axis head CTA demonstrates the right posterior cerebral artery (P1 segment) was slender and poorly developed (Fig. 4.6b).
C-D. Curved planar reformation (CPR) demonstrates mid-to-severe stenosis of the proximal common carotid artery (Fig. 4.6c–d).
E-F. E-F. Curved planar reformation (CPR) demonstrates the lesion of the left side was obvious (Fig. 4.6e–f).

Discussion

Aorto-arteritis, also known as Takayasu arteritis (TA), is a chronic, autoimmune, granulomatous, and inflammatory dis-

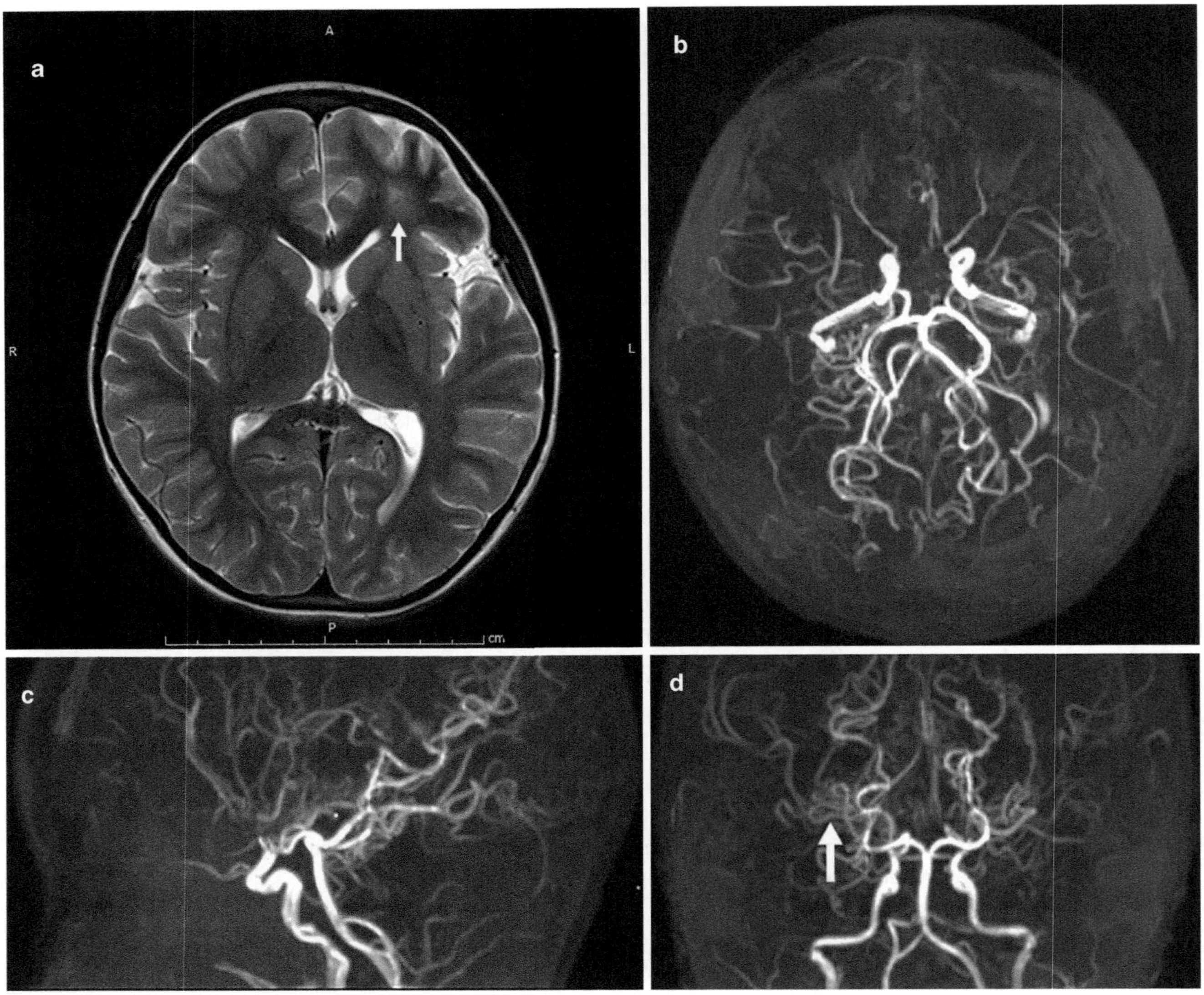

Fig. 4.5 Moyamoya disease

ease of the aorta and its major branches at their origin, which results in dilatation, occlusion, stenosis, and/or aneurysm formation of the affected arteries [18].

Although widely considered as a rare disease primarily affecting Asian women, TA can affect people of any ethnicity, with prevalence of disease varying by geographical location. The etiology of TA is unknown; however, several studies have demonstrated an association with human leukocyte antigens, suggesting a genetic predisposition for the immune-mediated process. In pediatric and adult patients of TA, common clinical manifestations include headache, fever, difficulty breathing, weight loss, and vomiting. TA classification is usually divided into five types.

Although there are no reliable clinical signs or laboratory parameters, and no ready-made tissue biopsy, imaging technology is the most important diagnostic tool in diagnosis. Conventional angiography, Magnetic Resonance Angiography (MRA), CTA, or Ultrasound can be used to diagnose TA [19].

Traditional angiography is still considered the gold standard diagnosis of TA. However, considering its invasiveness, exposure to significant radiation doses and the need for iodine contrast agents, apart from relying on professional knowledge, this can be a challenging procedure for children. In TA, the utility of noninvasive MRA is particularly high. MRA has been used in identifying stenosis, fusiform dilatations, aortic wall thickening (best demonstrated by axial T1WI), mural thrombi, and pulmonary artery involvement. A bright T2WI is obtained in inflammatory edema of the vessel wall. Vessel wall irregularity is clearly visualized with contrast-enhanced MRA. The advantage of multi-planar capability of MRI is useful in assessment of the extent of the aortic lesions in a longitudinal plane. The major disadvantages of MRI include its limitation in visualizing small branch vessels and poor visualization of vascular calcification CTA can show changes in lumens such as stenosis, occlusion, and calcification. Because it not only has the advantage of being able to observe the thickening of the vessel wall, but also can determine whether the blood vessel wall has blood supply by enhanced scanning. Besides, image post-processing technology plays an important role in daily clinical applications. For example, multi-planar recombination (MPR) technology allows to adjust the display angle at will, achieving a longitudinal axis along the vessel. The section simultaneously shows changes in the vessel lumen and vessel wall. Compensating for the limitations of cross-sectional observation, it is very suitable for evaluating changes in the blood ves-

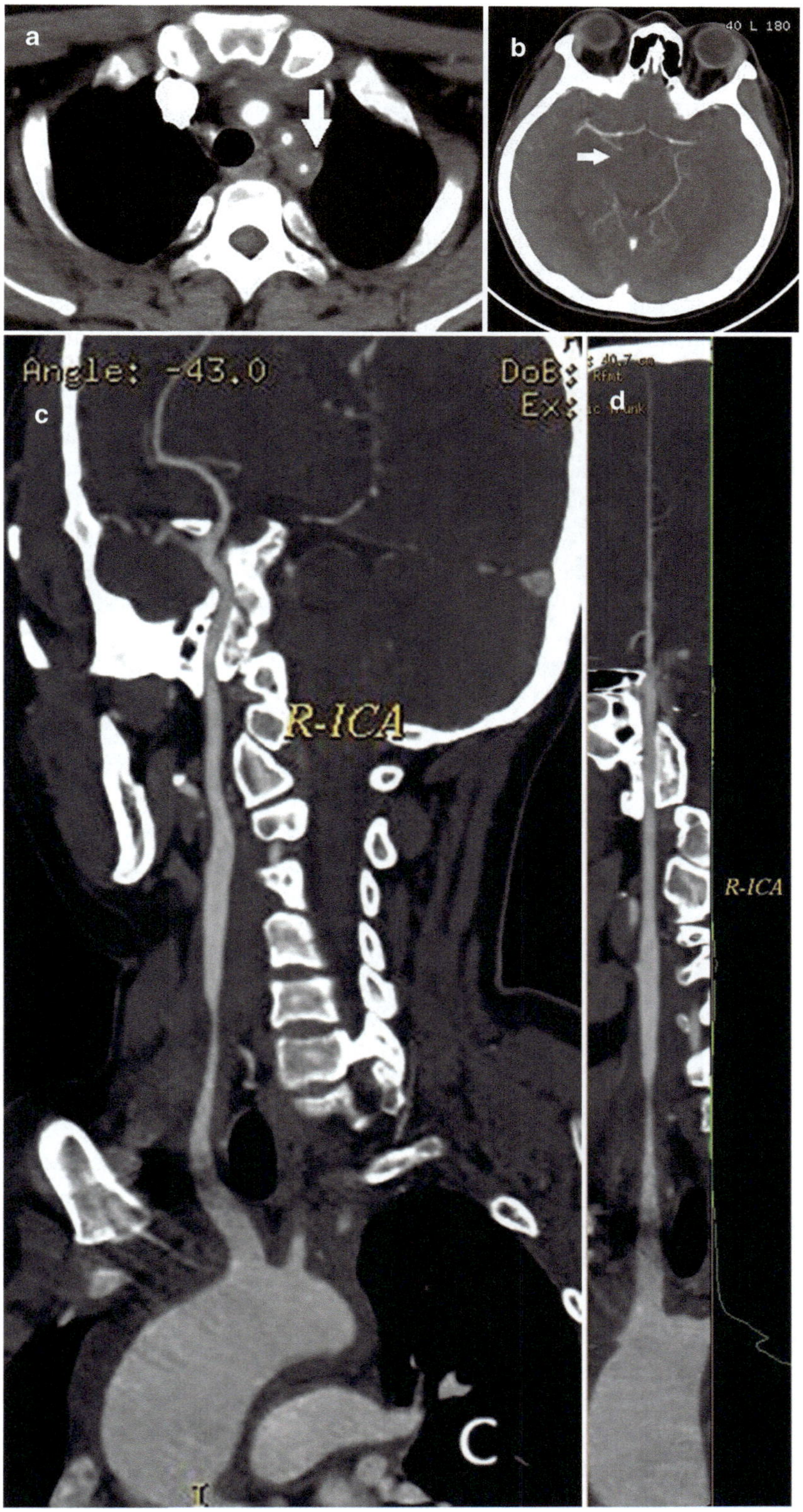

Fig. 4.6 Aorto-arteritis

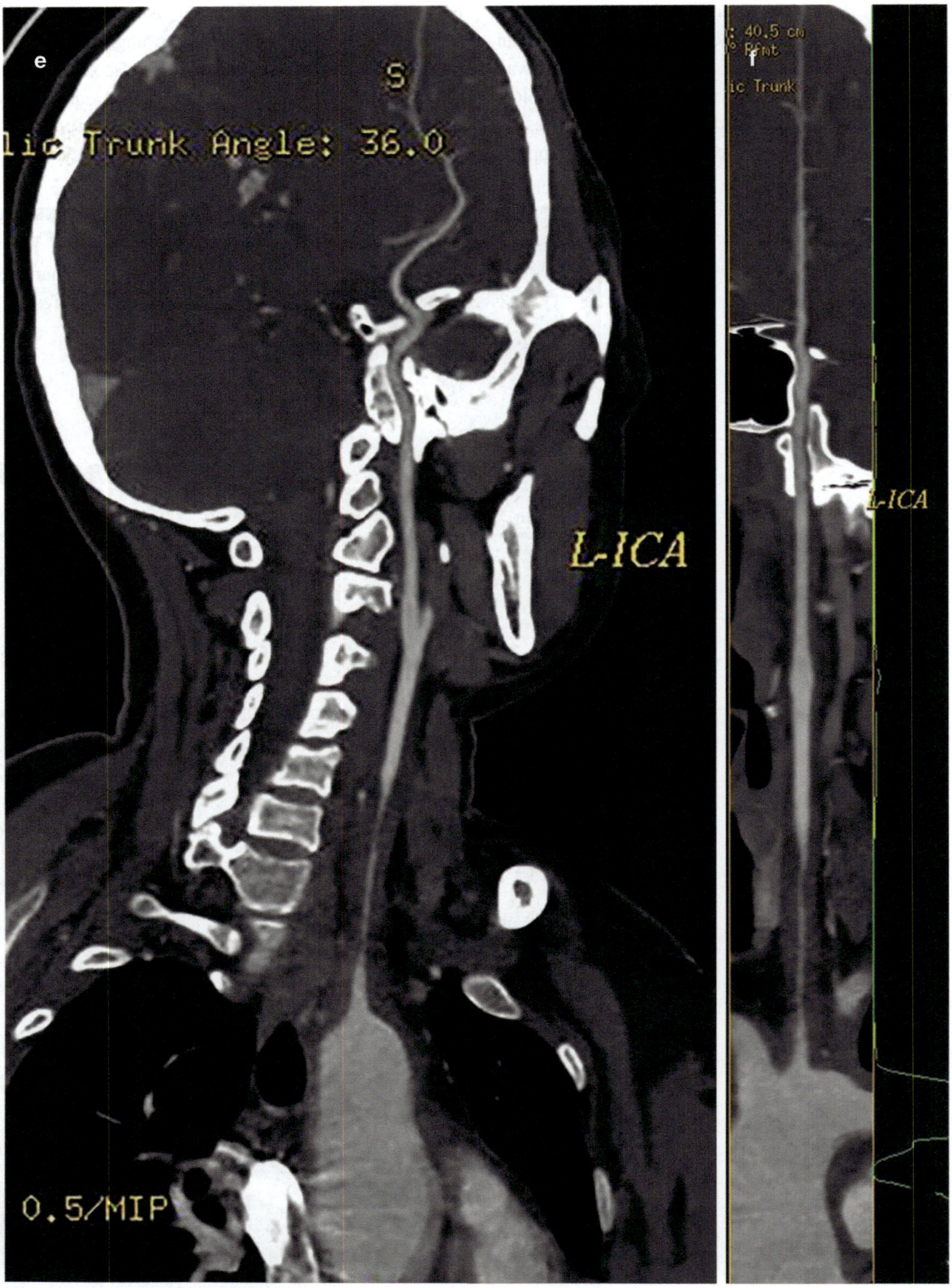

Fig. 4.6 (continued)

sel walls. The main disadvantage of CT is the large amount of radiation and great harm, especially for growing children. Ultrasound can directly measure the thickness of the blood vessel wall, so the sensitivity and specificity of evaluating the blood vessel wall are very high, especially in the evaluation of the common carotid artery. In addition, ultrasound can indirectly measure the stiffness of the arterial wall. However, the disadvantage of ultrasound is that its quality control relies on the professional knowledge of the researcher. Children's non-cooperation also limits its use in routine clinical practice.

Case 4.5 Vein of Galen Malformation

Clinical Presentation

An 11-month-old girl suffered from poor reaction with fever for more than half a day and convulsed for 30 min.

Half a day ago, the child developed crying and restlessness, difficulty to appease, poor response, vomiting once, non-ejective, milk, convulsions when seeing a doctor, characterized by angular arch, ankylosis, eyes closed, no response, unconsciousness, no cyanosis, and no foaming in the mouth. At that time, the body temperature was 39.5 °C, denied the history of glucose-6-phosphate dehydrogenase deficiency, denied the history of trauma, denied the history of surgery. Deny the history of blood transfusion.

Imaging Findings

A-B. Axial T2-weighted image and Axial T1-weighted image demonstrate the oval dilated empty blood vessels in the cistern of the great cerebral vein, surrounded by multiple flow empty vessels (Fig. 4.7a–b).

C. Axial T1-weighted image demonstrates ventricular dilatation (iso-T1 signal mass) and intracerebral hemorrhage (parietal-occipital high signal shadow) (arrow) (Fig. 4.7c).

D-E. MRA demonstrates the right posterior cerebral artery entering the venous aneurysm and forming an aneurysm adjacent to it (Fig. 4.7d–e).

F. Enhanced image demonstrates thick blood vessels converging into the cistern of the great cerebral vein (Fig. 4.7f).

G-H. Enhanced image demonstrates the venous tumor was connected with the straight sinus, and the straight sinus, sinus confluence, and transverse sinus were obviously dilated (Fig. 4.7g–h).

Discussion

Vein of Galen malformation (VGM), also known as the vein of Galen aneurysmal malformation (VGAM). VGM is a choroidal type of arteriovenous malformation and a rare congenital intracranial venous malformation, which often occurs from 6 to 11 weeks of pregnancy. It is one or more arteriovenous fistulas that divert blood to the forebrain vein of Markowski, the embryonic precursor of Galen vein [20]. This abnormal shunt can lead to progressive dilatation of the vein, which then develops into the Galen vein [20, 21]. Children born with this malformation may have clinical manifestations of congestive heart failure with high infusion volume, stunting, hydrocephalus, or epilepsy [20, 21]. The incidence is twice as high in men as in women, estimated at 1 in 1/10000 to 250, 000. Its severity and tolerance are related to the vascular architecture of VGAM and the age of children.

According to the characteristics of fistula, the vascular architecture of VGM can be divided into two types: the mural or choroidal type [22]. The mural type is supplied by the collicular and posterior choroidal arteries and converges into the aneurysm wall of the median forebrain vein. The choroid type is an extensive arterial network formed by the anastomosis between the arterial supply arteries supplied by the choroidal artery, the subfornical artery, or the external foramen artery of the thalamus and the venous aneurysm. Generally, the mural type is clinically well tolerated, while the choroid type often leads to more serious symptoms [22].

Magnetic resonance imaging (MRI) can distinguish the location of fistula, whether there are other lesions, venous thrombosis, and the number and type of arterial blood supply [22, 23]. MR imaging is the first choice to evaluate the damage of the ventricular system and brain parenchyma, which is critical to the choice of treatment and prognosis [24]. The middle forebrain vein (MPV) of Markowski and its surrounding feeding arteries form flow cavities. Intracranial T1WI hyperintense lesions showed calcification and ischemia, but ischemic lesions were rare in infants without myelin formation. Thrombus may show high signal on T1WI. When acute ischemia or infarction occurs, diffusion is limited on DWI. The best imaging examination for this disease is MR plus MRA/MRV sequence, because MRA can show the feeding artery, and MRV can show the anatomical relationship between MPV and vein.

Differential diagnosis should be made from Galen venous aneurysmal dilatation (VGAD) and dural arteriovenous fistula (DAVF) in children. VGAD generally does not have any clinical symptoms before the age of three. MRV shows that AVM can return to the real Galen vein, which is more rare [23]. For DAVF, when it is associated with high flow fistula, the appearance on MRI is similar to that of varicose veins and giant aneurysms that are common in VGAM. The external carotid artery can directly enter the sinus confluence, transverse sinus, or superior sagittal sinus [24].

The purpose of VGM treatment is to improve existing clinical symptoms, so there are different treatment goals for patients of different ages. For newborns, the purpose of treatment is to improve heart failure, while in older children, neurological symptoms are mainly prevented [22].

Case 4.6 Developmental Venous Anomalies

Clinical Presentation

A 7-year-old boy presented to the neurology clinic for paroxysmal convulsions for more than 4 years.

Imaging Findings

A-B. Axial T2-weighted image and Axial T1-weighted image demonstrate the oval dilated empty blood vessels in the cistern of the great cerebral vein, surrounded by multiple flow empty vessels (Fig. 4.8a–b).

C. Axial T1-weighted image demonstrates ventricular dilatation (iso-T1 signal mass) and intracerebral hemorrhage (parietal-occipital high signal shadow) (arrow) (Fig. 4.8c)

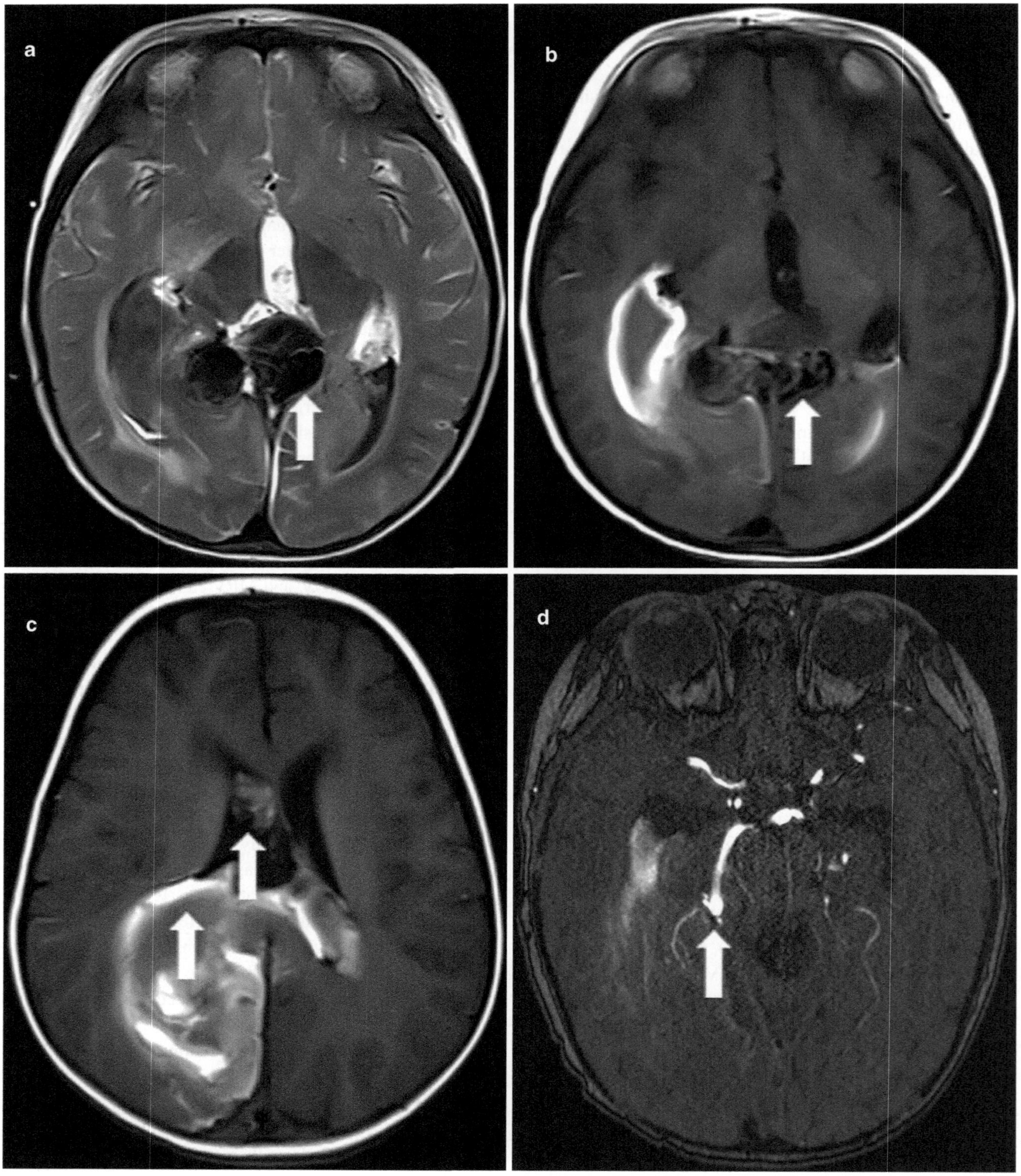

Fig. 4.7 Vein of galen malformation

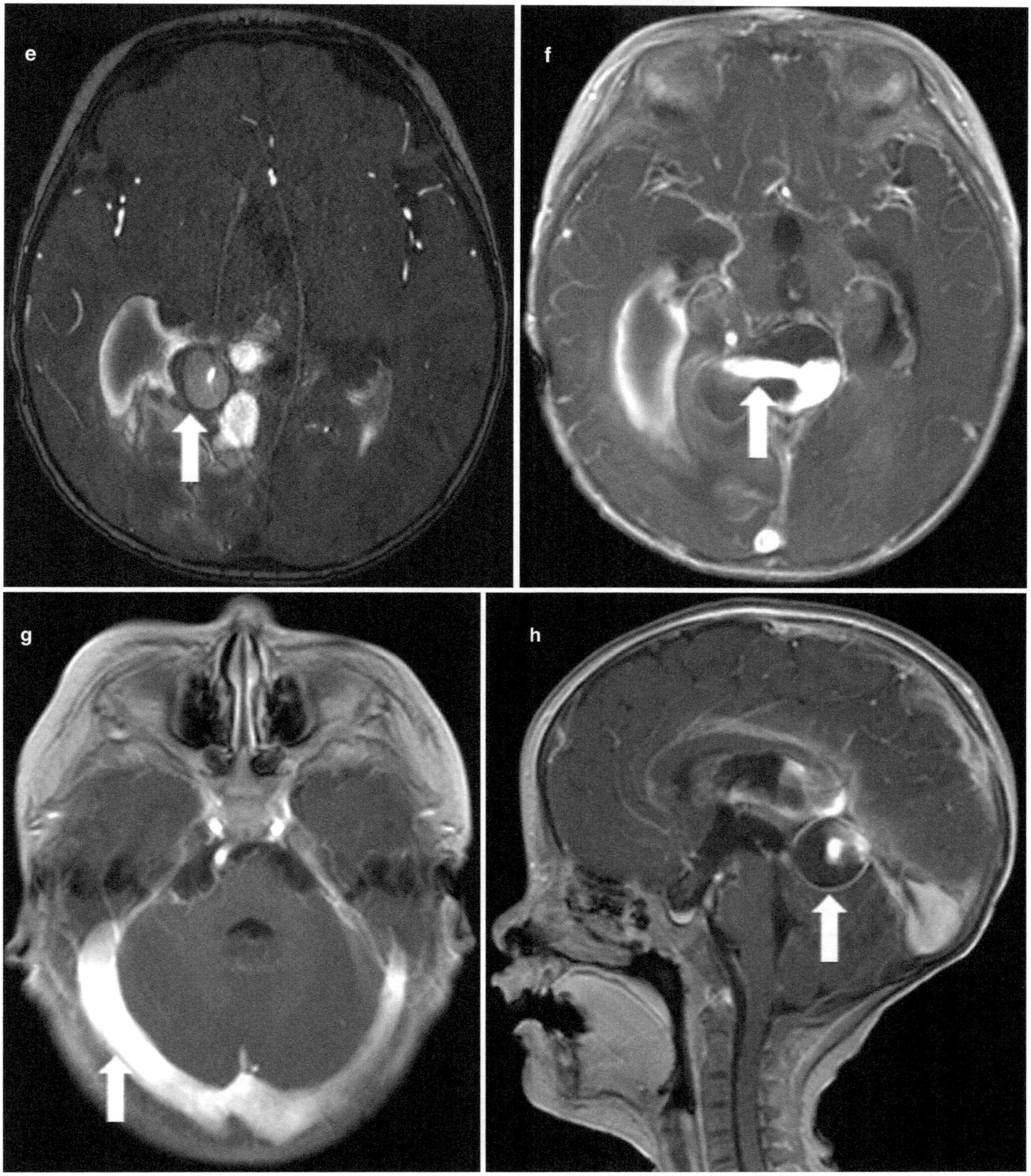

Fig. 4.7 (continued)

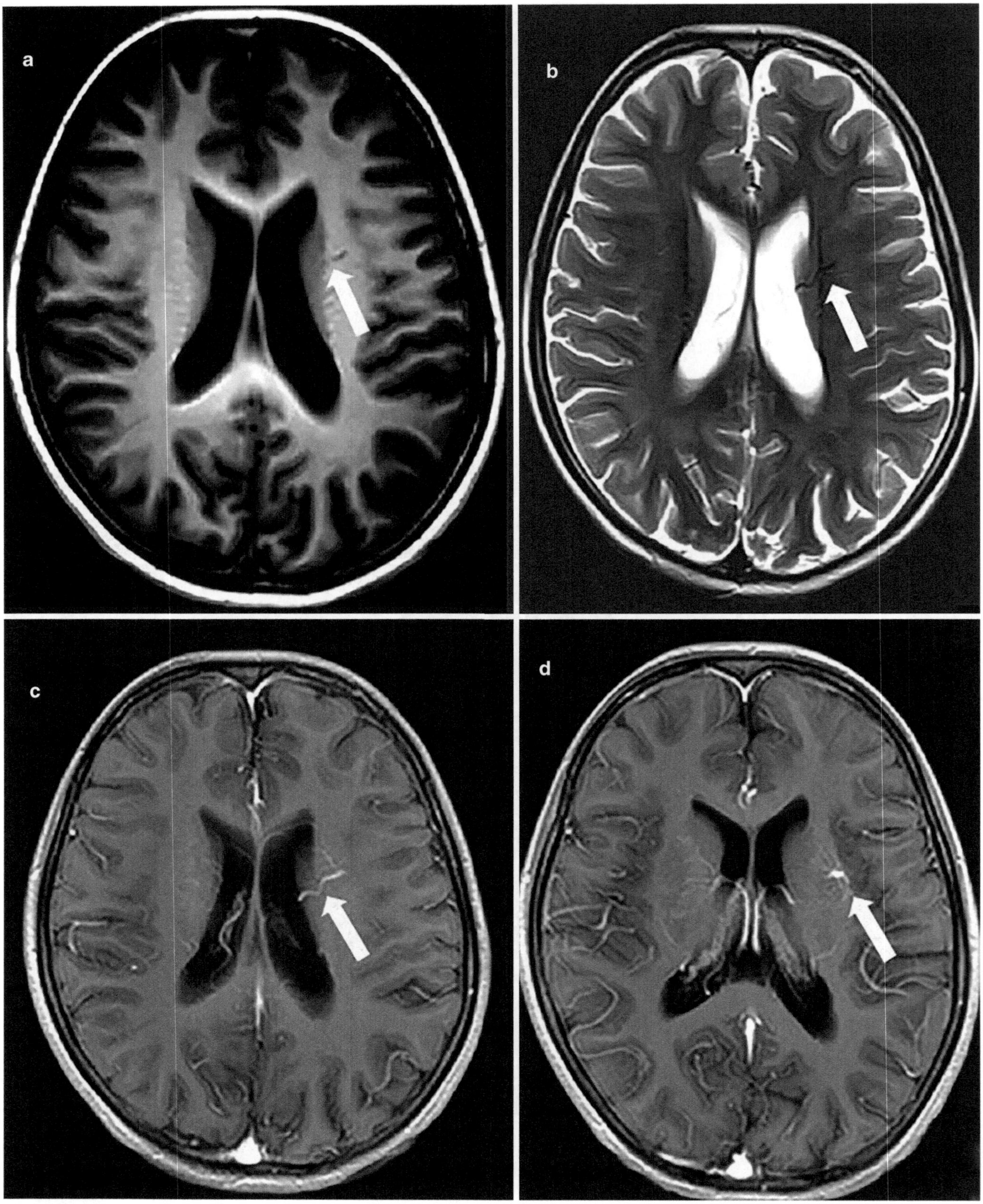

Fig. 4.8 Developmental venous anomalies

D-E. MRA demonstrates the right posterior cerebral artery entering the venous aneurysm and forming an aneurysm adjacent to it (Fig. 4.8d–e).

F. Enhanced image demonstrates thick blood vessels converging into the cistern of the great cerebral vein (Fig. 4.8f).

G-H. Enhanced image demonstrates the venous tumor was connected with the straight sinus, and the straight sinus, sinus confluence, and transverse sinus were obviously dilated (Fig. 4.8g–h).

Discussion

Developmental venous malformations (DVAs) are relatively common lesions that occur in up to 3% of the population. A DVA is composed of multiple radiating medullary veins converging centripetally into a single larger collecting vein, which ultimately drains into either superficial or deep cerebral venous system [25]. The exact mechanism and time of the development of DVAs remain unclear. The unifying theme of most current theories is that changes in venous drainage during fetal development led to the formation of DVA.

The natural history of DVAs is benign. With the widespread use of MRI, DVAs are now more frequently discovered and asymptomatic thus providing the normal venous drainage to the cerebral territory in which they reside. Therefore, neurological symptoms in patients seen are often due to the coexistence of an adjacent pathology, most commonly a cavernoma, fistula, or aneurysm when the underlying cause is intracranial hemorrhage (ICH) [26]. DVAs may also present symptoms due to mechanical or blood flow-related mechanisms. In cases of DVAs associated with hemorrhage, the most often cause are cavernous malformations (CMs) rather than DVAs themselves. The coexistence of CM and DVA is common. Because of the contribution to normal venous drainage and the risk for venous infarction, DVAs should never be surgically obliterated. It is recommended conservative management for all DVAs [27]. When resection is necessary for a cavernous malformation associated with a DVA, the surgical approach must consider how best to preserve the DVA.

At present, DVAs are often reported as incidental findings during routine diagnostic imaging procedures. DVAs occur as individual lesions and often occur in the frontoparietal region, with a reported range of 36–64%, whereas in the cerebellum this has been reported to be 14–27% [28]. Regardless of the imaging modality that is used, DVA diagnosis is dependent on identifying the area of caput medusa that drains into a common collecting vein. The gold standard for the diagnosis of DVA is cerebral digital subtraction angiography. In a CT without contrast, the collecting vein appears isodense and the acute thrombosis becomes hyperdense. It is also helpful in detecting calcifications, white matter lesions, atrophy, and hemorrhage associated with DVA. Flow voids in the white matter and connect to a venous sinus, and deep or cortical veins are typical appearances of a DVA on unenhanced T1W and T2W sequences. It has been found that contrast-enhanced CT or gadolinium administration with MRI was to demonstrate DVAs by showing marked enhancement of the radial veins and the main collecting vessel, giving rise to the classic "caput medusae" or "palm tree" appearance [26]. Mixed lesions are best diagnosed with magnetic resonance imaging [29]. In cases with an associated cavernoma, susceptibility-weighted sequences are most useful in the detection of such lesions due to blooming artifacts and can exhibit punctate or popcorn calcifications. Susceptibility weighted imaging (SWI) signal is not compromised by low-velocity venous flow and therefore is well demonstrated.

If the diagnosis of a simple DVA has been confirmed, it is not necessary to do follow-up imaging. In cases where an associated vascular abnormality has been identified (e.g., a cavernous malformation), follow-up is recommended on the basis of the associated lesion [27].

Case 4.7 Cavernous Malformation

Clinical Presentation

A 1-year-old boy who had cerebral hemorrhage for more than 1 month with altered mental status and seizure-like activities, transferred from the local hospital. He had no head injuries recently.

Imaging Findings

A. Computed tomography (CT) demonstrates a lobular hyperattenuation in the right temporal region, including a small and more pronounced density with 130HU, suggestive of focal calcification (arrows) (Fig. 4.9a).

B. AAxial T2-weighted image demonstrates the lesion with mixed-signal core of hemosiderin rim (arrows) (Fig. 4.9b).

C-D. Susceptibility-weighted imaging (SWI) of the same lesion demonstrates small multilocular areas of hyperintense core suggestive of subacute (extracellular methemoglobin) blood products, rimed with surrounding hypointensity (arrows). Numerous additional lesions were detected on SWI (Fig. 4.9c–d).

Discussion

Cavernous malformations (CMs) are low-flow vascular malformations found in both the supratentorial and the infratentorial regions of brain, and rarely in the spinal cord. They are also called as cavernous angiomas, cavernous hemangiomas, or cryptic vascular malformations, cavernomas. They are the second most common type of vascular lesion in the central nervous system, accounting for 10–15% of all vascular malformations. The majority of CMs are sporadic, but up to 20% follow a familial, autosomal dominant inheritance pattern, which is characterized by the presence of multiple CCMs in a single patient. They occur from autosomal dominant muta-

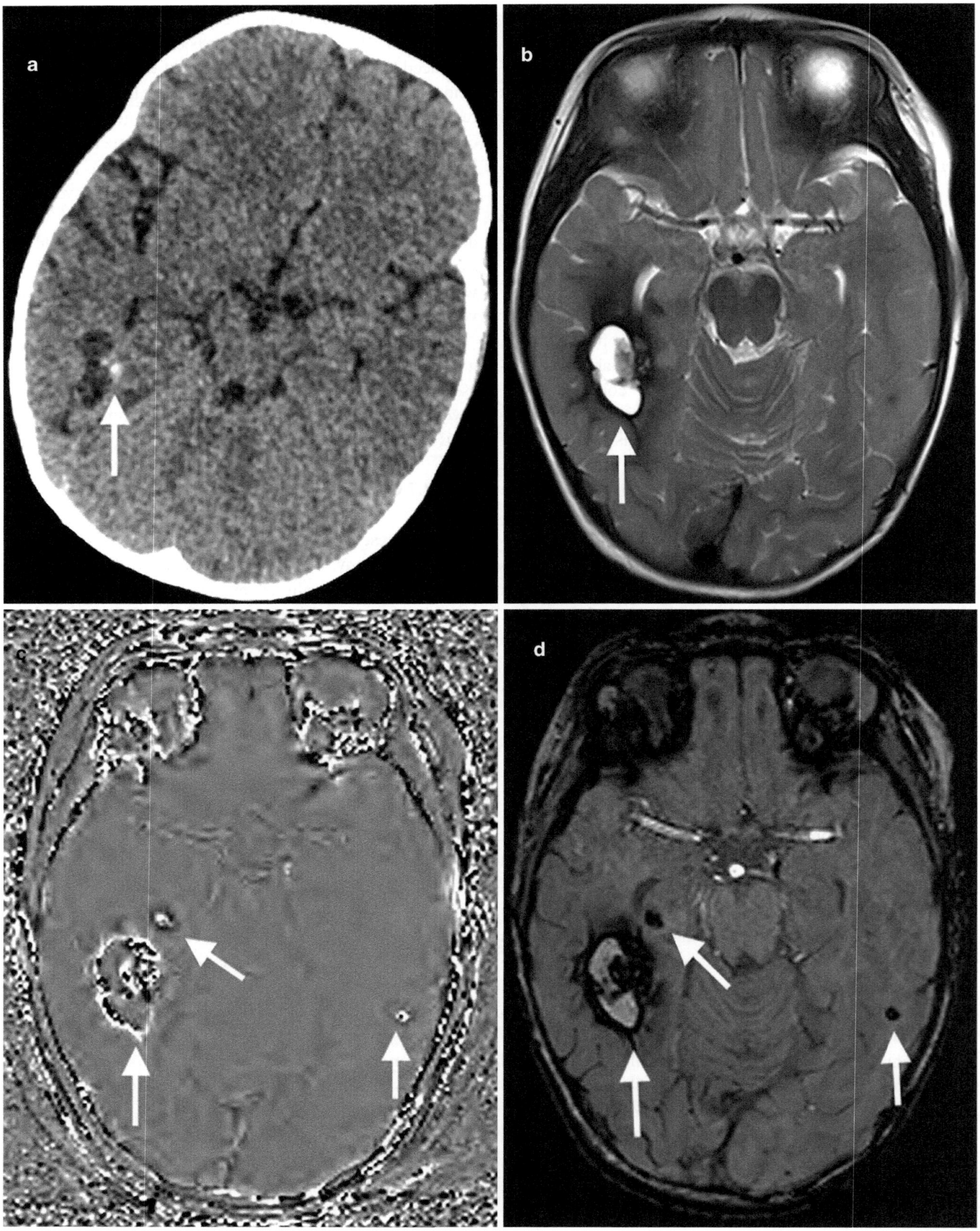

Fig. 4.9 Cavernous malformation

tion of 3 genes CCM1, CCM2, and CCM3. Sporadic CMs are rare, present as a single lesion, usually asymptomatic, and may be related to DVA [30].

CMs are vascular spaces lined by a single layer of endothelin without intervening brain parenchymal tissue within them. There is low pressure and slow flow of blood within the lesion, which leads to thrombus formation, followed by its organization, and this occurs in a repetitive manner. These characteristics are roughly visualized as a typical "mulberry appearance." There is insufficiency of the tight and adhesive connections of the endothelial cells, leading to leakage and blood–brain barrier dysfunction [31]. CMs can have different presentations depending on the location of the lesion. They can be supratentorial, which affects the cerebral cortex, and infratentorial, affecting the cerebellum or the brainstem; however, most of them are supratentorial lesions. When these lesions become symptomatic, a series of clinical manifestations may appear, including seizures, bleeding, headaches, and focal neurological deficits. Supratentorial lesions have been found to present more commonly with seizures, whereas infratentorial malformations are manifested as focal neurological deficits [32].

CT scans can detect lesions that are complicated by hemorrhage or calcification, but lack the sensitivity and specificity to detect smaller lesions; hence, it is not the main way to diagnose these lesions. Features on MRI are highly characteristic and diagnostic for CMs. A classification system was proposed by Zabramski et al. [33] with four different categories based on spin echo and GRE features and histopathologic correlation. The characteristics of Type I lesions are a hyperintense core on T1WI and a hypo- or hyperintense core on T2WI depending on the intracellular or extracellular stage of methemoglobin, and are intended to reflect CMs complicated by subacute hemorrhages. The characteristics of Type II lesions are features that are now commonly ascribed in the literature as being pathognomonic of the MRI features of CMs, and entail a mesh core with high and low T2 signal intensity with a surrounding low signal ring, which are considered pathologically related to ongoing thrombosis and hemorrhages of different ages. Type III lesions are characterized by noticeable hypointensity on T2WI and magnification of size of the hypointensity on GRE, with iso- or hypointensity seen on T1WI, and aims to reflect chronic hemorrhage with hemosiderin remaining in and around the lesion. Type IV lesions are not yet known, and are poorly visualized on traditional spin echo sequences. They appear as small punctate hypointense lesions on GRE, which are thought to reflect small hemosiderin deposits in either minute CMs or perhaps capillary telangiectasias. Due to its high sensitivity to deoxyhemoglobin and iron content, SWI is more precise in detecting vascular malformations. This is the only imaging method that can detect capillary telangiectasias and cavernomas that are nonhemorrhagic. It has not been proven superior to T2/GRE MRI although it can detect multifocal familial CMs.

Case 4.8 Arteriovenous Malformation (AVM)

Clinical Presentation

A 6-year-old boy presented to the pediatric clinic for paroxysmal dysesthesia.

Imaging Findings

A. Axial T1-weighted image demonstrates the "honeycomb" flow voids in the right parietal lobe (red arrow) and punctate high signal considered as hemorrhage (Fig. 4.10a).

B-D. Axial T2-weighted image, T2-FLAIR image and DWI demonstrate the "honeycomb" flow voids (red arrows) and drainage vein (white arrow) (Fig. 4.10b–d).

Discussion

Brain arteriovenous malformations (AVMs) were a tangle of dysplastic blood vessels in which the feeding arteries are directly connected to a venous drainage network with no interposed capillary system [34]. AVMs are the most common type of vascular malformations and the etiology and natural history are unclear [34], which have been regarded as congenital lesions that resulted from errors in embryonic vascular morphogenesis.

Brain AVMs are usually found in young adults aged between 20 and 40 years. Headache with hemorrhage, seizure, and focal neurologic deficit are the most common symptoms. The overall prevalence of AVM in children is estimated to be approximately 1–3 per million, but hemorrhagic presentation is disproportionately more frequent than that in adults.

Angioarchitecture features, including deep venous drainage pattern or deep AVMs location, venous ectasia, or stenosis, have been related to a higher risk of hemorrhage early in life [35]. Different from adults, brain AVMs in neonates and infants are rare, and the manifestations were arteriovenous fistulas with no intervening vascular network or nidus which can easily be detected by MRI and magnetic resonance angiography (MRA) [36]. CT and CT angiography are needed when hemorrhage is suspected and an accurate bleeding source needs to be found. Digital subtraction angiography (DSA) is not typically performed unless endovascular treatment or surgery is needed. In children and young adults, true AVMs with arteriovenous connection through an abnormal vascular network appear in addition to the arteriovenous fistulas.

MRI is the imaging modality of choice to screen or electively investigate the presence of arteriovenous malformations. In conventional T1WI sequence, signal varies with flow rate, direction, presence/age of hemorrhage. Both in T1WI and in T2WI, the low signal intensity of "honeycomb" flow voids can be seen. Perinidal gliosis is characterized by an increased signal on T2-weighted and fluid-attenuated inversion recovery (T2 FLAIR) imaging. If hemorrhage is present, T_2* GRE shows "blooming" sign. Post-contrast injection demonstrates strong enhancement of nidus as well

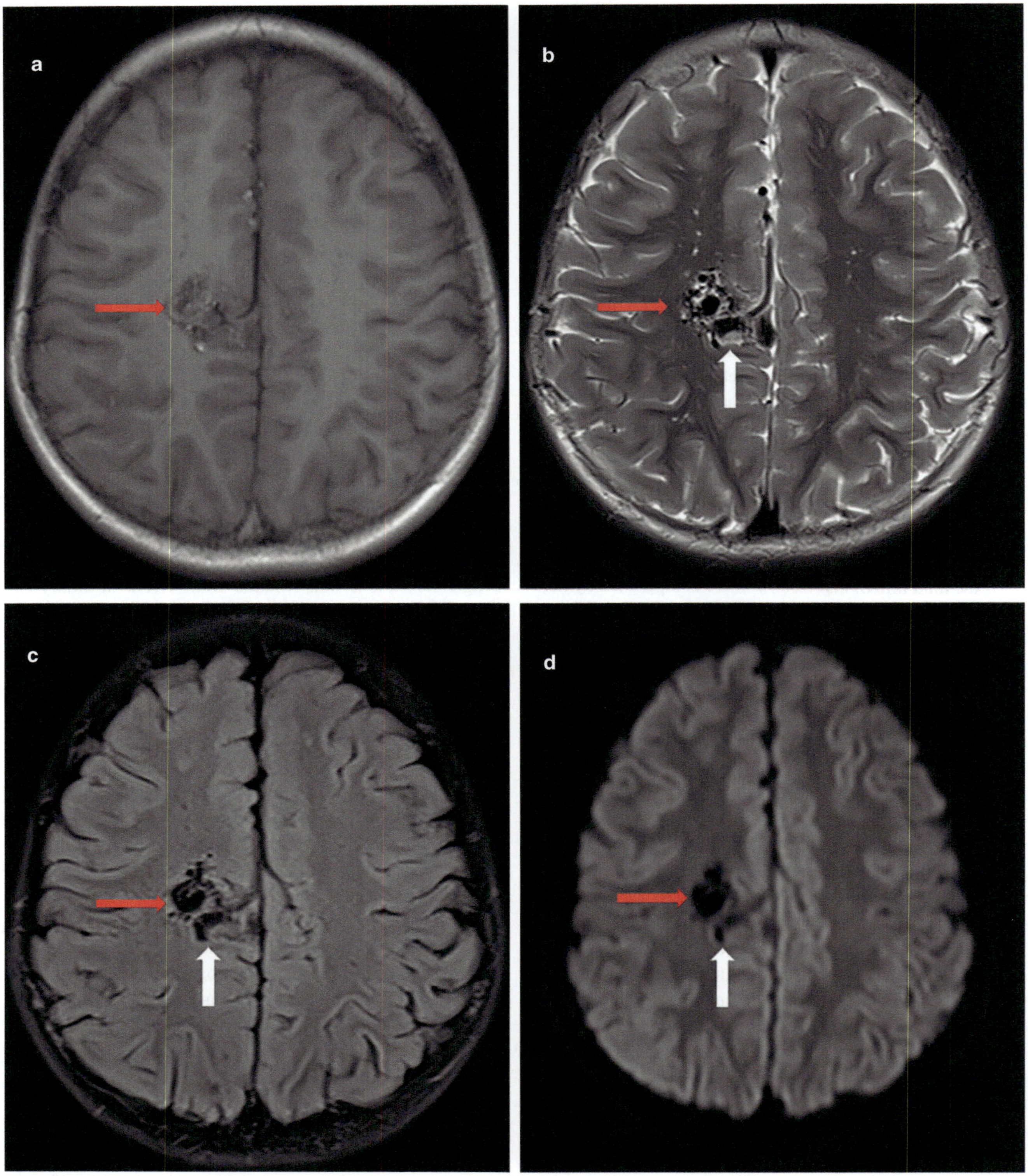

Fig. 4.10 Arteriovenous malformation

as draining veins. MRA can show varying degrees of dilatation of the arterial feeders as well as draining veins but does not depict detailed angioarchitecture.

Brain AVMs were classified into four types according to Spetzler–Martin (SM) grading system which is clinically useful because of its simplicity and practicability. Patients with low-grade AVMs (SM Grades I and II) usually have low morbidity rates, and high-grade AVMs (SM Grades IV and V) are associated with high morbidity rates [37].

Grade III AVMs were classified into the four subtypes according to Lawton's modified SM grading scale as follows: Grade III—(S1V1E1), Grade III (S2V1E0), Grade III+ (S2V0E1), and Grade III* (S3V0E0), where S1 indicates small-sized, 3 cm in diameter; S2, medium-sized, 3–6 cm;

S3, large-sized 6 cm; V0, superficial venous drainage; V1, deep venous drainage; E0, non-eloquent adjacent brain tissue; and E1, eloquent adjacent brain tissue [38].

The disease needs to be differentiated from cavernous hemangioma and intracranial aneurysm. On T1WI, cavernous hemangioma shows isointense or slightly hyperintense, and it is obviously hyperintense when bleeding; for T2WI, it is inhomogeneous hyperintense mixed with partial hypointense; both on T1WI and on T2WI, there is a ring-shaped low signal area around the lesion, which is caused by hemosiderin deposition caused by chronic hemorrhage. The lesions can be enhanced. There is no draining vein in the intracranial aneurysm.

Case 4.9 Intracranial Aneurysm

Clinical Presentation

A 3-month-old boy, admitted to the hospital with brain injury syndrome and high muscle tone.

Imaging Findings

A-C. Axial T2-weighted image, T2-FLAIR and DWI demonstrate abnormal airflow signal in the left thalamus and the hindlimb of the internal capsule (arrow). No significant abnormalities were found on T1-weighted image (Fig. 4.11a–c).

D. MRA image demonstrates a saccular aneurysm (Fig. 4.11d).

Discussion

Intracranial aneurysm (IA) in children is rare, accounting for 1–4% of all IA in the general population [39]. Although women are suffering from this disease among adults, boys are more common among children with IA group [40]. It is generally believed that the formation of Intracranial aneurysm is caused by chronic hemodynamic stress in the area of sudden changes in arterial bifurcation or arterial curvature. Some of the risk factors that exist in adults are missing in children, such as hypertension, obesity, high cholesterol, diabetes, alcohol abuse, and smoking. Children's IA may be related to underlying genetic abnormality or defects in arterial tissue development. The incidence of traumatic aneurysms is also higher. There are more dissecting aneurysms before the age of 5 years, while saccular aneurysms are more common in children over 6 years of age [41]. Intracranial aneurysms in childhood are different from adult saccular aneurysms in morphology, including a large number of fusiform shape, giant size, and de novo formation. The size and location of aneurysms in children are different from those in adults. Children's IA is mainly located in the anterior circulation, especially the internal carotid artery (ICA), and the posterior circulation is higher than that of adults (21% vs. less than 5%) [40]. However, some studies have shown that the most common site of intracranial aneurysms is MCA, and the frequency of MCA is significantly higher than that of ICA [42].

Subarachnoid hemorrhage (SAH) is the main clinical presentation of IA in children, accounting for more than 70% of the clinical presentation, followed by headaches, seizures, and focal deficit. SAH occurs in a lower proportion of children compared to adults, with about 80–90% of adults having SAH in IA. A large intracranial aneurysm in a pediatric population causes mass effect and is diagnosed as headache. Seizures in IA patients are also more common in childhood than in adulthood [40]. Some researchers believe that people with a family history of intracranial aneurysms should be screened, but this idea is controversial. Generally speaking, the incidence of SAH is 6–7/100,000 person/year, 85% of aneurysm rupture factors, and 60% of SAH pediatric patients are known to have IA. Compared with adults, pediatric patients are more tolerant of SAH and its complications and have better clinical outcomes.

The three most commonly used techniques for diagnosing intracranial aneurysms are DSA, MRA, and CTA. DSA is the "gold standard" for diagnosing unruptured IA and formulating treatment plans [43]. CT scanning should be the first diagnostic method to assess the possibility of subarachnoid hemorrhage. CT scans are very sensitive in detecting acute hemorrhage. If the patient receives a scan within 24 h after bleeding, the positive rate can reach 90–95%. As the time of subarachnoid hemorrhage increases, the detection efficiency of CT decreases. If a subarachnoid hemorrhage is strongly suspected clinically, but the CT scan is normal, it can be further verified by a lumbar puncture. CT scanning can provide important clues to the location of the aneurysm rupture based on the distribution of blood. The diagnostic accuracy of CTA for UIA is about 90%, especially for UIA larger than 3 mm in diameter [43]. UIAS on MR scanning can show the effect of flow void. MRI is insensitive in the detection of acute hemorrhage, so its usefulness in the early assessment of subarachnoid hemorrhage is limited. However, it is very useful in confirming subacute or chronic subarachnoid hemorrhage. In recent years, there have been studies on the use of ultra-high resolution MRA to estimate aneurysm wall thickness, combined with contrast-enhanced "black blood" MRI to measure the permeability of contrast agent to aneurysm wall to predict aneurysm status [43]. No other test provides the same detailed information as the DSA in measuring aneurysm size, location, and vascular branching patterns.

Case 4.10 Dural Arteriovenous Fistulae

Clinical Presentation

A month ago, a 3-month-old girl developed an abnormally large head circumference and intermittent vomiting.

Imaging Findings

A. Axial T2-weighted image demonstrates the right transverse sinus was dilated and the left transverse sinus showed nodular dilatation (Fig. 4.12a).

B, D. MRA image demonstrates abnormal tortuous vessels appeared in the cavernous segment of the bilateral

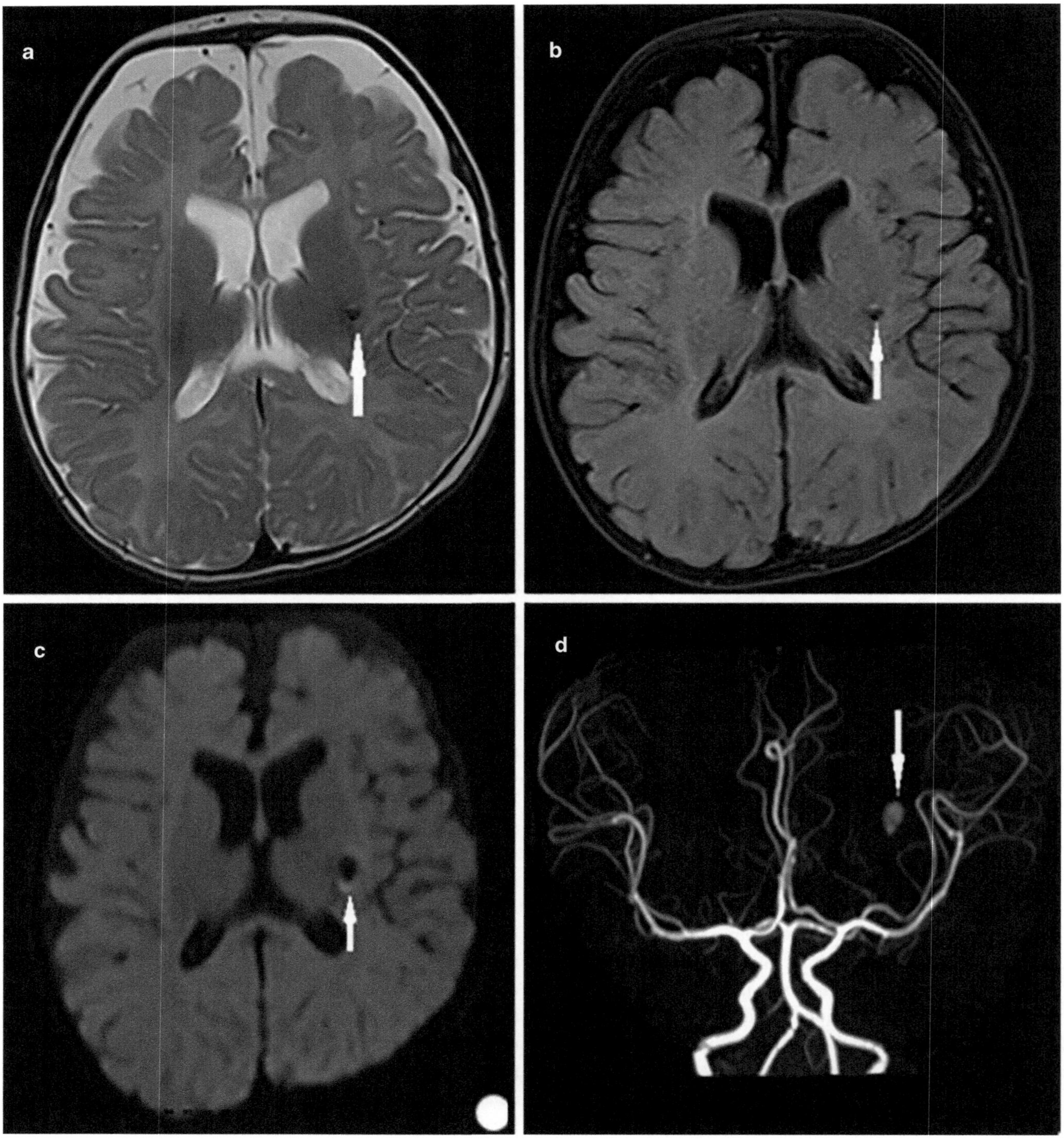

Fig. 4.11 Intracranial aneurysm

internal carotid artery, especially at the left side (Fig. 4.12b, d).

C. MRV image demonstrate the left transverse sinus showed nodular dilatation (Fig. 4.12c).

Discussion

Dural arteriovenous fistulas (DAVF) account for about 10% of all intracranial shunts in children [44]. It is a rare vascular lesion of the CNS with significant morbidity and mortality [45]. DAVF is a direct arteriovenous connection within the dura to drain into the dural sinus or pia cortical vein. While these rare lesions may be congenital, some studies suggest many are acquired [44]. Pediatric DAVF are usually caused by excessive growth of venous sinus wall, abnormal development of sigmoid sinus and transverse sinus cavity, and torcular herophili [46]. In children, symptomatic DAVF may present as high-output heart failure, cranial malformation, developmental delay, cognitive impairment, epilepsy, and focal neurological deficits, with or without hemorrhagic venous infarction secondary to venous outlet limitation [45].

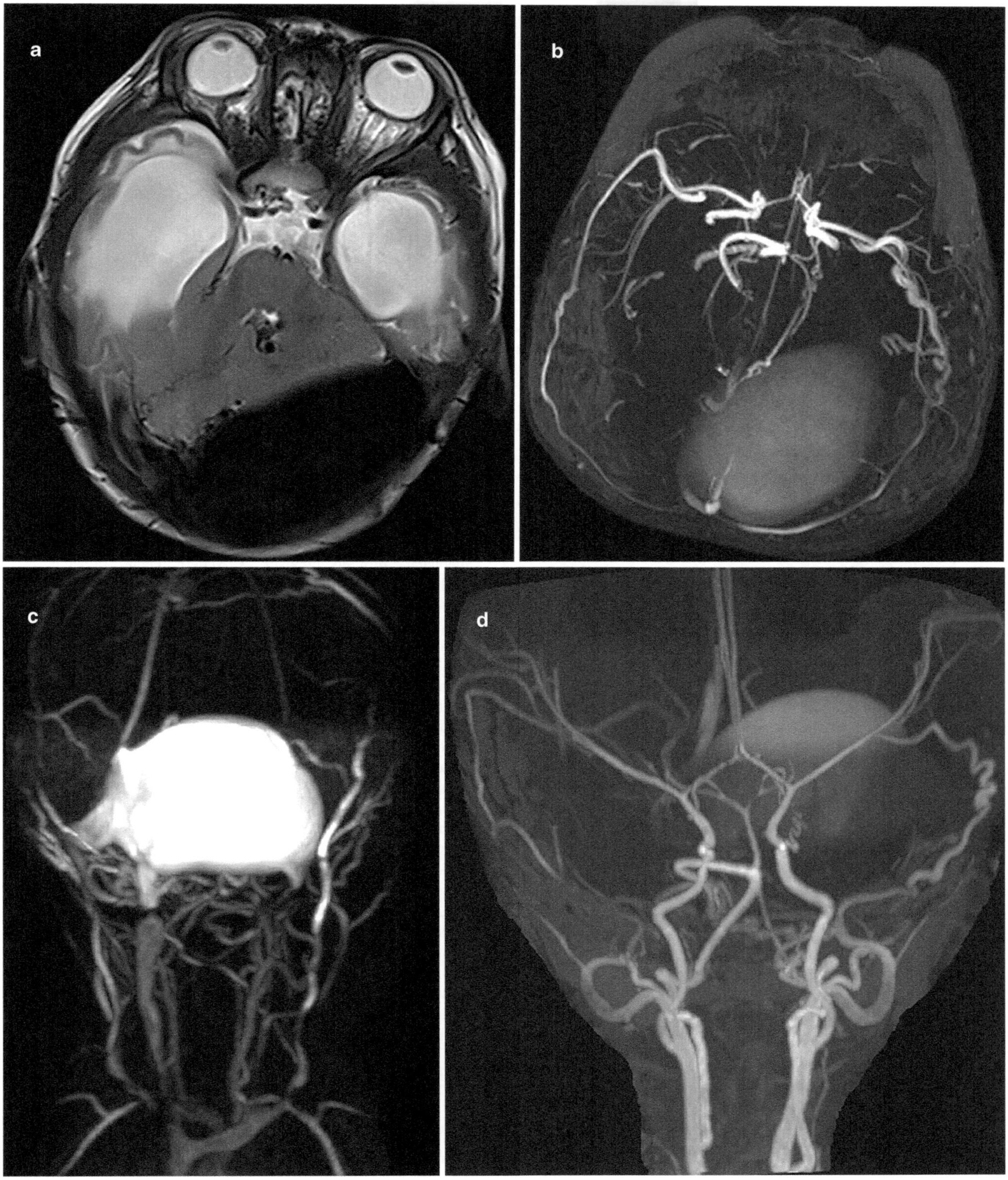

Fig. 4.12 Dural arteriovenous fistulae

Pediatric DAVF is divided into three types: dural sinus malformation (DSM), infantile DAVF, and adult-type DAVF [46]. At present, the most commonly used method in clinical practice is the classification by drainage vein proposed by Cognard et al.

Cognard Classification: I: Venous drainage into dural sinus with normal antegrade flow.IIa: Venous drainage into dural sinus with retrograde flow.IIb: Venous drainage into dural sinus with normal antegrade flow and CVD.IIa 1 b: Venous drainage into dural sinus with retrograde flow and

CVD.III: Venous drainage directly into a subarachnoid vein (CVD only).IV: Venous drainage directly into subarachnoid vein with venous ectasia.V: Venous drainage directly into spinal perimedullary vein [47].

Imaging findings of DVAF:

Cranial CT scans and contrast-enhanced scans can reveal some secondary changes in DAVF. The most common manifestations are hemorrhage, including subarachnoid hemorrhage and cerebral hemorrhage, as well as subdural hematomas. Contrast-enhanced scan showed tubular, nodular, and patchlike contrast enhancement, as well as decreased white matter density, venous sinus thrombosis, and hydrocephalus. CTA can show abnormally thickened arteries, dilated veins, and venous sinuses, but it cannot show fistulas and small supplying arteries, and it cannot determine the direction of blood flow and the situation of blood flow. Therefore, it cannot play a role in angiographic classification diagnosis and guiding treatment [48].

MRI plain scan showed a large number of vascular emptiness phenomenon, severe cerebral cortical venous earthworm extensive tortuosity. MRA can show abnormally thickened and tortuous vessels and can clearly show the fistula. MRV is also helpful in the diagnosis of venous sinus thrombosis [48].

Selective angiography is currently the gold standard for the diagnosis of DAVF. (1) Selective internal carotid and vertebral angiography: to exclude intracerebral arteriovenous malformations and to confirm whether meningeal branches originating from these arteries participate in blood supply. (2) Superselective angiography of the external carotid artery: show the supplying artery of the meninges, look for the best treatment route, sometimes after the main supplying artery embolization, the secondary supplying artery can appear. (3) To study the affected drainage vein, the direction of drainage, and the disorder of cerebral circulation [48].

The difference between DAVF and intracerebral arteriovenous malformations is as follows: (1) The blood supply artery is from meningeal artery (mainly external carotid artery) rather than intracerebral artery; (2) Abnormal blood vessels are not in the brain, but in the dura mater, so it is arteriovenous malformation outside the brain; (3) Due to the increased venous sinus pressure, cerebral veins are secondary to congestion and dilation, so there is no "stealing blood." In conclusion, DSA can clearly show the supplying artery, draining vein, and lesion site of DAVF, which is the gold standard for diagnosis [48].

References

1. Kobayashi Y, Yahikozawa H, Takamatsu R, et al. Left upper lung lobectomy is an embolic risk factor for cerebral infarction. J Stroke Cerebrovasc Dis. 2017;26(9):e177–9.
2. Arboix A, Alioc J. Cardioembolic stroke: clinical features, specific cardiac disorders and prognosis. Curr Cardiol Rev. 2010;6(3):150–61.
3. May AA, de Elizabeth KV, Irving RJ, et al. Atrial standstill presenting as cerebral infarction in a 7-year-old girl. Sage Open Med Case Rep. 2019;7:2050313X19827735.
4. Fang Y, Junliang H. Imaging features of cardiogenic cerebral infarction. Chin J Stroke. 2014;9(7):596–9.
5. Pauley R, Mercier E, Kumar A, Trescher W, Mainali G. Infant stroke associated with left atrial thrombus and supraventricular tachycardia. Child Neurol Open. 2021;8:2329048X21995296.
6. Wintermark M, Hills N, DeVeber G, Barkovich A, Bernard T, Friedman N, Mackay M, Kirton A, Zhu G, Leiva-Salinas C, et al. Clinical and imaging characteristics of arteriopathy subtypes in children with arterial ischemic stroke: results of the VIPS study. AJNR Am J Neuroradiol. 2017;38(11):2172–9.
7. Kaseka M, Slim M, Muthusami P, Dirks P, Westmacott R, Kassner A, Bhathal I, Williams S, Shroff M, Logan W, et al. Distinct clinical and radiographic phenotypes in pediatric patients with moyamoya. Pediatr Neurol. 2021;120:18–26.
8. Boulouis G, Hak J, Kerleroux B, Benichi S, Stricker S, Gariel F, Alias Q, Bourgeois M, Meyer P, Kossorotoff M, et al. Hemorrhage expansion after pediatric intracerebral hemorrhage. Stroke. 2021;52(2):588–94.
9. Bavle A, Srinivasan A, Choudhry F, Anderson M, Confer M, Simpson H, Gavula T, Thompson J, Clifton S, Gross N, et al. Systematic review of the incidence and risk factors for cerebral vasculopathy and stroke after cranial proton and photon radiation for childhood brain tumors. Neurooncol Pract. 2021;8(1):31–9.
10. Sirachainan N, et al. Incidences, risk factors and outcomes of neonatal thromboembolism. J Matern Fetal Neonatal Med. 2018;31(3):347–51.
11. Saracco P, Bagna R, Gentilomo C, et al. Clinical data of neonatal systemic thrombosis. J Pediatr. 2016;171:60–66.e1.
12. Kalita J, et al. Predictors and outcome of status epilepticus in cerebral venous thrombosis. J Neurol. 2018;266(2):417–25.
13. Fan Y, et al. Chinese Stroke Association guidelines for clinical management of cerebrovascular disorders: executive summary and 2019 update of clinical management of cerebral venous sinus thrombosis. Stroke Vasc Neurol. 2020;5(2):152–8.
14. Dlamini N, Muthusami P, Amlie-Lefond C. Childhood moyamoya: looking back to the future. Pediatr Neurol. 2019;91:11–9. https://doi.org/10.1016/j.pediatrneurol.2018.10.006.
15. Shang S, Zhou D, Ya J, et al. Progress in moyamoya disease. Neurosurg Rev. 2018; https://doi.org/10.1007/s10143-018-0994-5.
16. Piao J, Wu W, Yang Z, et al. Research progress of moyamoya disease in children. Int J Med Sci. 2015;12(7):566–75. https://doi.org/10.7150/ijms.11719.
17. Zhang H, Zheng L, Feng L. Epidemiology, diagnosis and treatment of moyamoya disease. Exp Ther Med. 2019;17(3):1977–84. https://doi.org/10.3892/etm.2019.7198.
18. Mathew AJ, Goel R, Kumar S, et al. Childhood-onset Takayasu arteritis: an update. Int J Rheum Dis. 2016;19(2):16–26.
19. Dejaco C, Ramiro S, Duftner C, et al. EULAR recommendations for the use of imaging in large vessel vasculitis in clinical practice. Ann Rheum Dis. 2018;77(5):636–43.
20. Society for Maternal-Fetal Medicine, Monteagudo A. Vein of galen aneurysmal malformation. Am J Obstet Gynecol. 2020;223(6):B27–9.
21. Karl K, Heling KS, Chaoui R. Ultrasound of the fetal veins part 3: the fetal intracerebral venous system. Ultraschall Med. 2016;37:6–26.
22. Alvarez H, et al. Vein of galen aneurysmal malformations. Neuroimaging Clin N Am. 2007;17(2):189–206.
23. Recinos PF, Rahmathulla G, Pearl M, et al. Vein of Galen malformations:epidemiology, clinical presentations, management. Neurosurg Clin N Am. 2012;23:165–77.
24. Gailloud P, et al. Diagnosis and management of vein of galen aneurysmal malformations. J Perinatol. 2005;25(8):542–51.
25. Aoki R, Srivatanakul K. Developmental venous anomaly: benign or not benign. Neurol Med Chir (Tokyo). 2016;56:534–43.

26. Marzouk O, Marzouk S, Liyanage SH, Grunwald IQ. Cerebellar developmental venous anomaly with associated cavernoma causing a hemorrhage—a rare occurrence. Radiol Case Rep. 2021;16:1463–8.
27. Mooney MA, Zabramski JM. Developmental venous anomalies. Handb Clin Neurol. 2017;143:279–82.
28. Brzegowy K, Kowalska N, Solewski B, Musial A, Kasprzycki T, Herman-Sucharska I, Walocha JA. Prevalence and anatomical characteristics of developmental venous anomalies: an MRI study. Neuroradiology. 2020;63(7):1001–8.
29. Idiculla PS, Gurala D, Philipose J, Rajdev K, Patibandla P. Cerebral cavernous malformations, developmental venous anomaly, and its coexistence: a review. Eur Neurol. 2020;83:360–8.
30. Idiculla PS, Gurala D, Philipose J, et al. Cerebral cavernous malformations, developmental venous anomaly, and its coexistence: a review. Eur Neurol. 2020;83(4):360–8.
31. Spiegler S, Rath M, Paperlein C, et al. Cerebral cavernous malformations: an update on prevalence, molecular genetic analyses, and genetic counselling. Mol Syndromol. 2018;9(2):60.
32. Whitehead MT, Cardenas AM, Corey AS, et al. ACR appropriateness criteria® headache. J Am Coll Radiol. 2019;16(11):S364–77.
33. Zabramski JM, Wascher TM, Spetzler RF, et al. The natural history of familial cavernous malformations: results of an ongoing study. J Neurosurg. 1994;80(3):422–32.
34. Rousseau PN, Piana RL, Chai XJ, et al. Brain functional organization and structure in patients with arteriovenous malformations. Neuroradiology. 2019;61(9):1047–54.
35. Hetts SW, Cooke DL, Nelson J, et al. Influence of patient age on angioarchitecture of brain arteriovenous malformations. AJNR Am J Neuroradiol. 2014;35(7):1376–80.
36. Lawton MT, Rutledge WC, Kim H, et al. Brain arteriovenous malformations. Nat Rev Dis Primers. 2015;1:15008.
37. Jeon HJ, Park KY, Kim SY, et al. Surgical outcomes after classifying Grade III arteriovenous malformations according to Lawton's modified Spetzler-Martin grading system. Clin Neurol Neurosurg. 2014;124:72–80.
38. Lawton MT. Spetzler-Martin Grade III arteriovenous malformations: surgical results and a modification of the grading scale. Neurosurgery. 2003;52(4):740–8. discussion 748-9
39. Kim M, Lee HS, Lee S, et al. Pediatric intracranial aneurysms: favorable outcomes despite rareness and complexity. World Neurosurg. 2019;125:1203–16.
40. Garrido E, Metayer T, Borha A, et al. Intracranial aneurysms in pediatric population: a two-center audit. Childs Nerv Syst. 2021;37(8):2567–75.
41. Gemmete JJ, Toma AK, Davagnanam I, et al. Pediatric cerebral aneurysms. Neuroimaging Clin N Am. 2013;23(4):771–9.
42. Chen R, Zhang S, You C, et al. Pediatric intracranial aneurysms: changes from previous studies. Childs Nerv Syst. 2018;34(9):1697–704.
43. Turan N, Heider RA, Roy AK, et al. Current perspectives in imaging modalities for the assessment of unruptured intracranial aneurysms: a comparative analysis and review. World Neurosurg. 2018;113:280–92.
44. Hetts SW, Moftakhar P, Maluste N, Fullerton HJ, Cooke DL, Amans MR, Dowd CF, Higashida RT, Halbach VV. Pediatric intracranial dural arteriovenous fistulas: age-related differences in clinical features, angioarchitecture, and treatment outcomes. J Neurosurg Pediatrics. 2016;18:602–10.
45. Walcott BP, Smith ER, Michael Scott R, Orbach DB. Dural arteriovenous fistulae in pediatric patients:associated conditions and treatment outcomes. J Neurointerventional Surg. 2013;5:6–9.
46. Lv X, Jiang C, Wang J. Pediatric intracranial arteriovenous shunts: advances in diagnosis and treatment. Eur J Paediatr Neurol. 2020;25:29–39.
47. Serulle Y, Miller TR, Gandhi D. Dural arteriovenous fistulae: imaging and management. Neuroimaging Clin N Am. 2016;26:247–58.
48. Zhou X, Wang J, Jianghe Kang CT. MRI and DSA imaging characteristics of dural arteriovenous fistula. China For Med Treat. 2020;17:192–5.

5 Metabolic Encephalopathy

Wangchun Dai, Bin Ai, Wen He, Zhenqing Liu, and Hongsheng Liu

Inherited metabolic encephalopathy refers to a group of diseases that cause the body's biochemical and metabolic disorders due to congenital metabolic defects, resulting in the accumulation of intermediate or bypass metabolites, or the lack of terminal metabolites, thereby causing symptoms and signs of the central nervous system. Although the incidence of a single disease of genetic metabolic encephalopathy is low, the overall incidence is not low, about 1/(2500–5000) [1]. Inherited metabolic encephalopathy often begins in infancy and childhood, and a few are delayed to adulthood. Inherited metabolic encephalopathy covers a wide variety of clinical manifestations, and is currently less than 1/2 of the diseases that can be diagnosed. The diagnosis of genetic metabolic encephalopathy relies on genetic testing, laboratory tests, clinical manifestations, and imaging examinations. MRI is the first and most important imaging method for genetic metabolic encephalopathy. MRI can help narrow the scope of the differential diagnosis of the disease, especially in the early diagnosis of important advantages. Although the imaging manifestations of each genetic metabolic encephalopathy have their own characteristics, most of the diseases show the common feature of symmetrical lesion distribution. Due to limited space, the following discussion will only cover some of the most common genetic metabolic encephalopathies.

W. Dai · B. Ai
Department of Radiology, Guangzhou Women and Children's Medical Center, Guangzhou City, Guangdong, China

W. He · Z. Liu
Division of Diagnostic, Guangzhou Women and Children's Medical Center, Guanzhou, Guangdong, China

H. Liu (✉)
Guangzhou Women and Children's Medical Center, Guangzhou City, Guangdong, China

5.1 Genetic Metabolic Encephalopathy

5.1.1 White Matter

Case 5.1.1.1 X-Linked Adrenoleukodystrophy

Clinical Presentation

A 7-year-old boy appeared mental regression under no obvious predisposing caused 20 days ago. He was distracted and had blank facial expressions. His character was changed, showed irritability. He also had a language barrier, assumed enunciation unclear and salivation. Meanwhile, he walked unstably. Fever and convulsion did not happen. No special disease history or personal history. Both parents are in good health. Specialist examination revealed weakness of all four limbs and muscular tension increased. Pathological reflex was not elicited. The level of plasma very long-chain fatty acid (VLCFA) was increased, C26:0;C26:0/C24:0. Adrenal insufficiency was found, characterized by ACTH increase and blood cortisol decrease.

Imaging Findings

A. Axial T2-weighted image demonstrates demyelinating in bilateral periventricular white matter, and parietal, occipital white matter. Splenium of corpus callosum were involved, including part of bilateral dorsal thalamus, the posterior limb of internal capsule and capsula externa. The arcuate fibers are not involved (Fig. 5.1a).
B. Axial T2-weighted image demonstrates that the corticospinal tracts in the pons and medulla are markedly affected (Fig. 5.1b).
C. Axial T1-weighted enhancement demonstrates no enhancement (Fig. 5.1c).
D. Relatively high Cho, low NAA were observed in 1H-MRS voxel located in the left periventricular white matter (Fig. 5.1d).

Discussion

X-linked Adrenoleukodystrophy is the most common peroxisomal disorder. It belongs to X-linked recessive inheritance. The

H. Liu, X. Zhang (eds.), *Pediatric Neuroimaging*, https://doi.org/10.1007/978-981-16-7928-5_5

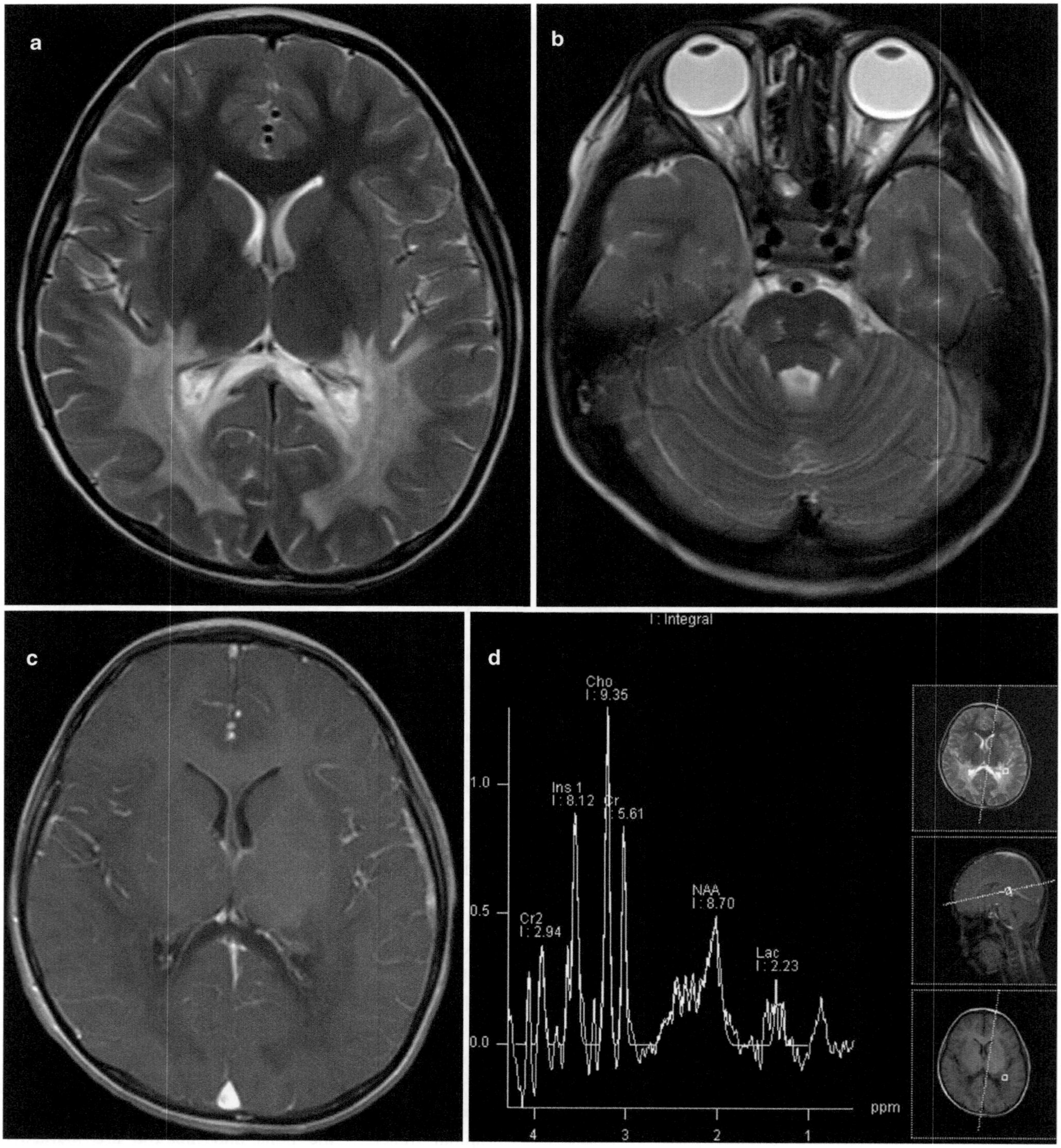

Fig. 5.1 X-linked adrenoleukodystrophy

disease gene is mapped on Xq28. Mutations in the ABCD1 gene affect the function of the encoded protein ALDP, which results in elevated levels of very long-chain fatty acids in plasma and tissues, that accumulate in the white matter of the brain, spinal cord, and adrenal cortex. It is clinically characterized by two main phenotypes: adrenomyeloneuropathy (AMN) and the cerebral demyelination form of X-ALD (cerebral ALD). A total of 35% of boys with ALD developed childhood cerebral ALD (CCALD), the most severe form of the disease [1].

X-ALD is most present in childhood, the patients were almost all men. The pathogenesis of that is undefined. Cognitive deficits at an early stage can lead to a decline in academic performance. As the disease progresses, more overt neurologic deficits become apparent, which include hearing impairment, visual loss, weakness of limbs, hemiplegia, cerebral ataxia, and epilepsy. At this stage, progression is extremely rapid and devastating. Affected boys can lose their ability to understand language and walk within a few weeks [2]. ALD has a poor prognosis and no remission, most died within a few years.

CCALD is characterized by inflammatory demyelination that spreads throughout the supratentorial and infratentorial white matter [3]. In 80% of patients, the initial demyelination lesion is localized in the splenium of the corpus callosum and progresses to involve the adjacent parieto-occipital white matter. A remarkable feature of imaging findings on CCALD is the lesion developed posterior to anterior gradually. Lesions were symmetrically localized in parieto-occipital white matter initially, progresses to involve temple and frontal lobe, and finally involve the centrum semiovale. They develop cerebral demyelination visible on brain MRI, as abnormal hypersignal of white matter on T2WI and T2WI-FLAIR, hyposignal of white matter on T1WI. In the peripheral area, no significant change was seen, and it shows an equal signal on T1WI. So, the scope of the lesions shown on T2WI is greater than T1WI. There is a significant correlation between enhancement and progression of disease. No enhancement was seen in the inactive stage. And circular enhancement can be seen in the active stage for the infiltration of inflammatory cells and destruction of the blood–brain barrier, it assumes that pathogenetic condition deteriorates further. The corticospinal tract of the ponsoblongata always was involved. This is the specific sign of the diagnosis of CCALD. MR spectroscopy shows a decrease of NAA and an increase of Cho in the demyelination lesions. The ratio of NAA/Cr and NAA/Cho are decreased, and Cho/Cr is increased. If the ratio of NAA/Cho is lower than five, it is strongly suggested that the area may be involved in a short time [4].

Case 5.1.1.2 Metachromatic Leukodystrophy (MLD)

Clinical Presentation

Patient, female, 8 years old, memory loss, learning disability for 6 months. At the same time, there are symptoms of motor function regression, such as slow walking and uncoordinated movements.

Imaging Findings

A. The axial T2WI showed periventricular symmetryobvious hyperintensity (Fig. 5.2a).
B. The axial T2-FLAIR showed periventricular symmetry-obvious hyperintensity (Fig. 5.2b).
C. The axial T1WI-enhanced images showed no enhancement in the lesion area (Fig. 5.2c).
D. The typical "Leopard skin sign" can be seen in the centrum semiovale. Subcortical U-fibers are not affected (Fig. 5.2d).

Discussion

Metachromatic leukodystrophy, MLD, is a common autosomal recessive disorder. Due to the defects of arylsulfatase A (ASA) in lysosomes, brain sulfur lipids cannot be degraded into cerebrosides. And sulfuric acid, a large amount of brain sulfur lipid deposits in tissues and organs, causing extensive demyelination of the white matter of the central nervous system in the brain. The incidence rate is 1/40,000 to 1/100,000 [5]. According to the age of onset and clinical manifestations, MLD is divided into late infantile type (1–2 years old), juvenile type (onset between 3 and 12 years), and adult type (after 16 years of age). Among them, late infantile type account for 50–80%, usually onset from 1 to 2 years old. The main clinical symptoms are gait instability, ataxia, quadriplegia, language disorder, and progressive mental retardation. Patients usually die within 4 months to 4 years.

The imaging features of Metachromatic leukodystrophy are as follows: (1) The white matter symmetry abnormal signal around the bilateral lateral ventricle, T1WI showed a slightly lower signal, and T2WI showed a high signal. Lesions do not involve subcortical white matter in the early onset. The abnormal signs of early cases appear in the anterior horn and/or posterior horn of the lateral ventricle. The lesions are further enlarged, merged into pieces, and developed to the centrum ovale. Finally, the subcortical white matter and cerebellar white matter are involved, and brain atrophy occurs. Most patients follow the order of white matter invading the brain from front to back. Enhanced scans are generally not enhanced. (2) The lesion T2WI of the centrum ovale showed an uneven high signal, and there was a scattered low-signal area in the high-signal area, which was called "leopard pattern." (3) Corpus callosum involvement is another important sign. MLD can involve the carcass early, especially in the knee and/or splenium of the corpus callosum. (4) MR spectroscopy shows reduced *N*-acetyl aspartate (NAA) peaks, increased choline peaks, increased lactate peaks in the affected white matter [6]. (5) Diffusion is restricted in the lesion area, and ADC shows low signal, suggesting cytotoxic edema [6, 7].

MLD needs to be differentiated from other white matter diseases such as adrenal white matter dystrophy (ALD) and Alexander disease. Although ALD also involves the corpus callosum, the enhancement of the white matter lesion area is helpful for identification. Alexander's disease white matter lesions can also be enhanced, and often accompanied by an increase in head circumference, which is helpful for identification.

Case 5.1.1.3 Alexander's Disease

Clinical Presentation

A 7-months-old girl presented to the neurology department for epilepsy and hepatic dysfunction. The laboratory examination discovered the GFAP mutation in gene detection.

Imaging Findings

A. T2WI shows high signal in bilateral semioval center and frontal white matter (Fig. 5.3a).
B. T2WI shows high signal in bilateral semioval center and frontal white matter (Fig. 5.3a).
C. CE-T1WI sequence shows no enhancement in bilateral semioval center and frontal white matter (Fig. 5.3c).

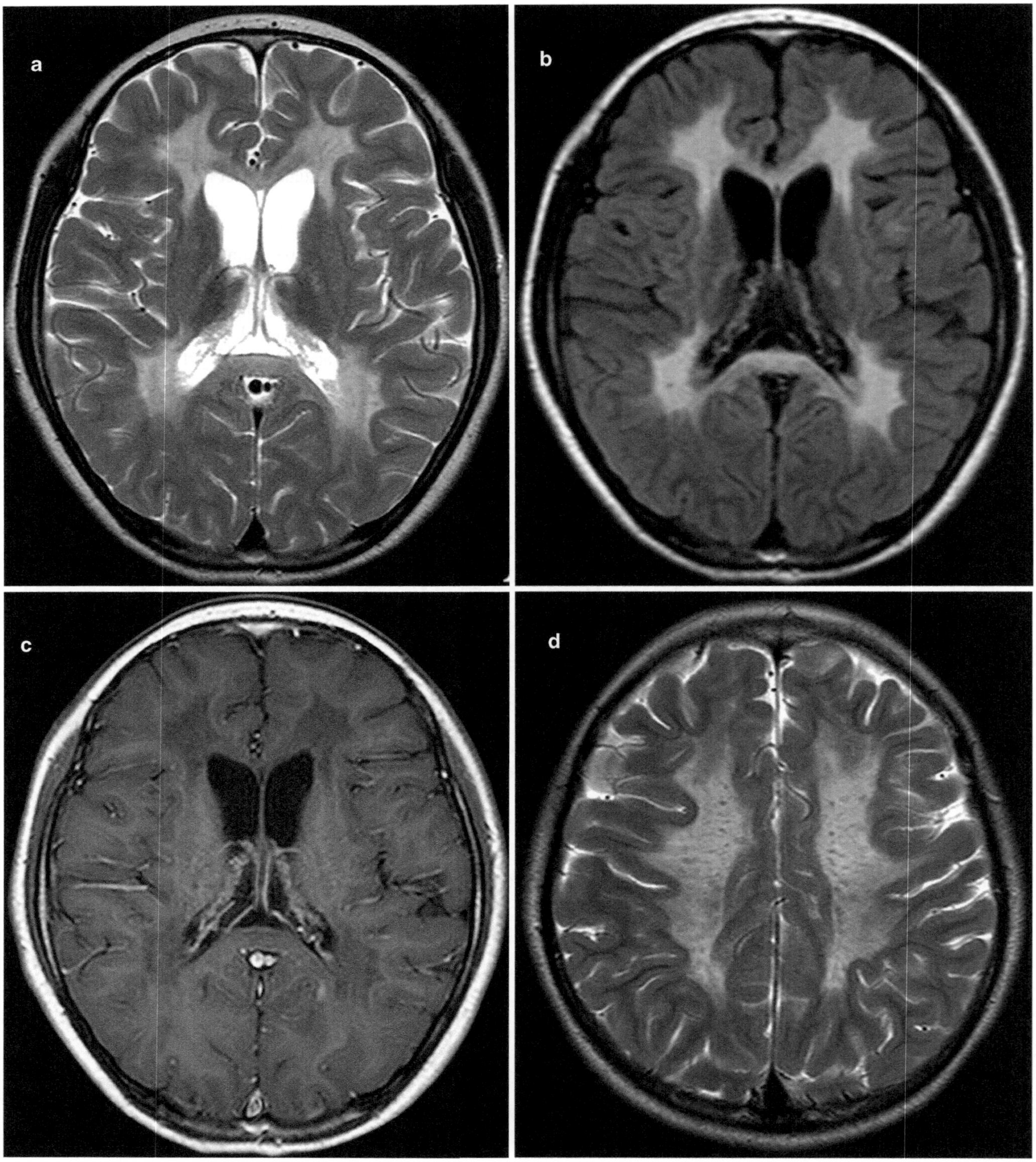

Fig. 5.2 Metachromatic leukodystrophy, MLD

D. T2WI-FLAIR show high signal in bilateral semioval center and frontal white matter (Fig. 5.3d).
E. DWI sequences show low signal in bilateral semioval center and frontal white matter (Fig. 5.3e).
F. ADC sequences show high signal in bilateral semioval center and frontal white matter (Fig. 5.3f).

Discussion

Alexander's Disease is also known as fibrinoid leukodystrophy, is a rare progressive degenerative disease of the central nervous system caused by astrocytic dysfunction.

Alexander's Disease is a retrogression caused by the deposition of Rosenthal fibers (RF) in the brain due to

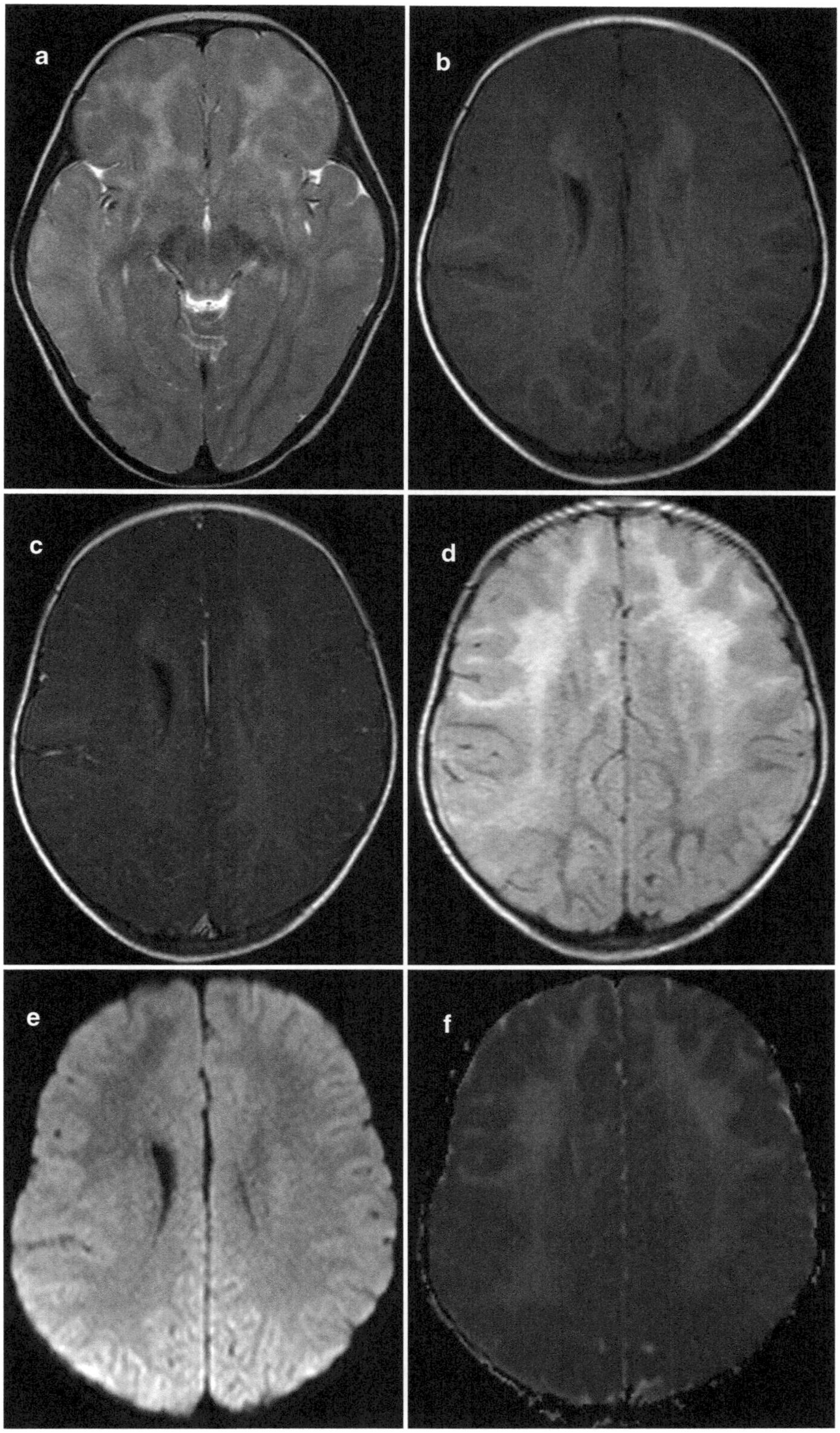

Fig. 5.3 Alexander's disease

abnormal astrocyte function. More RF could be found in the white matter, especially in basal ganglia, thalamus, hypothalamus, and frontal lobe. Recently, almost all patients have shown GFAP mutations encoding glial fibrillary acidic protein, which is the main intermediate filament protein in astrocytes. But the studies have not discovered other genetic causes. Although previous studies have a family history with the genetic homogeneity, there are a broad range of disease expression without exact mechanisms of mutations [8].

According to the age of onset and clinical manifestations, it can be divided into infantile type, juvenile type, and adult type. The infantile type is the most common type, often onset at 2 years old. The infantile type mainly characterized by symptoms of macrocephaly, psychomotor retardation, progressive central nervous system dysfunction, epilepsy, and died before pre-teen. The juvenile type often began at 4–14 years old. This type mainly manifested as rare seizures and macrocephaly, relatively slow development, severe brain stem lesions, and bulbar paralysis. The adult type is rare and characterized by pyramidal signs, cerebellar signs and systemic myoclonus. A few patients have autonomic dysfunction, short nuchal, and kyphosis appearance.

Alexander's Disease is characterized by abnormal symmetric signal area in white matter of cerebral hemisphere diffusely, which frontal lobe and periventricular white matter were mostly involved, together with basal ganglia, thalamus, and brainstem white matter. T1WI sequence shows low signal, T2WI and T2WI-FLAIR sequences show high signal, and enhancement after administration of contrast in the early disease. The Brain atrophy, softening focus, and frontal angle and body of lateral ventriculomegaly can be often found in the disease. Meanwhile, MRS reveals abnormal levels of the Lac peak and decreased NAA peak.

The disease needs to be differentiated from Canavan disease. Canavan disease is characterized by symmetrical abnormal signal area in white matter of cerebral hemisphere diffusely, which subcortical white matter was mostly involved, and the boundary between the gray matter (GM) and white matter (WM) was blurring, even involved the deep white matter, and the NAA peak obvious increased on the MRS.

Case 5.1.1.4 Canavan Disease

Clinical Presentation

An 8-months-old girl presented to the neurology department for macrocephaly, psychomotor retardation, and severe hypertonia. The laboratory examination show *N*-acetyl aspartate (NAA) in urine. She was full-term normal delivery.

Imaging Findings

A. T2WI shows high signal in the white matter of the cerebral hemisphere showed diffusely symmetrical abnormal signal area.there was no slightly low signal in the anterior limb of internal capsule (IC), posterior limbs of IC, genu of corpus callosum (CC), and the splenium of CC (Fig. 5.4a).
B. T1WI show low signal in the white matter of the cerebral hemisphere showed diffusely symmetrical abnormal signal area.there was no slightly high signal in the anterior limb of internal capsule (IC), posterior limbs of IC, genu of corpus callosum (CC), and the splenium of CC (Fig. 5.4b).
C. T2WI-FLAIR show high signal in the white matter of the cerebral hemisphere showed diffusely symmetrical abnormal signal area.there was no slightly low signal in the anterior limb of internal capsule (IC), posterior limbs of IC, genu of corpus callosum (CC), and the splenium of CC (Fig. 5.4c).
D. T2WI shows high signal in the white matter of the cerebral hemisphere showed diffusely symmetrical abnormal signal area (Fig. 5.4d).
E. T1WI show low signal in the centrum ovale showed diffusely symmetrical abnormal signal area (Fig. 5.4e).
F. T2WI-FLAIR in the centrum ovale showed diffusely symmetrical abnormal signal area (Fig. 5.4f).

Discussion

Canavan Disease is a rare neurodegenerative disease of autosomal recessive inheritance, which is also known as spongiform leukodystrophy. The disease is caused by mutations in the aspartoacylase gene (ASPA), leading to a lack of aspartoacylase activity and increased concentrations of the substrate *N*-acetyl-aspartate (NAA) in the blood, cerebrospinal fluid, and urine. Accumulation of NAA leads to spongiform degeneration of white matter and serious impairment of psychomotor development [9].

Canavan disease leads to brain edema, aberrant myelination, and gross morphological changes in the white matter of cerebral hemisphere diffusely, and its clinical sequelae included macrocephaly, serious cognitive and motor delay, and epilepsy, death usually occurred by the third decade.

The clinical classification of Canavan disease can be divided into neonatal type, infantile type, and adolescent type. The neonatal type, also known as congenital type, is rare and mainly characterized by symptoms of hypomyotonia, poor absorption ability and dysphagia, and death usually within postnatal weeks. The infantile type is the most common type, mainly occurring in Jewish infants. This type is mainly manifested as psychomotor retardation and macrocephaly within postnatal 6 months, often accompanied by optic nerve atrophy and blindness, hypertonia, and spastic paralysis. The clinical symptoms deteriorate progressively and die at young. The onset of juvenile type often began at 5 years old, presenting with progressive mental retardation, motor impairment, decreased vision, and epilepsy. Some children did not have macrocephaly or mental retardation [10].

Canavan disease is characterized by symmetrical abnormal signal area in white matter of cerebral hemisphere diffusely, which subcortical white matter were mostly involved, and the boundary between the gray matter (GM) and white matter (WM) was blurring. T1WI sequence shows low signal, T2WI and T2WI-FLAIR sequences show high signal, and no enhancement after administration of contrast. The characteristic manifestation is that the NAA peak obviously increased, and Cho and Cr peak decreased on the MRS. The early disease is mainly located in subcortical white matter and arcuate fibers. The progressive stage involved deep white matter, such as the internal capsule (IC) and corpus callosum (CC). Other affected sites currently reported include gray matter structures, such as the thalamus, globus pallidum, dentate nucleus, and a few involve the brainstem and spinal

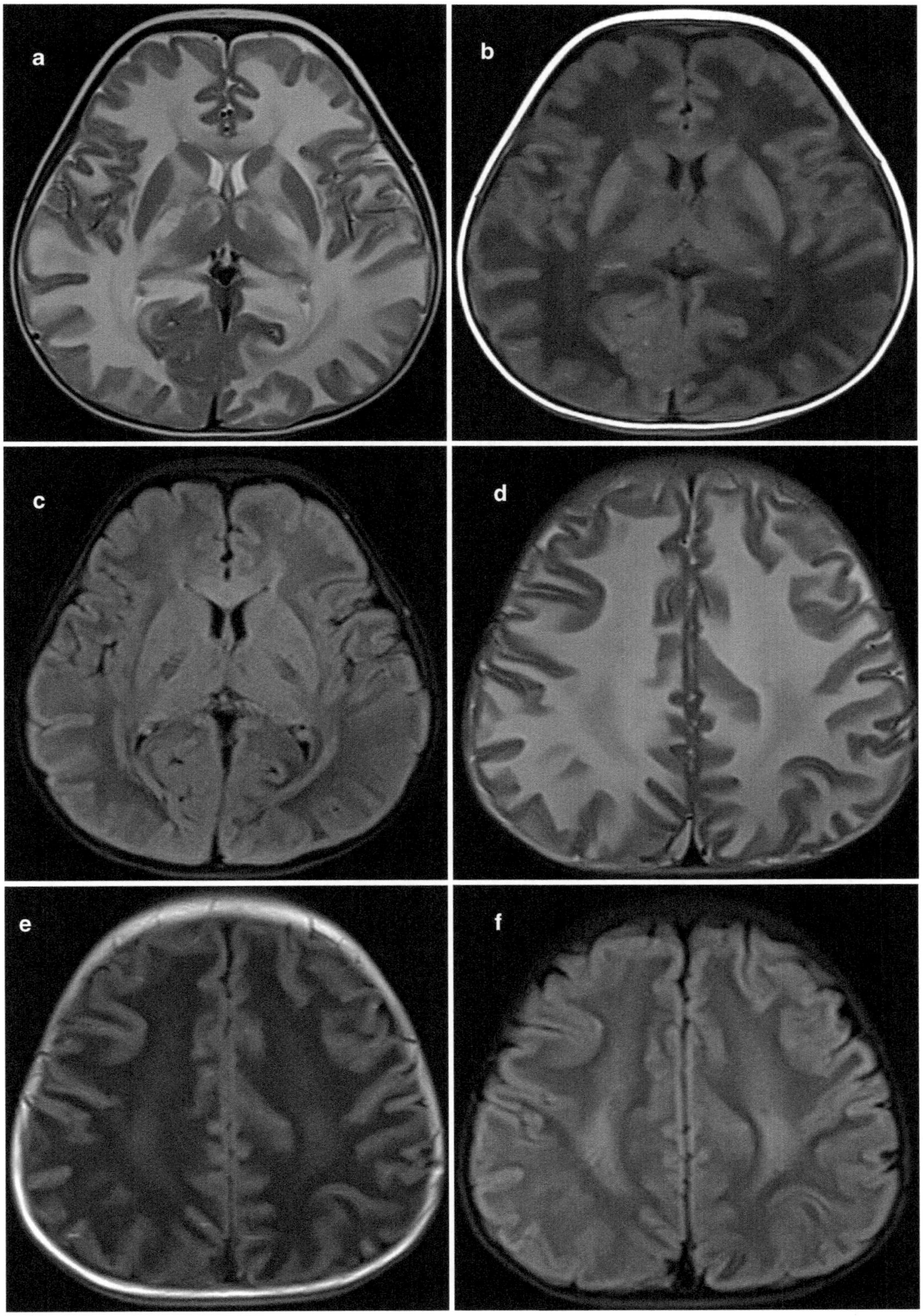

Fig. 5.4 Canavan disease

cord. The late stage is atypical, mild atrophy with macrocephaly, involving all white matter, showing bilateral symmetry and centripetal progression.

The disease needs to be differentiated from Pelizaeus-Merzbacher disease and Alexander's Disease. Pelizaeus-Merzbacher disease is characterized by myelination behind their peers, the same as infantile appearance, and without myelinoclasis. Alexander's Disease is characterized by abnormal signal area in white matter of cerebral hemisphere diffusely, which frontal lobe and periventricular white matter were mostly involved, and the NAA peak obvious decreased on the MRS.

Case 1.1.5 Globoid Cell Leukodystrophy (Krabbe's Disease)

Clinical Presentation

The boy, 3-years old, has a motor function that has gone backward for 6 months. Growth and development are normal within 2 years of age, but from the age of 2 years and a half, running, cycling, and other sports are gradually weakened compared with children of the same age. At present, children have abnormal gait, unclear speech, and visual impairment. No history of seizures or difficulty eating. No family history of genetic diseases.

Imaging Findings

A. Axial T2WI showed symmetry hyperintensity in deep white matter of the parietal and occipital lobes (Fig. 5.5a).
B. Axial T2-FLAIR showed symmetry hyperintensity in deep white matter of the parietal and occipital lobes (Fig. 5.5b).
C. Axial T1WI showed symmetry slightly lower signal in deep white matter of the parietal and occipital lobes (Fig. 5.5c).
D. Coronal T2WI showed the corticospinal tract (arrow) is involved (Fig. 5.5d).

Discussion

The globoid cell leukodystrophy (GLD), also known as Krabbe disease, is an autosomal recessive disorder that affects the central and peripheral nervous systems. Caused by mutations in the galactocerebrosidase (GALC) gene, which accumulates the central nervous system galactocerebroside and sphingosine galactosides, proliferating astrocytes replacing damaged oligodendrocytes and leading to demyelination change. The incidence of this disease is about 1/100,000. The prominent pathological features of GLD are microglia proliferation and peripheral macrophage infiltration into the CNS parenchyma and transformation into highly active multinuclear phagocytic cells, characteristic "spheroid cells." Krabbe disease is more common in infants and young children. It can be divided into four subtypes (early infantile-onset (<6 months) form, late infantile (onset from 7 months to 3 years) form, juvenile (onset from 3 to 8 years). Form, and adult (onset after 9 years) form.). Among them, the early infantile-onset form is the most common. In the early stage, there are clinical symptoms such as irritability, crying, feeding difficulty, muscle tension reduction, and developmental delay. Then, symptoms such as increased muscle tone and hyperreflexia can occur. Followed by infant and adult subtypes, characterized by visual impairment, can be associated with cognitive disorders, dementia, ataxia, and slower progression of the lesion.

MRI is the best image inspection method for GLD. GLD is mainly characterized by abnormal white matter signal, T1WI is slightly lower signal, T2WI and T2WI-FLAIR are high signal changes. However, there are five different manifestations of white matter changes [11]. The first type is a diffuse symmetry distribution of bilateral cerebral hemisphere white matter lesions. The corpus callosum, corticospinal tract, and posterior sac of the internal capsule are involved. The deep white matter and dentate nucleus of the cerebellum are also affected. The second type is mainly caused by white matter involvement in the occipital lobe, accompanied by corticospinal tract and corpus callosum involvement. The cerebellum is not involved. The third is the involvement of only the corticospinal tract. The fourth type is bilateral cerebral hemispheres with white matter scattered in the patch. The fifth brain is normal. The first three types are the most common. Enhanced scanning Most GLD lesions are not enhanced. Some patients can see the Thickening of the Optic nerve. Thickening of the cauda equina roots is another common finding in Krabbe disease [12]. MRS may show reduced *N*-acetyl aspartate and elevation in choline and myoinositol peaks.

CT has limited diagnostic value for Krabbe's disease, mainly showing a decrease in the density of the above lesions. But it can specifically show that the bilateral thalamus, caudate nucleus, corona radiata, posterior limb of the inner capsule, cerebellum, and cerebral cortex are scattered in small calcifications.

At present, there is no specific treatment for Krabbe's disease, mainly supportive and symptomatic treatments. Some patients can undergo hematopoietic stem cell transplantation (HSCT) before neurological symptoms appear.

Case 5.1.1.6 Pelizaeus-Merzbacher Disease

Clinical Presentation

A 1-year-old boy presented to the neurology department for motor retardation. He had been seen gait instability at 4 months old. His little brother has a history of similar motor retardation. He has no history of premature delivery and perinatal asphyxia.

Imaging Findings

A. T2WI shows diffusely symmetrical high signal in centrum ovale, and shows distribution feature alternate with the myelin deletion zone and myelin intact area, which looks like a leopard print (Fig. 5.6a).
B. T1WI shows diffusely symmetrical low signal in centrum ovale (Fig. 5.6b).
C. T2WI shows diffusely symmetrical high signal in the anterior limb and posterior limb of internal capsule and genu of corpus callosum (CC) (Fig. 5.6c).
D. T1WI shows diffusely symmetrical low signal in the anterior limb and posterior limb of internal capsule and genu of corpus callosum (Fig. 5.6d).
E. T2WI shows diffusely symmetrical high signal in white matter area of temporo-occipital region (Fig. 5.6e).
F. T1WI shows diffusely symmetrical low signal in white matter area of temporo-occipital region (Fig. 5.6f).

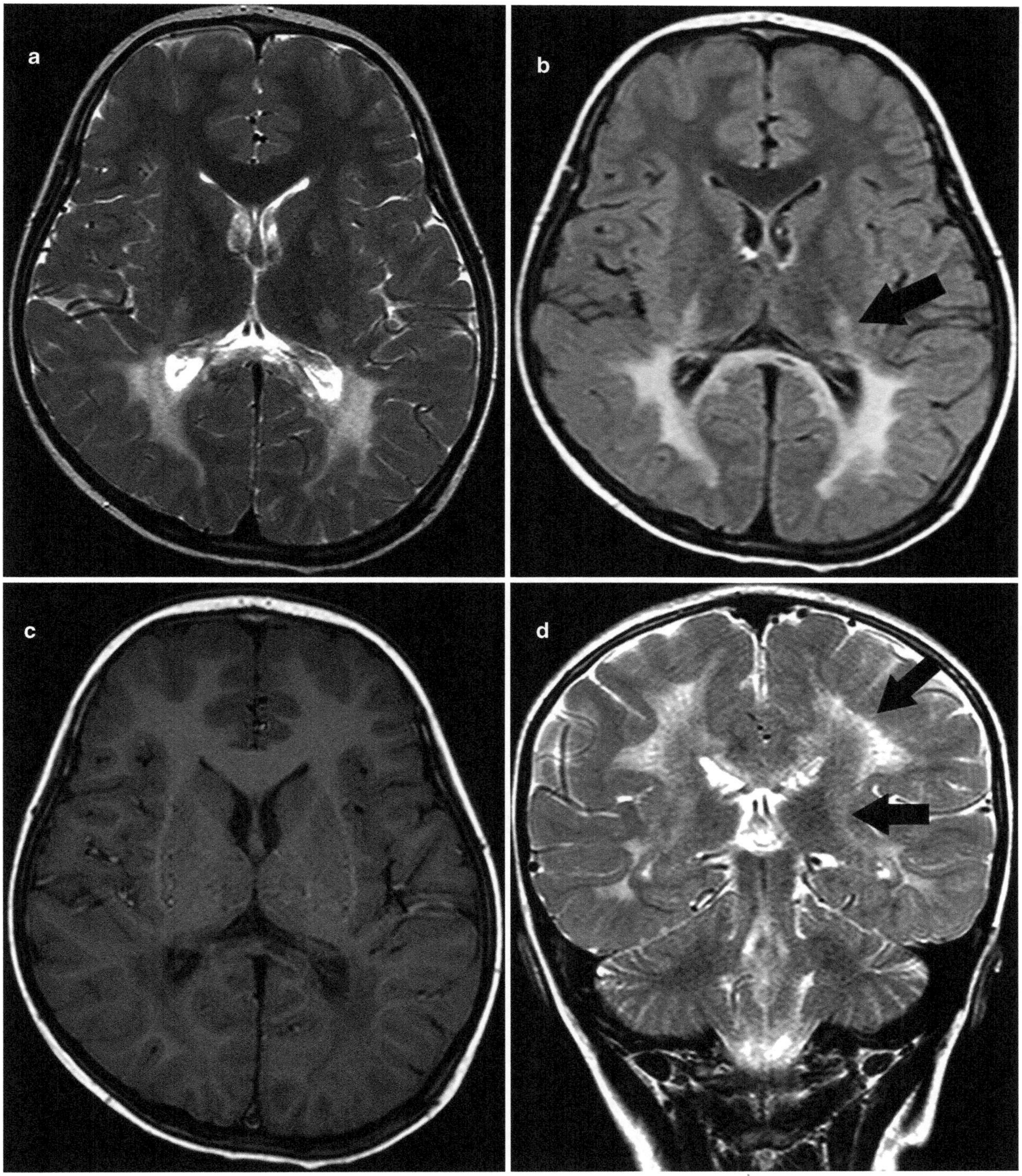

Fig. 5.5 Globoid cell leukodystrophy

Discussion

Pelizaeus-Merzbacher disease is a rare recessive X-linked leukoencephalopathy, which is diagnosed by gene defect in proteolipid protein (PLP) 1 caused by Xq 22.2 [13], leading to dysmyelination.

Whole exome sequencing (WES) discover the possible duplicates of Xq 22.2 contains the PLP and inherited from the mother, and also carried by the younger brother, which is consistent with the characteristics of the disease.

Pelizaeus-Merzbacher disease is divided into four types: classical type, connatal type, transitional type, and adult type [14]. The prognosis of classical type is best, then is transitional type, and connatal type is the worst. The classical type is mainly characterized by symptoms of nystagmus, ataxia, retard of motor development, and often misdiagnosed as cerebral palsy. The connatal type is rare and characterized by severe clinical symptoms, which mainly manifested as extrapyramidal symptoms, pendulum nystagmus, spasm, optic

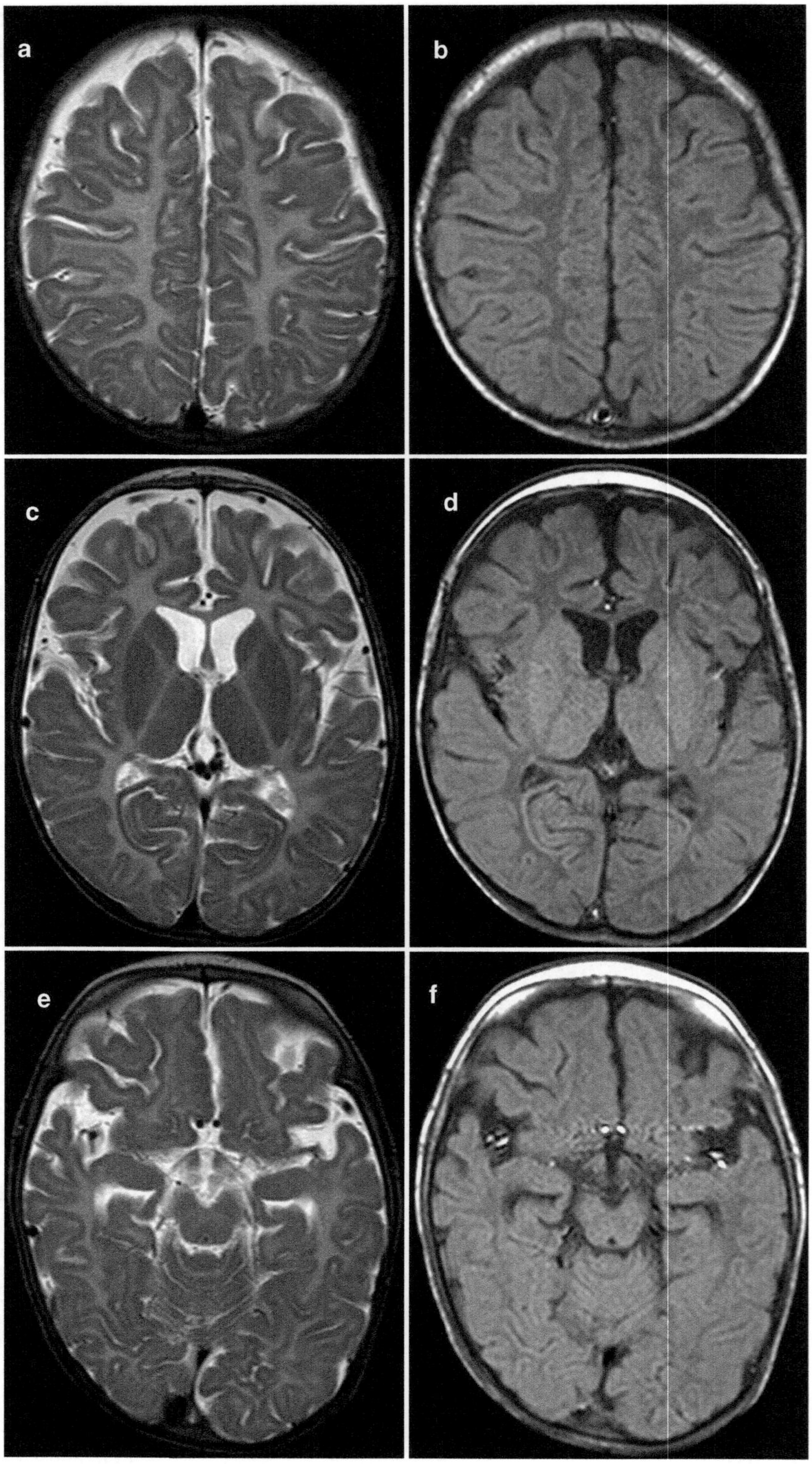

Fig. 5.6 Pelizaeus-Merzbacher disease

atrophy, and even epilepsy. Most patients died in infants and young children.

Pelizaeus-Merzbacher disease has characteristic imaging performance, is characterized by that myelination is poorer than their peers, similar to those seen in newborns. T1WI sequence shows low signal in most of cerebral white matter, expert for optic tract, optic radiation of internal capsule (IC) and posterior limb of IC, and T2WI and T2WI-FLAIR sequences show high signal. The brain appears distribution feature alternate with the myelin deletion zone and myelin intact area, which looks like a leopard print. The characteristic manifestation is that MRS reveals the decreased NAA peak.

The disease needs to be differentiated from Pelizaeus-Merzbacher like disease (PMLD) and vanishing white matter disease (VWM). PMLD is an autosomal recessive inheritance disease without gender difference. The diagnose between these two diseases can only rely on gene detection. VWM is mainly characterized by symptoms of liquefaction and cystic degeneration on the periventricular white matter. There were no clinical manifestations of nystagmus.

Case 5.1.1.7 Megalencephalic Leukoencephalopathy with Subcortical Cysts

Clinical Presentation

A 5-year-old boy presented to the emergency department for fever and poor mental response. He has no history of premature delivery and perinatal asphyxia.

Imaging Findings

A. T2WI show high signal in bilateral subcortical white matter of cerebral hemisphere diffusely, mainly in the deep white matter, involved in the pons, periventricular and temporal lobe,and the characteristic symmetrical subcortical cysts were found in bilateral temporal lobe (Fig. 5.7a).
B. T1WI show high signal in bilateral subcortical white matter of cerebral hemisphere diffusely, mainly in the deep white matter, involved in the pons, periventricular and temporal lobe,and the characteristic symmetrical subcortical cysts were found in bilateral temporal lobe (Fig. 5.7b).
C. T2WI-FLAIR show high signal in bilateral subcortical white matter of cerebral hemisphere diffusely, mainly in the deep white matter, involved in the pons, periventricular and temporal lobe, and the characteristic symmetrical subcortical cysts were found in bilateral temporal lobe (Fig. 5.7c).
D. T2WI show low signal in bilateral subcortical white matter of cerebral hemisphere diffusely, mainly in the deep white matter, involved in the corpus callosum, periventricular and temporal lobe (Fig. 5.7d).
E. T1WI show high signal in bilateral subcortical white matter of cerebral hemisphere diffusely, mainly in the deep white matter, involved in the corpus callosum, periventricular and temporal lobe (Fig. 5.7e).
F. T2WI-FLAIR show high signal in bilateral subcortical white matter of cerebral hemisphere diffusely, mainly in the deep white matter, involved in the corpus callosum, periventricular and temporal lobe (Fig. 5.7f).

Discussion

Megalencephalic Leukoencephalopathy with Subcortical Cysts (MLC) is a rare neurodegenerative disease of autosomal inheritance, which is also known as van der Knaap disease. The disease is caused by mutations in the 22qtel of MLC1 [15], leading to a large number of spongy vacuolar structures in subcortical white matter.

Seventy-five percent of MLC is related to the mutations in MLC1, and its clinical sequelae included walk unsteadily, easy to fall, and epileptic. The giant brain is present at birth, and the increase in head circumference tends to be normal within postnatal 1 year. The imaging findings were severe while the clinical symptoms were relatively mild.

The clinical classification of MLC can be divided into the classical and the improving type. This classical type mainly manifested as increased head circumference and dyskinesia. The clinical manifestations of improving type were similar to those of classical cranial MLC at 1 year of age, but clinical manifestations gradually improved after 1 year of age.

The symmetrical abnormal signals were found in bilateral subcortical white matter and corona radiata, accompanied by mild brain white matter swelling and ventriculi lateralis lightly enlarging. T1WI sequence shows low signal, T2WI, T2WI-FLAIR, and DWI sequences show high signal, and no enhancement after administration of contrast. The characteristic manifestation is that the subcortical cysts in the bilateral temporal lobe, prefrontal lobe, and parietal junction. On the MRS showed that the NAA peak and Cho peak decreased.

The disease needs to be differentiated from Canavan disease and Alexander's Disease. Neither had typical bilateral temporal lobe cysts. The Canavan disease without decreased NAA peak and without involved thalamus and globus pallidus. The MLC lesion is widespread and involves white matter in the parietal occipital lobe and u-shaped fibers, but no enhancement after administration of contrast, which can be differentiated from Alexander's disease.

Case 5.1.1.8 Phenylketonuria

Clinical Presentation

A 10-month year girl presented red rash on limbs and back at 3-month, and hair were fade. Growth was delayed, mainly manifested as sit unsteady alone and can't speak. She smells like rat urine slightly. There was not any abnormality at birth, full-term normal delivery, and no history of asphyxiation. The neonatal screening showed elevated blood phenylalanine. A qualitative analysis of urinary organic acid using Gas Chromatography Mass Spectrometry (GCMS) showed elevated urinary levels of phenylpyruvic acid.

Imaging Findings

A. Axial T2-weighted image demonstrates abnormal high signals in the cerebral white matter of posterior horn of bilateral ventricles (Fig. 5.8a).
B. Axial T2-weighted fluid-attenuated inversion recovery image demonstrates high signals in the cerebral white matter of posterior horn of bilateral ventricles (Fig. 5.8b).
C. Axial T1-weighted image demonstrates low signals in the cerebral white matter of posterior horn of bilateral ventricles (Fig. 5.8c).

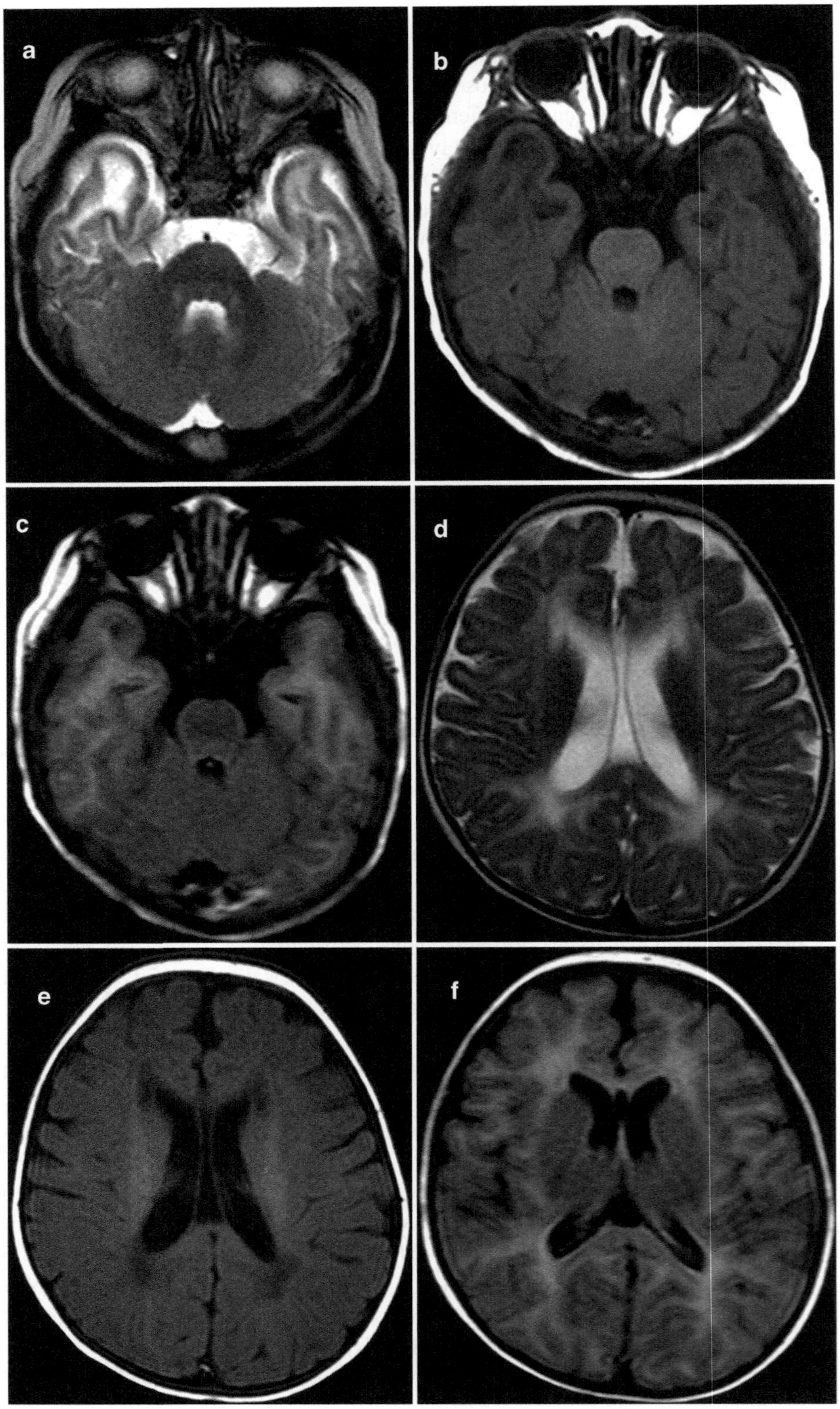

Fig. 5.7 Megalencephalic leukoencephalopathy with subcortical cysts

D. Axial T1-weighted enhancement image demonstrates no enhancement (Fig. 5.8d).

Discussion

Phenylketonuria (PKU) is an autosomal recessive attributed to phenylalanine hydroxylase deficiency for the mutations of the gene, result in that phenylalanine can't be metabolized to tyrosine [16]. It is considered to be a rare inborn error of metabolism, with an estimated prevalence of 1: 11,000.

PKU is characterized by mental retardation, microcephaly, depigmentation of hairs, and specific odor caused by the presence of keto acids in urine [17]. In some studies, epileptic seizure and extrapyramidal symptoms were also reported, including tremor, tendon hyperreflexia, hyperactivity, or hypoactivity [16]. Among that, mental retardation is the most

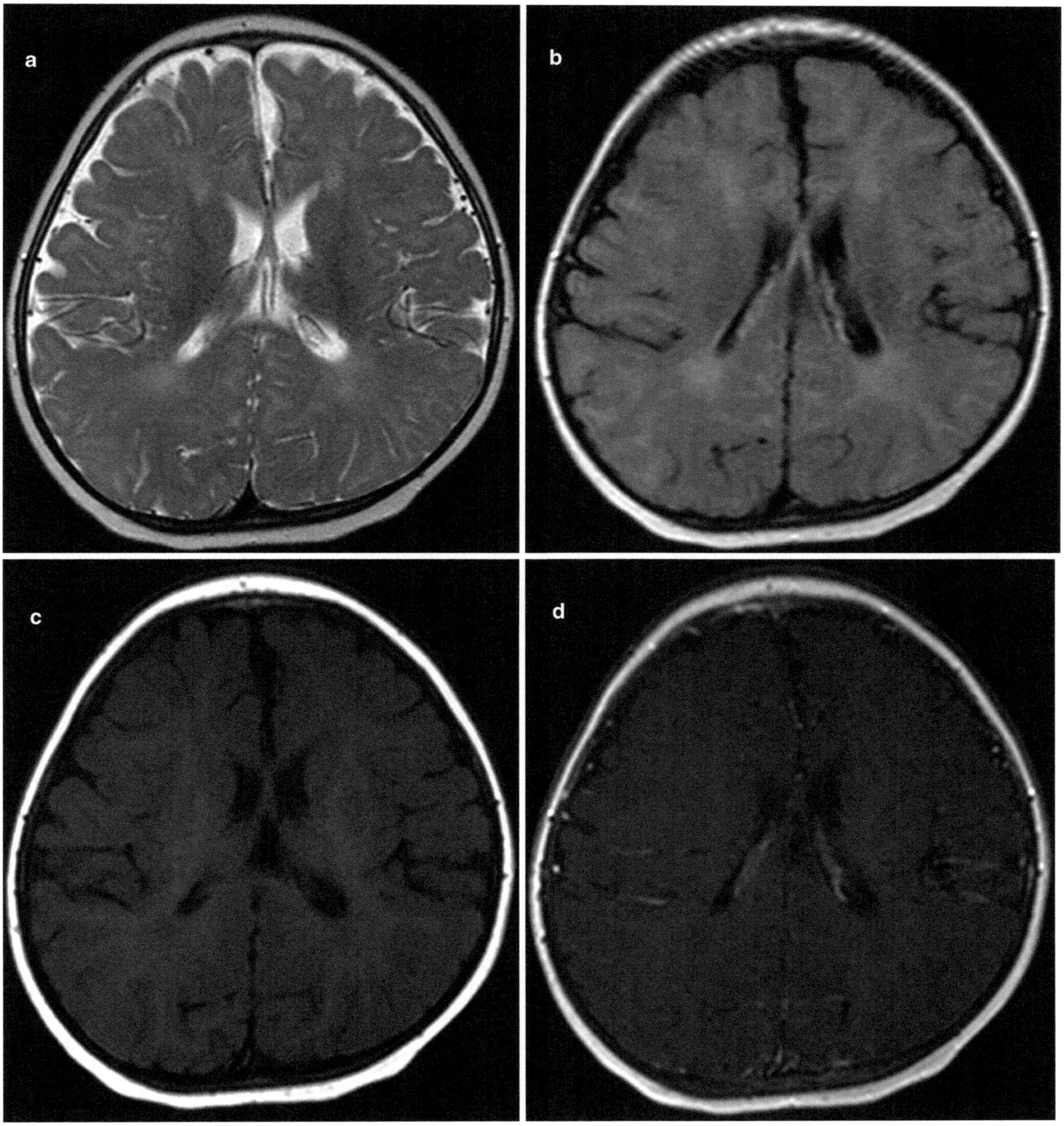

Fig. 5.8 Phenylketonuria

typical clinical symptom. The main cause of mental retardation is the deficiency of the neurotransmitter dopamine, which depending on the reduction of brain tyrosine levels. And the deficiency of serotonin results in depigmentation of hairs. Phenylacetic acid is the metabolite of phenylalanine's second metabolic pathway. It is excreted in urine, caused the patient to smell like rat urine [16].

High concentration of phenylalanine can affect the synthesis of oligodendrocytes and the stability of the myelin sheath. So, MRI findings of PKU indicated white matter involvement, mainly located in the occipital region. It shows a high signal on T2WI and FLAIR sequences. And severity of white matter involvement was not related to the initial phenylalanine levels or to the duration of dietary therapy. According to the study, there is a statistical correlation between MRI involvement and mean 1-year phenylalanine level of patients. So, brain MRI and white matter involvement can be utilized to the evaluation of long-term control of phenylalanine levels in PKU cases [18]. The follow-up of MRI indicated that the process of myelination was improved after low phenylalanine diet [19]. Meanwhile, MRS shows a decrease in NAA, but no significant change in Cho [20]. These results assume that the white matter involvement of PKU may be related to the disorder of myelin sheath formation, not demyelination.

5.1.2 Gray Matter

Case 5.1.2.1 Mitochondrial Encephalopathy with Lactic Acidosis and Stroke-Like episodes (MELAS)

Clinical Presentation

A 7-year-old girl began to have limb weakness and reduced exercise from a year ago, accompanied by repeated dizziness, headache, and recent blurred vision. Laboratory studies reveal blood lactate levels of 2.4 nmol/L.

Imaging Findings

A. Axial T1WI showed the left occipital lobe brain atrophy, multiple cortical cerebellar softening lesions and cortical necrosis (Fig. 5.9a).
B. Axial T2WI sequences showed swelling of the right occipital lobe and focal abnormal hyperintensity (Fig. 5.9b).
C. Axial T2WI-FLAIR sequences showed swelling of the right occipital lobe and focal abnormal hyperintensity (Fig. 5.9c).
D. Transverse axial T1WI showed no enhancement in the right occipital lobe (Fig. 5.9d).
E. MRA showed a decrease in the occipital artery branch of the left occipital lobe, while the branch of the right occipital cerebral artery was dilated and increased (Fig. 5.9e).
F. After a year of follow-up, Axial T2WI-FLAIR sequences showed the right occipital lobe (arrow) evolved into brain atrophy, enephalomalacia, and new lesions of the left temporal lobe (triangle) were seen (Fig. 5.9f).

Discussion

Mitochondrial myopathy, encephalopathy, lactic acidosis, and stroke-like episodes (MELAS) is a type of mitochondrial disorder that was first described by Pavlakis et al. in 1984 [21]. And it is the most common maternal-inherited mitochondrial disease. Approximately 80% of MELAS cases have an A3243G mutation, and various other mutations have been reported. MELAS syndrome is a multi-organ disease with broad manifestations including stroke-like episodes, recurrent headaches, epilepsy, lactic acidemia, dementia, myopathy, hearing impairment, and short stature. Patients with MELAS syndrome frequently present with more than one clinical manifestation. Childhood is the typical age of onset with 65–76% of affected individuals presenting at or before the age of 20 years. Only 1–6% of individuals were present after the age of 40 years and 5–8% before the age of 2 years. MELAS often shows elevated lactate concentrations on blood and spinal fluid examination.

The pathophysiology of stroke-like episodes is not fully understood, various hypotheses have been proposed: (1) ischemic vascular mechanism, (2) energy metabolism abnormality mechanism, and (3) nonischemic neurovascular cellular mechanism [22]. Ischemic vascular mechanism refers to ischemic change due to abnormal mitochondrial deposition of smooth muscle cells in the small arteries of the brain. However, it does not explain that the stroke-like lesions of the disease are inconsistent with the vascular distribution, and single-photon emission computed tomography (SPECT) shows hyperemia rather than ischemia. Energy metabolism abnormality mechanism suggested that Mitochondria are important organelles for intracellular energy production, and their dysfunction can lead to a decrease in ATP production, leading to apoptosis. The theory suggests that abnormal energy metabolism can lead to cell homeostasis and chronic lactic acidosis, which can induce stroke-like episodes when energy demand increases. The mechanism of nonischemic neurovascular cellular suggested that the stroke-like episodes may reflect neuronal hyperexcitability (epileptic activity), which increases energy requirements and creates an imbalance between energy requirements and the adequate availability of adenosine triphosphate (ATP) due to an oxidative phosphorylation defect.

CT has a limited value in the diagnosis of MELAS. The most common CT findings were focal low-density stroke-like lesions, cerebral and cerebellar atrophies, or bilateral basal ganglia and thalamic calcification [23].

MRI is the most valuable imaging method for diagnosing MELAS. The typical manifestation is a stroke-like lesion that is incongruent with vascular territories. SLL presented long T1 long T2 signals, mostly located in the posterior part of the cerebral hemispheres, i.e., the apical and occipital lobes. The shape, size, and extent of SLL vary with the condition of the disease, and are migratory; often multifocal distribution, not distributed according to the vascular dominating area, spanning different blood supply areas. In addition, the lesion mainly involves the cerebral cortex. In the acute phase, the cortical swelling is obvious, and the T2 signal is significantly increased. If not treated promptly, malacia and atrophy of the cerebral cortex will present in the advanced stage. Deep white matter is less affected. Rare brainstem and basal ganglia are involved. Enhanced scans of SLL are generally not enhanced.

The arterial spin labeling (ASL) sequence showed an increase in perfusion in the acute phase of SLL and a decrease in chronic phase perfusion. Because SLL shows an increase in perfusion in the acute phase, MRA or CTA can be characterized by thickening of blood vessels and increased branching in the lesion. This is clearly different from infarcts, and vascular imaging does not show stenosis or occlusion.

Diffuse weighted imaging (DWI) showed an increase in the apparent diffusion coefficient (ADC) of SLL, suggesting the presence of vasogenic edema [24], which is different

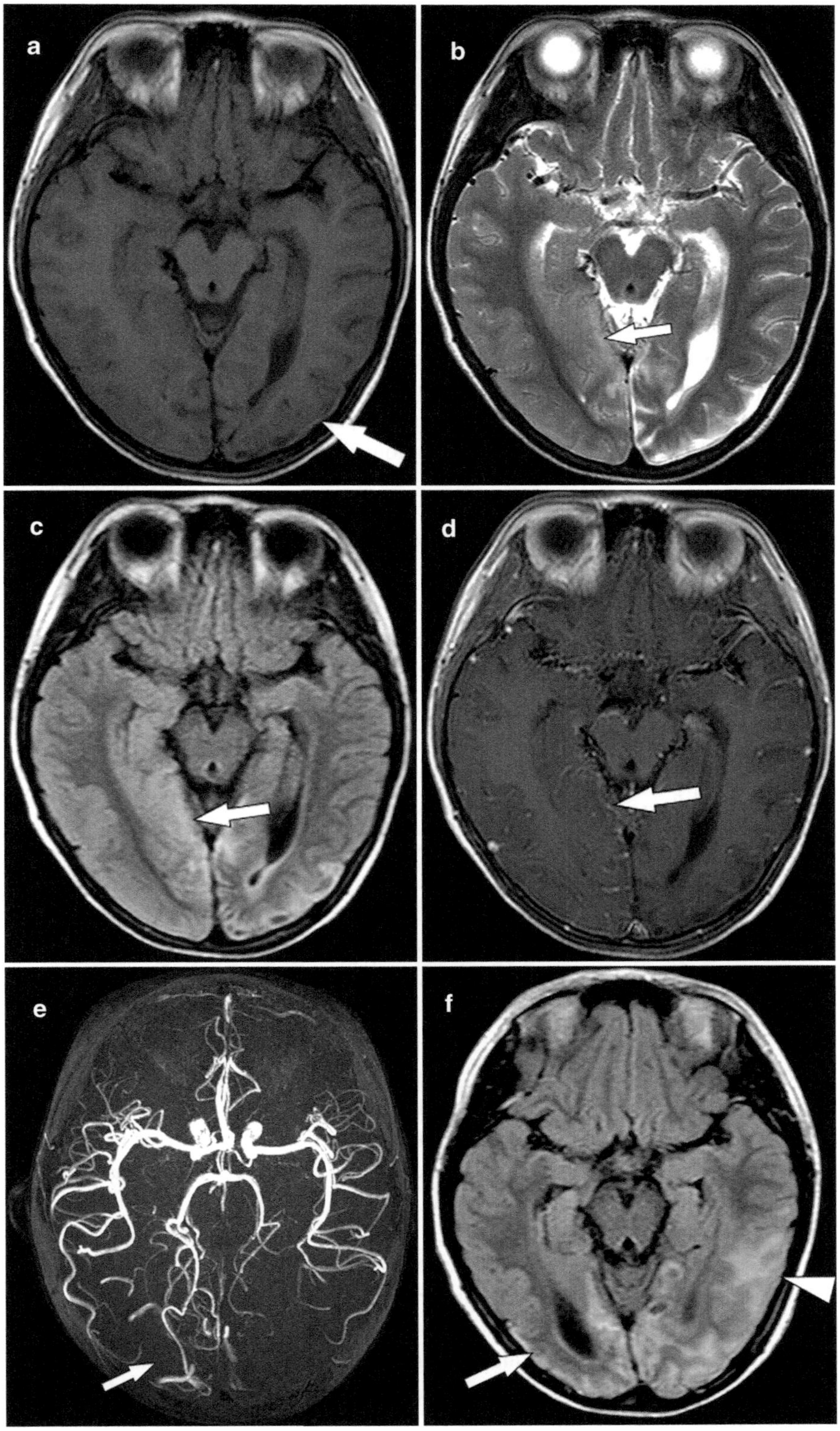

Fig. 5.9 Mitochondrial encephalopathy with lactic acidosis and stroke-like episodes

from the reduction in ADC values due to cytotoxic edema in acute cerebral infarction.

MRS is characterized by a decrease in NAA and an increase in lactic acid peak, but these changes are not specific.

Differential diagnosis: The conventional MRI of MELAS demonstrates abnormal signal involving both cortex and subcortical white matter, particularly in the occipital and parietal areas that strongly mimics ischemic stroke. However, the difference with cerebral infarction is: (1) SLL are incongruent with vascular territories, mainly involving cortical and subcortical white matter, while the deep white matter is not involved; (2) the lesion is not enhanced; (3) serial observation shows that SLL can change, sometimes even disappears, unlike cerebral infarction.

Case 5.1.2.2 Subacute Necrotic Encephalomyelopathy (Leigh Disease)

Clinical Presentation

A 2 year and 6 month old boy came to the hospital because of unstable walking. The mental development of the child lags behind that of the same age. There is a limb twitching 2 weeks ago, and there is a language disturbance, and the speech rate slows down. Physical examination: short height.

Imaging Findings

A. Axial T2WI showed symmetry distributed patchy T2WI high-signal lesions were seen in the dorsal part of the pons (Fig. 5.10a).
B. Axial T2WI showed symmetry distributed patchy T2WI high-signal lesions were around the central aqueduct (Fig. 5.10b).
C. Axial T2WI showed symmetry distributed patchy T2WI high-signal lesions were seen in the the putamen (Fig. 5.10c).
D. The sagittal T1WI showed that the dorsal lesions in the brainstem were more obvious (Fig. 5.10d).

Discussion

Leigh disease, also known as subacute necrotizing encephalomyelopathy, is an autosomal recessive disorder that is a defect of pyruvate and cytochrome c oxidase and is a common mitochondrial myopathy in infants and children. Leigh syndrome is more common before the age of 10 years, more common in infants and young children, no gender, and ethnic orientation. Symptoms such as low muscle tone, mental motor developmental disorders, ataxia, ptosis, and deterioration of language function often occur in children after onset [25].

The main pathological changes of Leigh's disease have the following characteristics: (1) the lesions are mostly distributed in the basal ganglia, thalamus, midbrain, and cerebellar dentate nucleus; (2) the lesions are multifocal and symmetric, and along the periaqueductal gray distribution is specific; and (3) small cystic cavities, vascular proliferation, neuronal loss, and demyelination [26].

The main examination methods are CT and MRI. CT has limited diagnostic value for this disease; MRI is the preferred method for examination of this disease.

Imaging findings correspond to pathological features. (1) The morphological and distribution characteristics of the brain lesions of Leigh disease are mostly bilateral symmetric distribution, irregular lesions, and plaque lesions of different sizes. (2) The lesion mainly involves the brain stem, basal ganglia, and thalamus. Brain stem lesions are mainly affected by dorsal involvement, especially along periaqueductal gray. (3) The MRI signal features of the lesions were hypointensity on T1WI and "javascript:;" hyperintensity on T2WI. The lesion signal of T2-FLAIR sequence is heterogeneous. DWI lesions were mostly diffusely restricted. Due to different pathological periods and different degrees of lesions, lesion signals were also heterogeneous on DWI images. When the lesion is in the acute phase and acute mitochondrial dysfunction occurs, the ^{1}H-MRS of Leigh syndrome patients may have an elevated lactate peak, and the NAA peak may decrease, but this is not specific [27].

The main symmetry of Leigh syndrome involves the putamen, globus pallidus, caudate nucleus, and periaqueductal gray. It needs to be differentiated from other diseases in the area. Hepatolenticular degeneration can also affect the above-mentioned areas, but the symmetry lesions in the basal ganglia are mainly, and the age of onset is relatively late, mainly in the 6–8 years old. In addition, the physical examination found that the appearance of K-F ring in the eye also helps identify. The typical manifestation of nuclear jaundice is the high signal of bilateral globus symmetry T2WI, which generally does not involve the brainstem and cerebellum for identification. In addition, patients with nuclear jaundice have a history of severe jaundice. Leigh syndrome has similar pathological changes and distribution characteristics to Wernicke encephalopathy, and it is difficult to differentiate from imaging. However, Wernicke encephalopathy has a clinical history of malnutrition or vitamin deficiency, which is helpful for differentiation with Leigh syndrome.

Case 5.1.2.3 Wilson Disease

Clinical Presentation

An 11-year-old boy was sent to the hospital for abdominal distention and anorexia. The physical examination found Kayser-Fleischer (K-F) ring in the boy's eyes corneal. He has no history of premature delivery and perinatal asphyxia.

Imaging Findings

A. T2WI show high signal in bilateral basal ganglia regions (Fig. 5.11a).
B. T1WI sequence shows low signal in bilateral basal ganglia regions (Fig. 5.11b).
C. T2WI-FLAIR shows low signal in bilateral basal ganglia regions (Fig. 5.11c).
D. CE-T1WI sequence shows no enhancementin bilateral basal ganglia regions (Fig. 5.11d).

Discussion

Wilson Disease is a rare abnormal copper metabolism of autosomal recessive inheritance, which is also known as hepatolenticular degeneration (HLD). The disease is caused by ketone metabolic disturbance, leading to the deposition of copper in the brain, liver, eyes corneal, and renal.

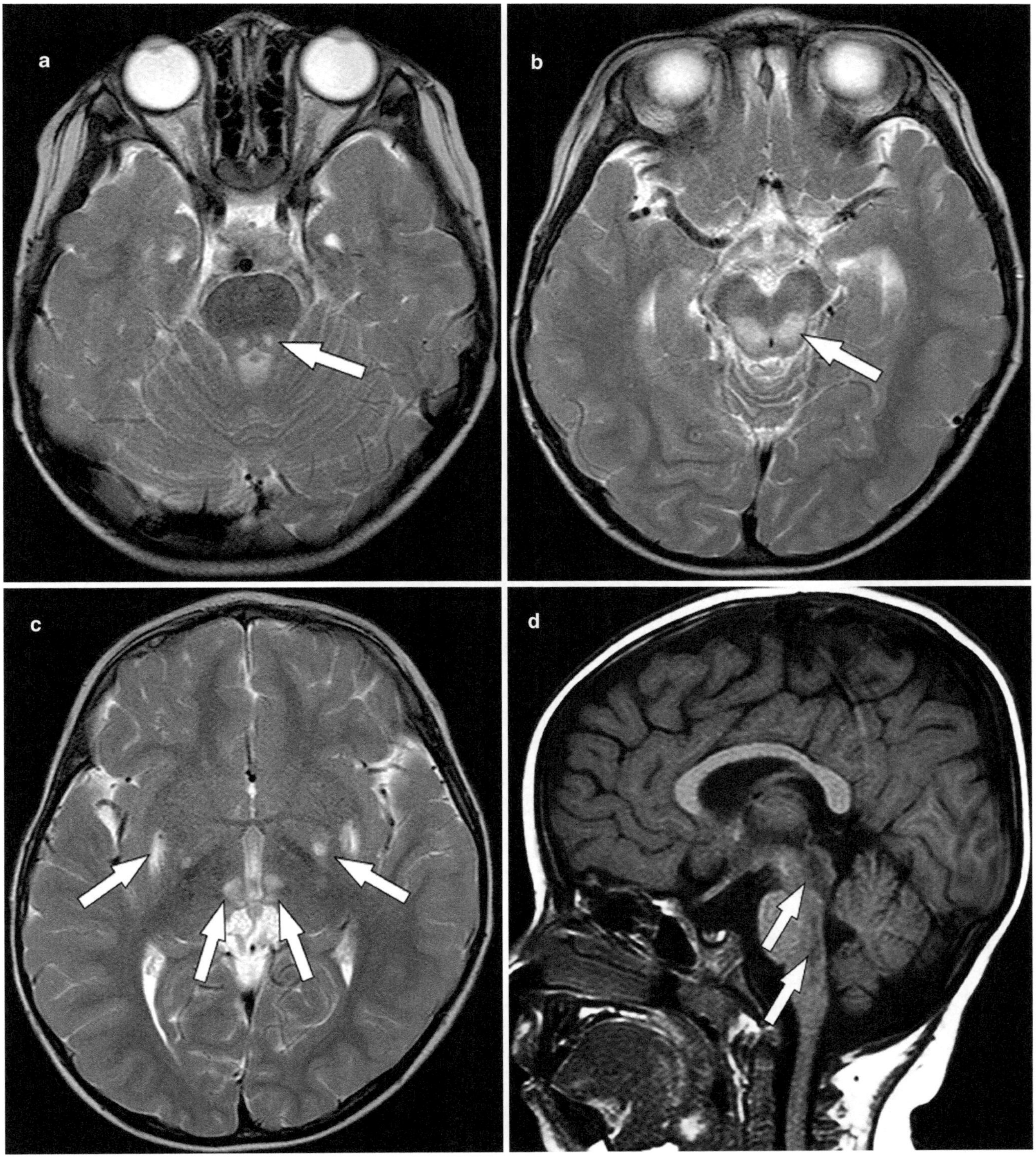

Fig. 5.10 Subacute necrotic encephalomyelopathy (leigh disease)

Wilson Disease is related to the main pathogenic genes of 13q14.3 between D13S31 and D13S59 [28, 29]. The HLD can cause damage to liver, brain, cornea, kidney, bone, and so on, but the severity of symptoms varies from person to person.

This disease mainly manifested as K-F ring in the eyes corneal, liver necrosis and sclerosis, impaired renal proximal tubular function, with intelligent degeneration, tremor, involuntary movement, ataxia, and myotonia. The copper and ceruloplasmin decreased in serum. The copper deposition is first seen in the liver. In the early stage of the disease, intrahepatic mitochondrial abnormalities are seen, and hepatomegaly and jaundice occur in the clinical, and in the advanced stage, it is characterized by fibrosis and cirrhosis. Subsequently, copper fibrosis and cirrhosis. The yellow

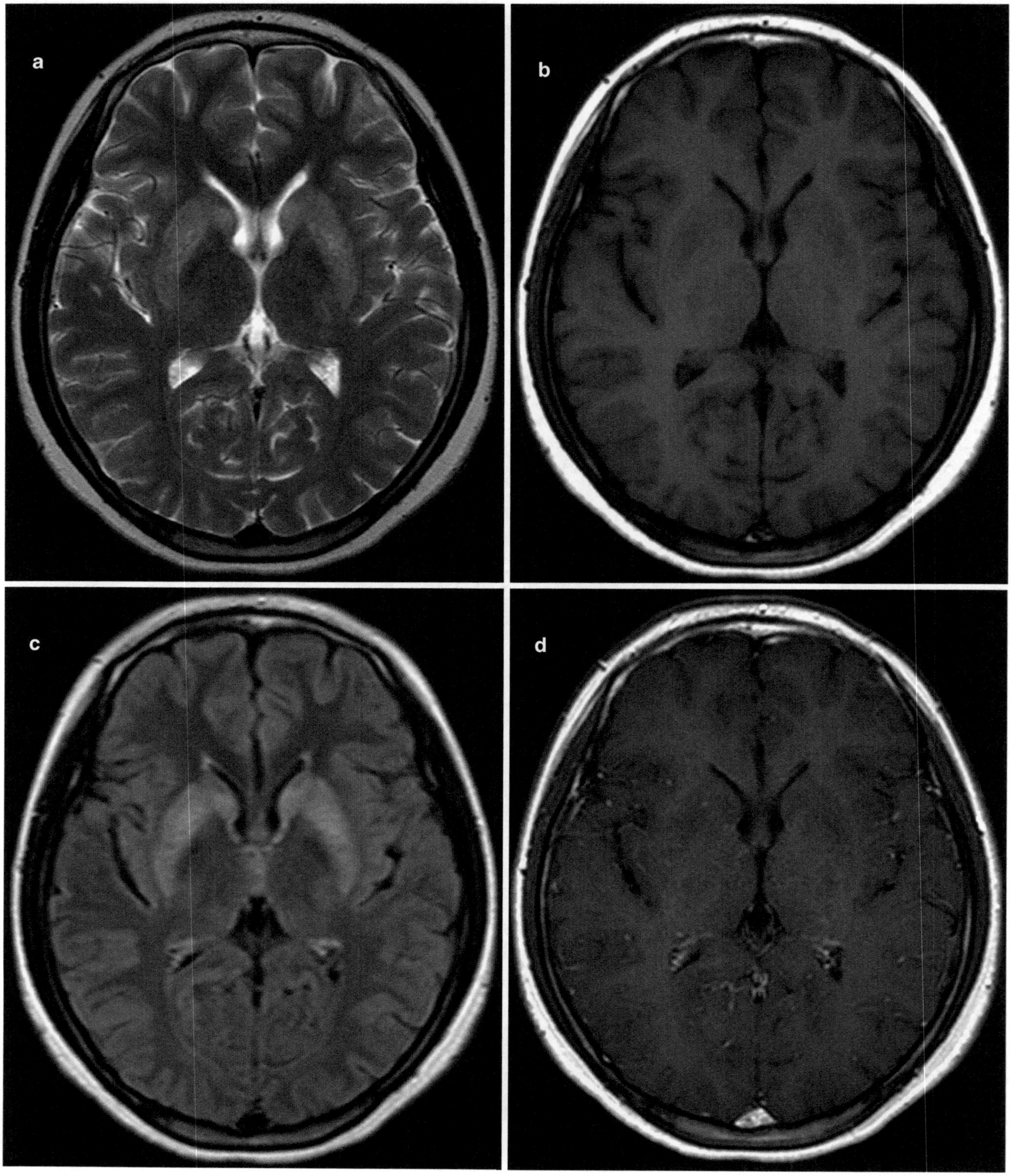

Fig. 5.11 Wilson disease

brown K-F ring in the cornea is the main diagnostic criteria. The decrease in serum ceruloplasmin is also a diagnostic criterion. The disease onset between 6 and 8 years old, and is usually admitted to hospital with similar manifestations of hepatitis. With timely and effective early treatment, patients can achieve a quality of life close to normal people.

The changes in magnetic resonance signals were mainly caused by glial proliferation and cell degeneration. T1WI sequence shows symmetrical low signal in bilateral basal ganglia regions, pons, dorsal thalamus, T2WI and T2WI-FLAIR sequences show high signal, and no enhancement after administration of contrast. The DWI shows high signal in the early stage of the disease, and the DWI shows low signal in the advanced stage. The basal ganglia region is expressed as "butterfly sign" or "八" sign. The asymmetric white matter lesions are located in the frontal lobe and are often accompanied by encephalatrophy.

The disease needs to be differentiated from Hallervorden-Spatz Disease. Hallervorden-Spatz Disease shows a symmetrical low signal on T1WI sequence and the high density on the CT in globus pallidus, substantia nigra, and putamen.

Case 5.1.2.4 Fahr Disease

Clinical Presentation

An 11-year-old girl presented to the hospital for head trauma and convulsion. She has no history of premature delivery and perinatal asphyxia.

Imaging Findings

A. CT shows the high density in bilateral basal ganglia regions, which suggested calcification (Fig. 5.12a).
B. Axial T2WI show high signal in bilateral basal ganglia regions, accompanied by mild brain atrophic (Fig. 5.12b).
C. T1WI show high signal in bilateral basal ganglia regions, accompanied by mild brain atrophic (Fig. 5.12c).
D. T2WI-FLAIR show high signal in bilateral basal ganglia regions, accompanied by mild brain atrophic. (Fig. 5.12d).
D. Coronal T2WI shows high signal in bilateral basal ganglia regions, accompanied by mild brain atrophic (Fig. 5.12e).

Discussion

Fahr Disease is a rare neurodegenerative disease of autosomal recessive inheritance, which is also known as familial basal ganglia calcification (FBGC) or idiopathic basal ganglia calcification (IBGC). The disease is caused by symmetrical diffuse calcinosis in terminal arterioles and venule of putamen, caudate nucleus, globus pallidus, dentate nucleus, and gray–white matter junction area of brain, which includes mucopolysaccharide, plumbum, phosphorus, iron, potassium, and so on, leading to non-arteriosclerosis angiolithic degeneration, softening focus in severely calcified regional and unusual widening of Virchow-Robin space.

Fahr Disease is related to SLC20A2, PDGFRB, PDGFB, XPR1 [30], and familial incidence. The clinical symptoms are varied, it often onset at adolescence or middle age, presenting with progressive mental disorder, hypophrenia, dementia, dysarthria, abnormal growth and development, extrapyramidal symptom and epileptic seizure, often accompanied by dizziness, headache, tetany, and so on. The Fahr Disease can be divided into mild cerebral calcification type, moderate cerebral calcification type, severe cerebral calcification type. The mild cerebral calcification type has no clinical symptoms. The moderate cerebral calcification type is mainly characterized by symptoms of headache, dizziness, epilepsy, and psychosis. The severe cerebral calcification type manifests hypophrenia, abnormal growth, and development, in addition to the above partial symptoms.

CT shows the high density in cerebral hemisphere diffusely, which suggested calcification, especially in the basal ganglia regions and cerebellum. The basal ganglia region's calcification is inverted V sign, thalamus calcification is symmetrical triangle and paraventricular white matter is "flame" shape or "bone spicule" shape calcification. MRI showed decreased signal intensity in T1WI and T2WI. T1WI sequence shows low signal, T2WI and T2WI-FLAIR sequences show hyper-hypo intense, and no enhancement after administration of contrast. It is often associated with cerebral atrophy.

The disease needs to be differentiated from hypoparathyroidism and tuberous sclerosis. The hypoparathyroidism showed decreased blood serum calcium and increased phosphorus. The nodular calcifications of tuberous sclerosis are mainly located in paraventricular matter, especially the foramen of Monro and subependymal.

Case 5.1.2.5 Hallervorden-Spatz Disease

Clinical Presentation

An 8-year-old boy presented to the hospital for hypophrenia and dyskinesia. He has no history of premature delivery and perinatal asphyxia.

Imaging Findings

A. T2WI show high signal in the bilateral globus pallidus, which appeared as the "eye of the tiger" sign (Fig. 5.13a).
B. T1WI shows low signal in the bilateral globus pallidus, which appeared as the "eye of the tiger" sign (Fig. 5.13b).
C. T2WI-FLAIR show high signal in the bilateral globus pallidus, which appeared as the "eye of the tiger" sign (Fig. 5.13c).
D. CE-T1WI shows no enhancement in the bilateral globus pallidus (Fig. 5.13d).
E. T2WI show high signal in the bilateral globus pallidus, which appeared as the "eye of the tiger" sign (Fig. 5.13e).

Discussion

Hallervorden-Spatz Disease is a rare neurodegenerative disease of autosomal recessive inheritance. The disease is caused by the iron salt deposition in globus pallidus, substantia nigra, and putamen, leading to neurodegeneration with brain iron accumulation.

Hallervorden-Spatz Disease is related to mutations in the pantothenate kinase 2 (PANK2) [31, 32], and its clinical sequelae included reticularis neural cells demyelination, iron accumulation, spheroplast swollen axonal, and glial proliferation in globus pallidus and substantia nigra.

The disease is characterized by pyramidal sign, hypophrenia, retinopathy, and extra pyramidal symptoms, such as dystonia, rigidity, bradykinesia, and resting tremor. The clinical symptoms deteriorate progressively. The clinical classi-

Fig. 5.12 Fahr disease

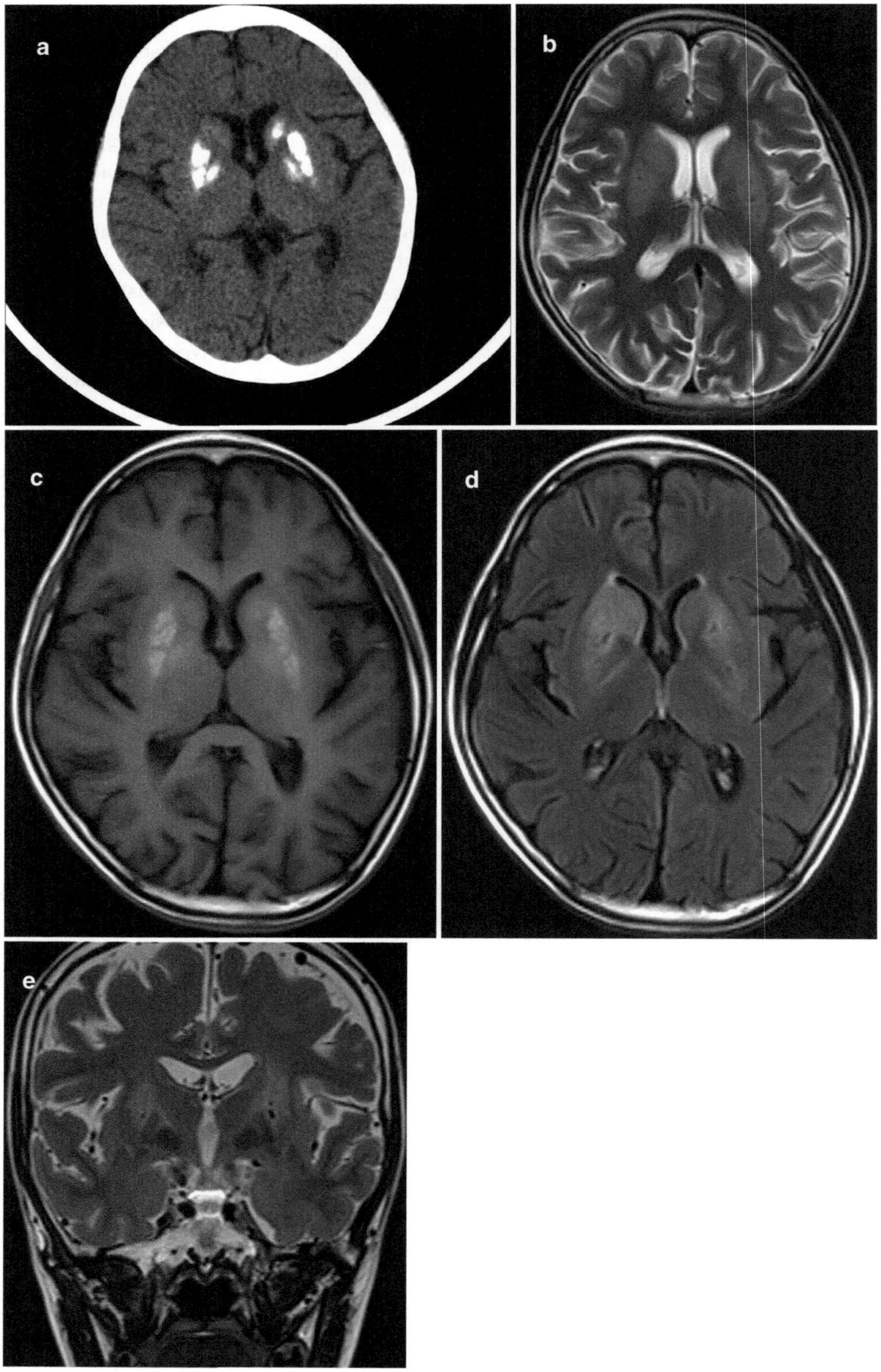

fication of Hallervorden-Spatz Disease can be divided into classic and atypical. The classic type is characterized with early onset associated with dystonia, rigidity, dysarthria and corticospinal system, and corticospinal system damage. The clinical symptoms progress rapidly and often lose the ability to walk independently after 10 years of onset. The atypical type is characterized by late onset associated with dysarthria, psychosis, dystonia and rigidity. The clinical symptoms progress slowly and often lose the ability to walk independently after 15 years to 40 years of onset.

Hallervorden-Spatz Disease shows a symmetrical low signal on T1WI sequence and CT shows the high density on globus pallidus, substantia nigra, and putamen. The characteristic manifestation is that MRI showed spotty low signal in T2WI

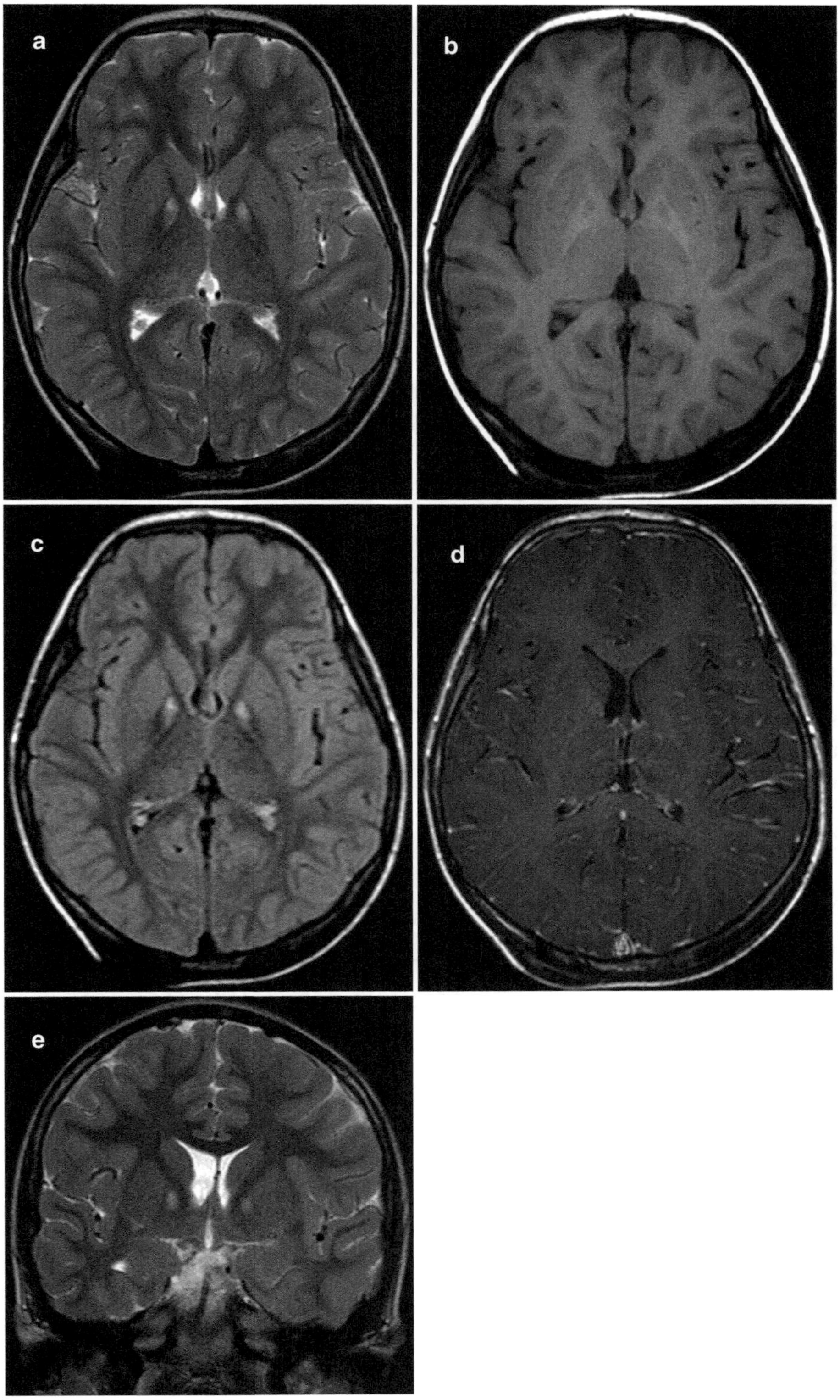

Fig. 5.13 Hallervorden-Spatz disease

in the globus pallidus and substantia nigra, surrounding by high signal, namely the "eye of the tiger" sign. MRS showed that a decreased NAA peak in the globus pallidus.

The disease needs to be differentiated from Parkinson's disease (PD). Hallervorden-Spatz Disease progresses rapidly and affects simultaneously almost all the organs and tissues of the body at the beginning of the disease, especially the lower extremities. The rigidity was more serious than the tremor. The hypophrenia was more early and severe than PD. MRI showed macula areas of low signal in T2WI in the globus pallidus and substantia nigra, surrounding by high signal, namely the "eye of the tiger" sign.

5.1.3 White and Gray Matter

Case 5.1.3.1 Cockayne Syndrome

Clinical Presentation

A 4-year-old boy presented to the neurology department for growth and developmental retardation. He had been seen photosensitivity in 40-day-old. The laboratory examination show the ERCC6 mutation in gene detection, which inherited from the mother and father, and also carried by his older brother. He was weak and prone to respiratory tract infection. He has no history of premature delivery and perinatal asphyxia.

Imaging Findings

A. CT shows the high density in bilateral basal ganglia regions which suggested calcification (Fig. 5.14a).
B. CT shows the high density in bilateral basal ganglia regions which suggested calcification (Fig. 5.14b).
C. T2WI shows high signal in periventricular white matter and semioval center white matter (Fig. 5.14c).

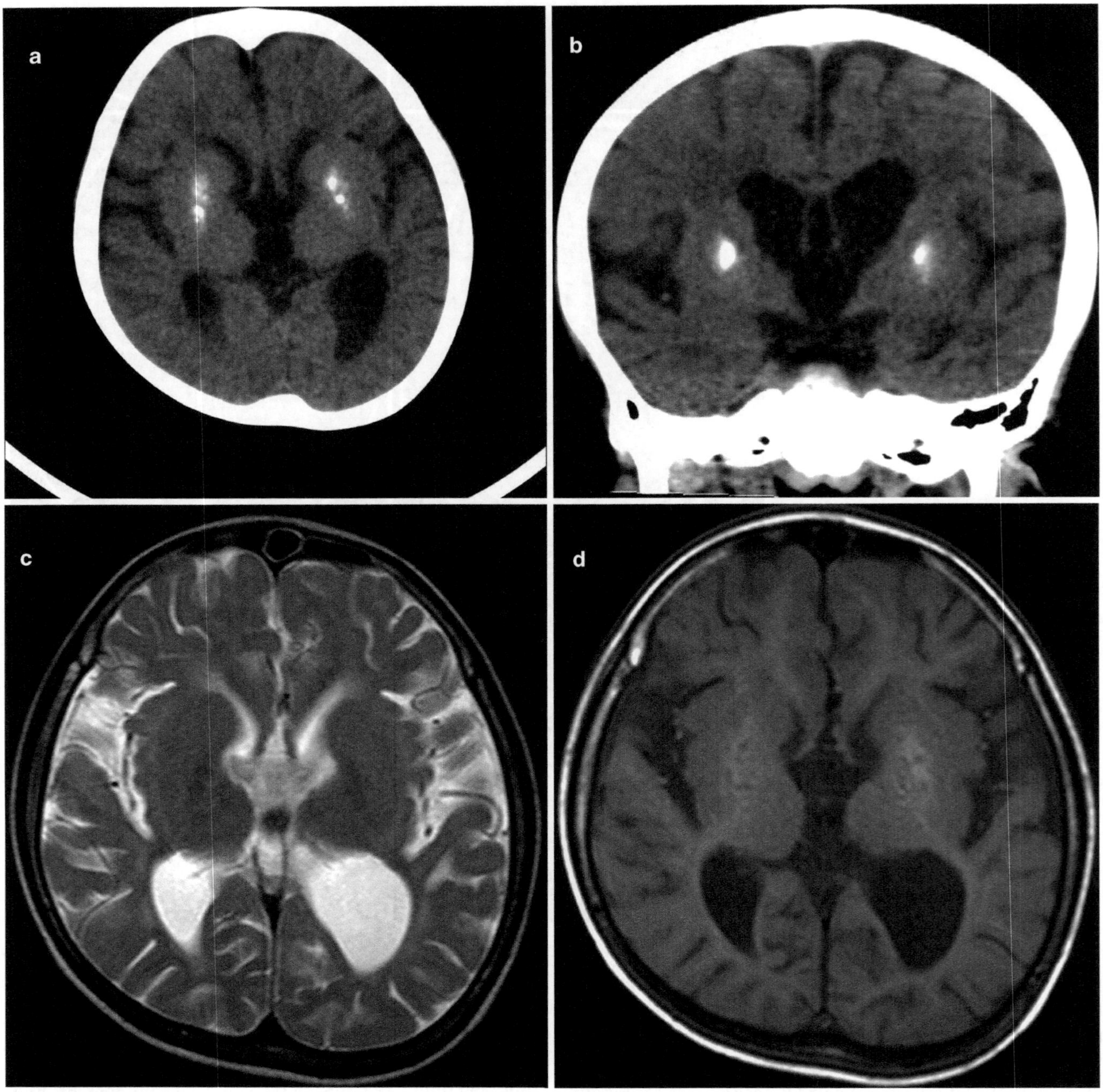

Fig. 5.14 Cockayne syndrome

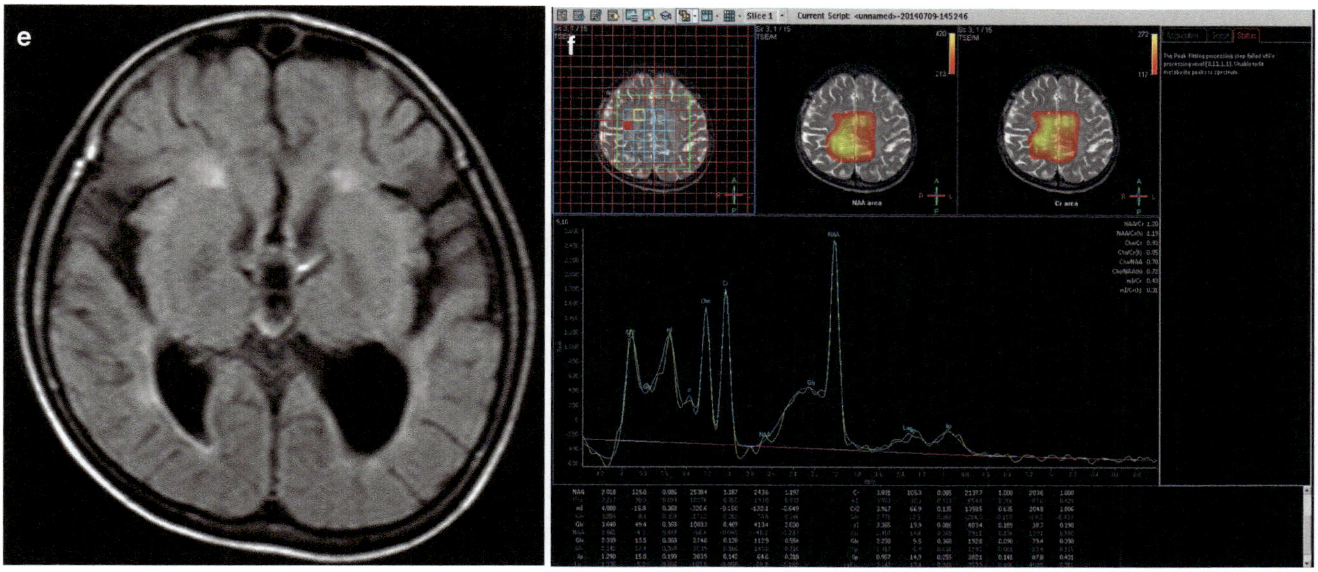

Fig. 5.14 (continued)

D. T1WI shows low signal in periventricular white matter and semioval center white matter (Fig. 5.14d).
E. T2WI-FLAIR shows high signal in periventricular white matter and semioval center white matter (Fig. 5.14e).
F. MRS reveals the decreased NAA peak (Fig. 5.14f).

Discussion

Cockayne Syndrome is a rare disease of autosomal recessive inheritance, which involved multiple systems. The disease is caused by the functional inactivation of familial hereditary excision repair mechanism, leading to repair deficiency and transcription deficiency.

Whole exome sequencing (WES) is used to diagnose Cockayne Syndrome, which is related to the main pathogenic genes of XPB, XPD, XPG, CSA (ERCC8), and CSB (ERCC6) [33]. The RNA synthesis defects of fibroblast cells in the skin after ultraviolet irradiation were served as the gold standard. The earlier the onset, the more severe the illness and the shorter the life span.

The characteristic manifestation is that developmental retardation, growth retardation, and microcephaly, often accompanied by photosensitivity, progressive retinopathy, enophthalmus, tooth enamel dysplasia, and progressive sensory deafness. Some literatures report that the disease is related to arthritis and atherosclerosis. The clinical classification of Cockayne Syndrome can be divided into Cockayne syndrome type I, Cockayne syndrome type II, and Cockayne syndrome type III. The Cockayne syndrome type I is classical and mainly characterized by symptoms of the circumferences of height, weight, and head are much smaller than healthy peers, abnormal growth and development, nervous system injury, and progressive visual impairment. Although most patients were normal at birth, and onset in within 2 years old, involving the brain, nerves, eyes, skin, and other systems. Cockayne syndrome type II is severe, early onset, progressive, and mainly characterized by postnatal development retardation, congenital cataract or other eye diseases, contracture of the spine, joints in the early disease, and died before 7 years old. Cockayne syndrome type III is mild and late onset, involving normal growth and development or developmental retardation in the advanced disease.

The characteristic manifestation is that CT shows the high density in bilateral basal ganglia regions which suggested calcification. T1WI sequence shows high signal, T2WI and T2WI-FLAIR sequences show low signal, often accompanied by encephalatrophy and white matter of cerebral hemisphere diffusely injury. The lipid peak elevation could be shown on the MRS.

The disease needs to be differentiated from congenital microcephaly and neuronal ceroid lipofuscinoses. The congenital microcephaly could been found immediately at birth, but Cockayne Syndrome appears after postnatal long time. Cockayne Syndromes showed decreased NAA peak and Cho peak, which is different from the neuronal ceroid lipofuscinoses.

Case 5.1.3.2 GM1 Gangliosides

Clinical Presentation

Female, 1 year and 8 months. The patient was unable to raise his head, had aphasia, and cannot control her body from prone to supine. Brief medical history: G2P2, the child has a full-term delivery, and exercise regression begins after 7–8 months. Her brother has a similar medical history.

Imaging Findings

A. Axial T2WI showed A diffuse hyperintensity of white matter in the bilateral cerebral hemisphere (Fig. 5.15a).
B. Coronal T2WI showed diffuse hyperintensity of white matter in the bilateral cerebral hemisphere (Fig. 5.15b).

C. Axial T1WI showed a diffuse slightly hypointensity of white matter in the bilateral cerebral hemisphere (Fig. 5.15c).
D. Axial T2WI-FLAIR image showed a hyperintensity of white matter in the bilateral cerebral hemisphere (Fig. 5.15d).

Discussion

Gangliosidosis comprises a group of lysosomal storage diseases characterized by the accumulation of complex glycosphingolipids in the nervous system and other tissues. It contains GM1 and GM2 gangliosidosis, two distinct groups

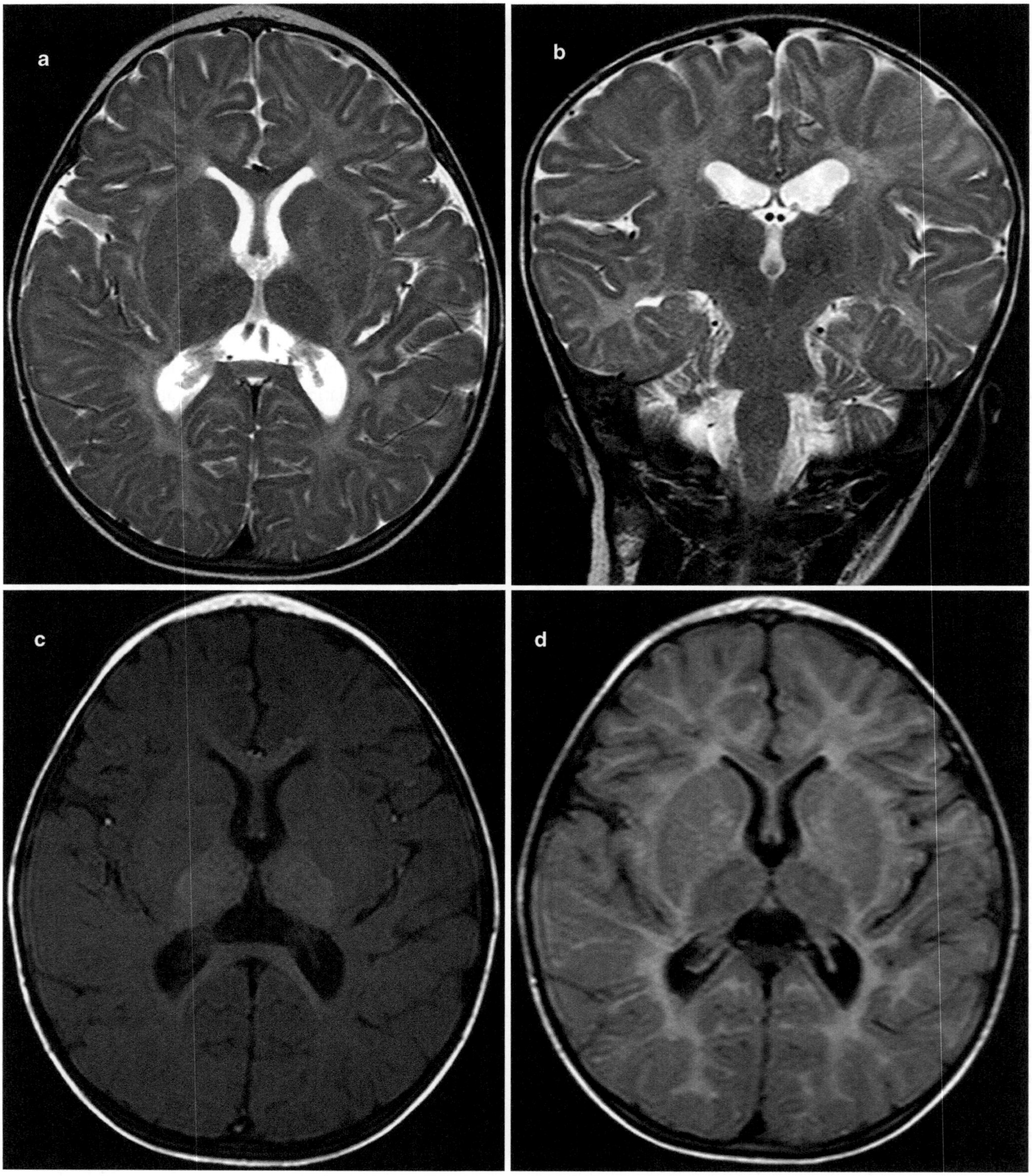

Fig. 5.15 GM1 gangliosides

of the gangliosidosis, and those associated with deficiency of β-galactosidase and β-hexosaminidase, respectively. GM1 gangliosidosis is more common in China than GM2. This section mainly discusses the clinical and imaging manifestations of GM1.

GM1 gangliosides are widely present in various cells of the human body and constitute an important part of the cell membrane, with the highest content in brain and nerve tissue. Ganglioside deposition disease is an autosomal recessive hereditary disease with a poor prognosis. So far, there is no effective treatment for this disease, and the prognosis is poor.

According to the clinical manifestations and age of onset, GM1 gangliosidosis is mainly divided into three types: infant type (type I), juvenile type (type II), and adult type (type III). Infant type is more common than others. Type I children start to onset mainly in 3–6 months, and a small number of onset in the neonatal period, mainly characterized by progressive neurological deterioration, developmental degeneration, sensorimotor, and mental retardation [34]. Typical manifestations are cherry erythema at the macula, facial deformity, hepatosplenomegaly, and skeletal dysplasia.

Image manifestations: Skeletal X-rays of patients with GM1 often show multiple bone dysplasia, osteoporosis, posterior kyphosis, and the anterior inferior border of the thoracic and lumbar vertebral bodies is a beak-like protrusion, similar to mucopolysaccharidosis. Brain MRI scan showed that the infant type was mainly characterized by diffuse demyelination of white matter, T2WI showed diffuse high signal, T1WI showed slightly lower signal; it could be accompanied by brain atrophy. The MRS examination showed a decrease in the NAA/Cr ratio and an elevation in the Cho/Cr ratio. Sometimes, the brain MRI of infantile and juvenile types shows symmetrical abnormal thalamus or globus pallidus signals [35, 36].

The main features of this disease are diffuse abnormal signals of brain white matter and brain atrophy-like changes. Combined with clinical psychomotor regression and bone changes, it is helpful for diagnosis. The disease needs to be differentiated from Pelizaeus-Merzbacher disease (PMD). The typical leopard sign of PMD and the characteristics of male onset are helpful for differential diagnosis.

Case 5.1.3.3 Fucosidosis

Clinical Presentation

The girl, 3-years old, began to have an abnormal walking posture 1 year ago. It is difficult to stand on her own after lying down, accompanied by a backward language ability. Laboratory tests indicate positive oligosaccharides in the urine. Her 2-year-old brother had similar features.

Imaging Findings

A. Axial T2WI showed diffuse blurred edges, high signal were observed in the deep white matter and subcortical white matter areas of bilateral cerebral hemispheres (Fig. 5.16a).
B. Coronal T2WI showed diffuse blurred edges, high signal were observed in the deep white matter and subcortical white matter areas of bilateral cerebral hemispheres (Fig. 5.16b).
C. Axial T1WI showed diffuse blurred edges, low signal were observed in the deep white matter and subcortical white matter areas of bilateral cerebral hemispheres (Fig. 5.16c).
D. There was no enhancement of the lesion (Fig. 5.16d).
E. The lateral radiograph of the spine (Fig.5.16e) showed a bullet-like change in the anterior border of the lower thoracic and lumbar vertebral bodies, which was prominent in the lumbar spine (Fig. 5.16e).

Discussion

Fucosidosis is caused by a mutation in the FUCA1 gene on chromosome 1p36-p34. It is a rare autosomal recessive lysosomal storage disease with low myelination and mucopolysaccharide metabolism disorder. Patients suffer from multisystemic symptoms, including progressive motor deterioration, hepatomegaly, splenomegaly, progressive neurological deterioration, seizures, recurrent sinopulmonary infections, dwarfism, and other musculoskeletal anomalies.

The disease is classified into type I (infantile type) and type II (adult type), according to the age at which the symptoms appear. Type I usually progresses rapidly and the child usually dies during infancy. Type II usually develops slowly and the symptoms are relatively mild.

Fucoside storage disease is a multisystem disease, and neurological symptoms are the most common and have certain characteristics in imaging. Fucosidosis storage disease lacks characteristics on CT, mainly characterized by a decreased density of radiation crown and globus pallidus. In addition, extensive atrophy of the brain and cerebellum can be shown later in the disease. MRI is the best method of examination to show the location of the lesion more accurately. The main feature of Fucosidosis is the low myelination of the white matter of the brain, which is characterized by extensive, progressive, and symmetrical signal abnormalities of the periventricular white matter and subcortical white matter. T2WI is a high signal and T1WI is an equal or slightly lower signal. In addition, Fucosidosis also causes signal abnormalities in the globus pallidus, which is manifested by the low signal of the T2WI sequence and the high signal of the T1WI sequence [37]. In addition, as the disease progresses, extensive brain and cerebellar atrophy will occur.

In the pediatric age group, this disease needs to be differentiated from GM1 gangliosidosis. Both are manifested as

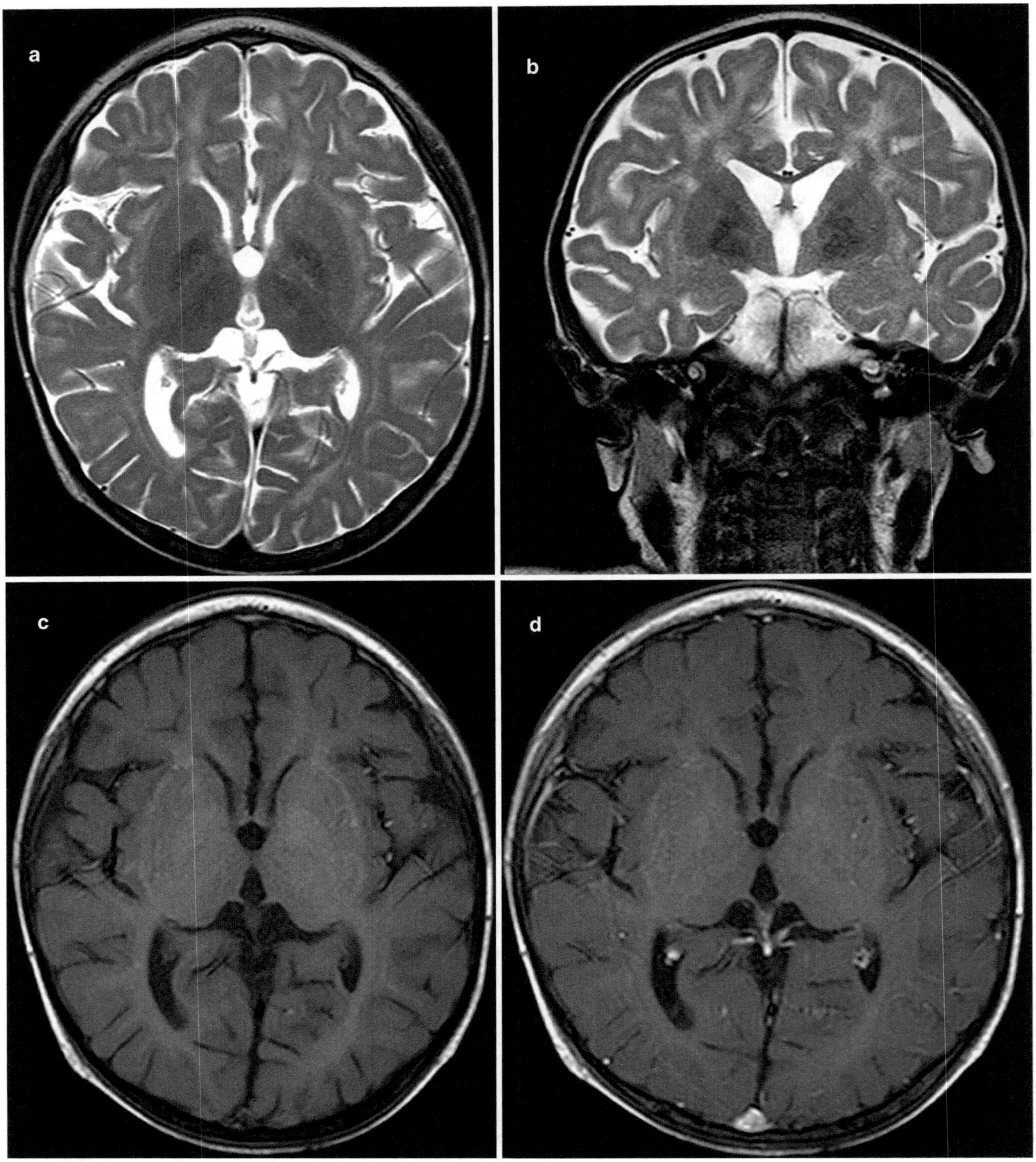

Fig. 5.16 Fucosidosis

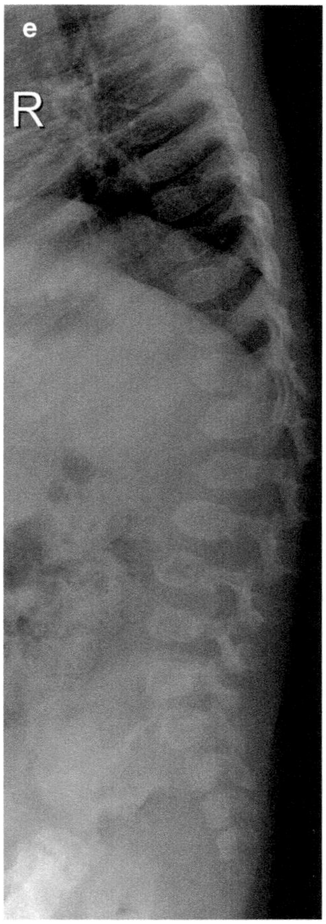

Fig. 5.16 (continued)

diffuse symmetrical abnormal signals in the white matter of the brain, but the T2WI signal of the bilateral basal ganglia decreased in this disease can help distinguish.

Case 5.1.3.4 Maple Syrup Urine Disease

Clinical Presentation

An 8-month-old boy has dyspnea and convulsive seizure at birth of 10 days. Now, he cannot raise his head and sit alone. His eyes cannot follow the light, and his ears cannot distinguish the source of the sound. Other clinical symptoms include drowsiness, unresponsiveness, and poor eating. Muscle tension is normal. There was not any abnormality at birth, full-term normal delivery, and no history of asphyxiation. A qualitative analysis of urinary organic acid using Gas Chromatography Mass Spectrometry (GCMS) showed elevated urinary levels of BCAAs.

Imaging Finding

A. Axial T1-weighted image demonstrates low signal in bilateral precentral and postcentral gyrus (Fig. 5.17a).
B. Axial T1-weighted image demonstrates low signal in bilateral inner capsule hindlimbs (Fig. 5.17b).
C. Axial T1-weighted image demonstrates low signal in bilateral ventrolateral thalamic nucleus (Fig. 5.17c).
D. Axial T1-weighted image demonstrates low signal in pons dorsal (Fig. 5.17d).
E. Axial T1-weighted image demonstrates low signal in bilateral cerebellar dentate nucleus (Fig. 5.17e).
F. Axial T2-weighted image demonstrates high signal in bilateral inner capsule hindlimbs and ventrolateral thalamic nucleus (Fig. 5.17f).
G. Axial T2-weighted image demonstrates high signal in bilateral precentral and postcentral gyrus. In addition, multiple circular high signals are detected on T2-weighted image in bilateral deep white matter of the frontal lobe and center semicircle (Fig. 5.17g).
H. Axial T2-weighted fluid-attenuated inversion recovery image demonstrates low signals in bilateral deep white matter of the frontal lobe and center semicircle (Fig. 5.17h).

Discussion

Maple syrup urine disease (MSUD) is caused by a deficiency of the branched-chain α-ketoacid dehydrogenase enzyme complex, leading to accumulations of the branched chain amino acids (leucine, isoleucine, and valine) and their toxic by-products (ketoacids) in the blood and urine [38, 39]. It is an autosomal recessive disorder. MSUD is divided into five different forms: classic, intermittent, intermediate, thiamine responsive, and dihydrolipoyl dehydrogenase (E3) deficient [40]. The relevant symptoms were shown on newborn, and it is usually classic form. However, it is difficult to diagnosis because patients with MSUD do not show any specific clinical manifestations except a maple syrup odor, nor specific routine laboratory findings. Other uncharacteristic clinical symptoms include convulsive seizure, feeding problems, lethargy, and so on. In recent years, different hypotheses have been proposed for the mechanism of brain injury in MSUD patients. Most studies reported that are the edema of brain cells and myelin production disorders [41]. The brain MRI of classic MSUD is specific. The regions of injury are in line with myelinization of white matter on the newborn. The concerned region mainly includes central part of the radial crown, posterior limb of the inner capsule, ventrolateral nucleus of thalamus, crus cerebelli, dorsal pontine, and cerebellar dentate nucleus. It shows normal myelinization of white matters (high signal) disappear on T1WI, and shows high signal on T2WI symmetrically [38–41].

Case 5.1.3.5 Methylmalonic Acidemia

Clinical Presentation

An 18-month-old girl, 1 year ago, she cannot raise her head stability, and bilateral moderate impairment was detected in auditory evoked potential. Then, she was diagnosed as Methylmalonic acidemia (MMA). Now, decreased strength and tension of the muscle.

Imaging Finding

A. Axial T2-weighted image demonstrates high signal in bilateral lenticular and caudate nucleus symmetrically (Fig. 5.18a).
B. Axial T2-weighted fluid-attenuated inversion recovery image demonstrates high signals in bilateral lenticular and caudate nucleus symmetrically (Fig. 5.18b).
C. Axial T1-weighted image demonstrates low signals in bilateral lenticular and caudate nucleus symmetrically (Fig. 5.18c).
D. Axial T1-weighted enhancement image demonstrates no enhancement (Fig. 5.18d).

Discussion

Methylmalonic acidemia (MMA) is the accumulation of acylcarnitine in blood and increased urinary methylmalonic acid excretion due to the decrease in the activity of methylmalonyl-coA mutase [42]. It is a neurometabolic disorder with autosomal recessive inheritance. MMA can present with neurologic deficits, metabolic acidosis, vomiting, lethargy, anorexia, respiratory distress, severe ketoacidosis, and hypotonia. If this disorder is not treated immediately, the patient may go into coma and die [42]. Organs involvement in methylmalonic acidemia includes central nervous system (CNS), bone marrow, and kidneys [42]. The basal ganglia were involved on MMA

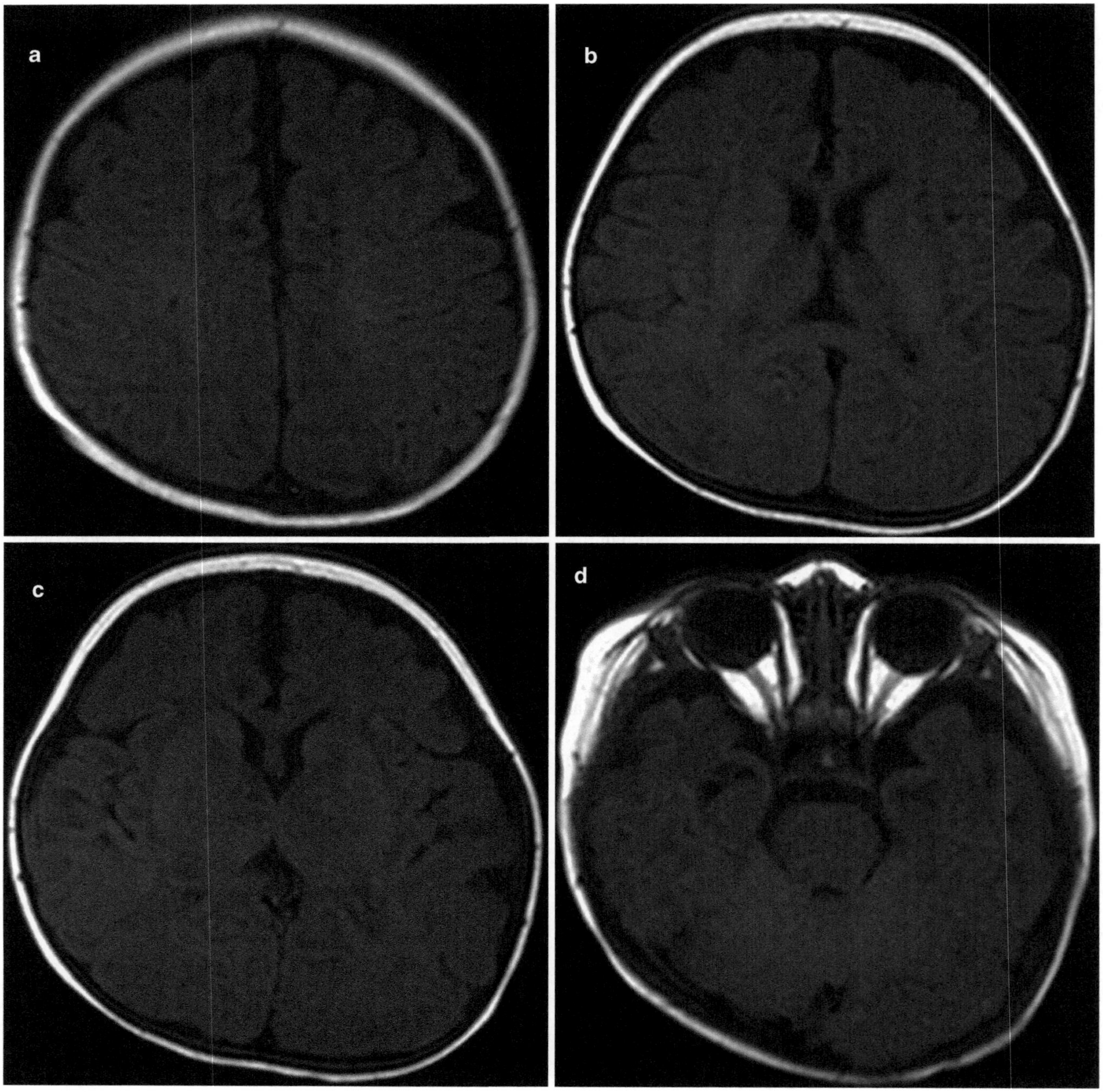

Fig. 5.17 Maple syrup urine disease

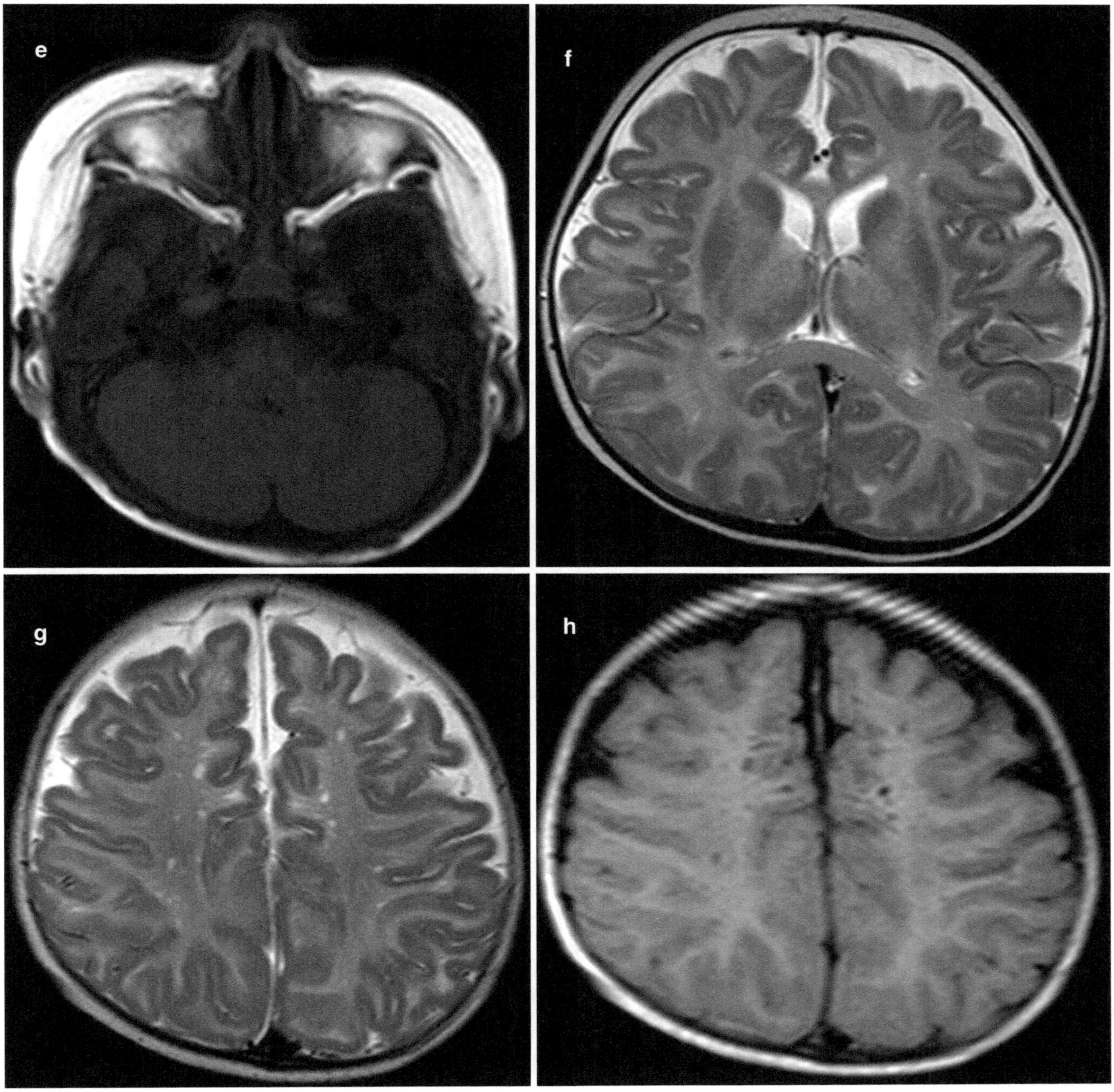

Fig. 5.17 (continued)

because the metabolism of basal ganglia is vigorous and sensitive to lack of energy [1, 2]. It shows high signals on T2-weighted and T2-weighted fluid-attenuated inversion recovery image, low signals on T1-weighted image, and no enhancement on T1-weighted enhancement image [43–44]. Due to the long-standing energy shortage, it maybe shows delayed myelinization or shrinking brain.

Case 5.1.3.6 Propionic Acidemia

Clinical Presentation

A boy was admitted at the age of 1 month. He had feeding problems after birth, which manifest as poor sucking reflex and milk was not increased. He also had repeated vomiting and a reduction of body weight. No fever or convulsion was mentioned. The color of skin and sclera were normal. There was no abnormality at birth, full-term normal delivery, and no history of asphyxiation. A qualitative analysis of urinary organic acid using Gas Chromatography Mass Spectrometry (GCMS) showed elevated urinary levels of lactic acid, 3-hydroxypropionic acid, propionylglycine, 3-hydroxyalanine, acetoacetic acid, methyl crozoyl glycine, and methyl citric acid.

Imaging Findings

A. Axial T2-weighted image demonstrates high signal in bilateral pallidus symmetrically (Fig. 5.19a).
B. Axial T1-weighted image demonstrates low signal in bilateral pallidus symmetrically (Fig. 5.19b).

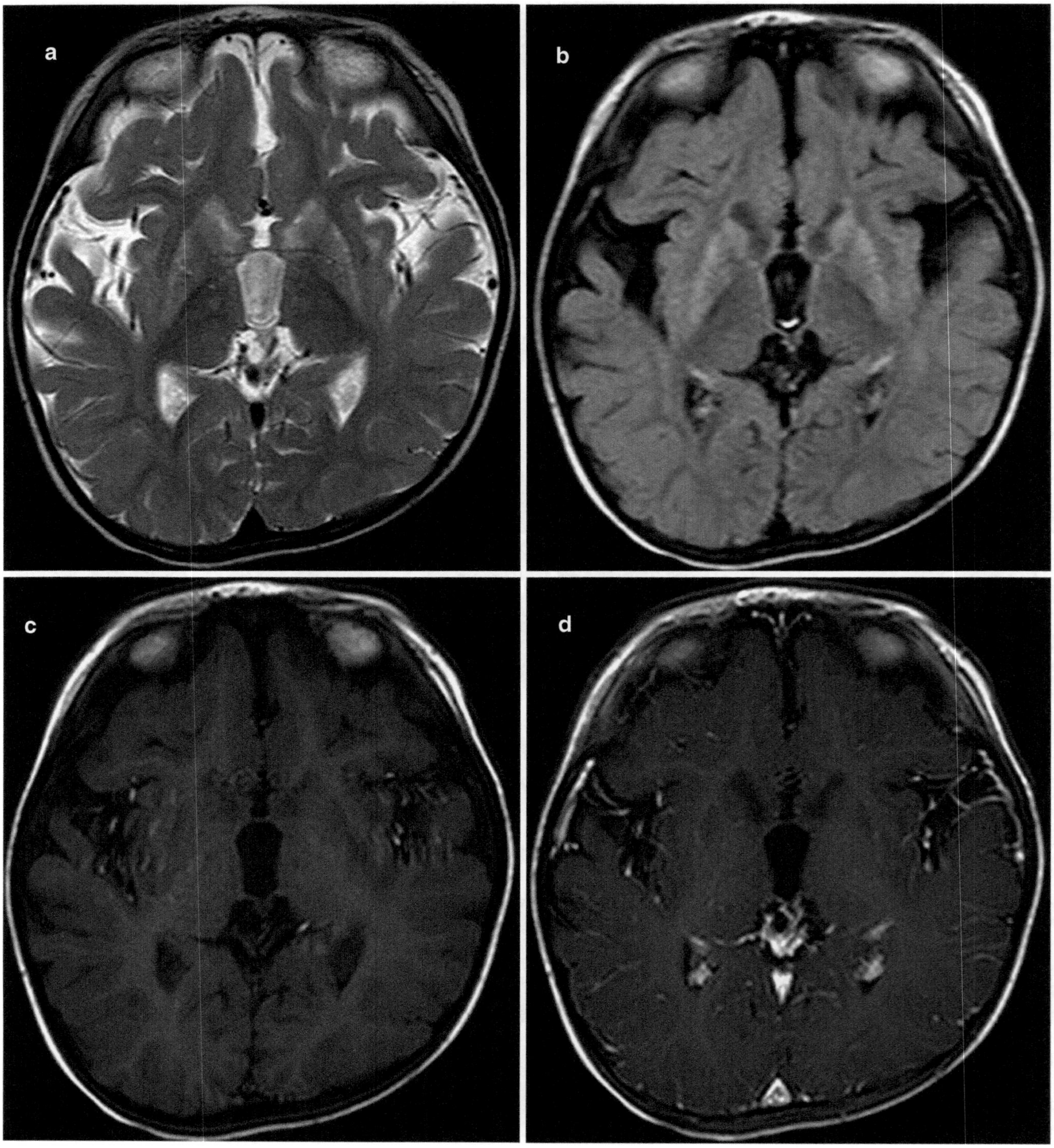

Fig. 5.18 Methylmalonic acidemia

C. Axial T1-weighted enhancement image demonstrates no enhancement (Fig. 5.19c).
D. Axial diffusion weighted image demonstrates high signal in bilateral pallidus symmetrically (Fig. 5.19d).

Discussion

Propionic Acidemia (PA) is the inborn deficiency of propionyl-CoA carboxylase that causes a failure in the catabolization of propionyl-CoA to methylmalonyl-CoA and subsequent accumulation of organic acids, and leads to multiple metabolic and neurologic abnormalities [45–47]. It is an autosomal recessive genetic disease. No special clinical manifestations were detected in PA. Most of them present in the neonatal period, and a less common group has a late-onset disease with the appearance of symptoms during the first years of life. Feeding refusal, vomiting, and abdom-

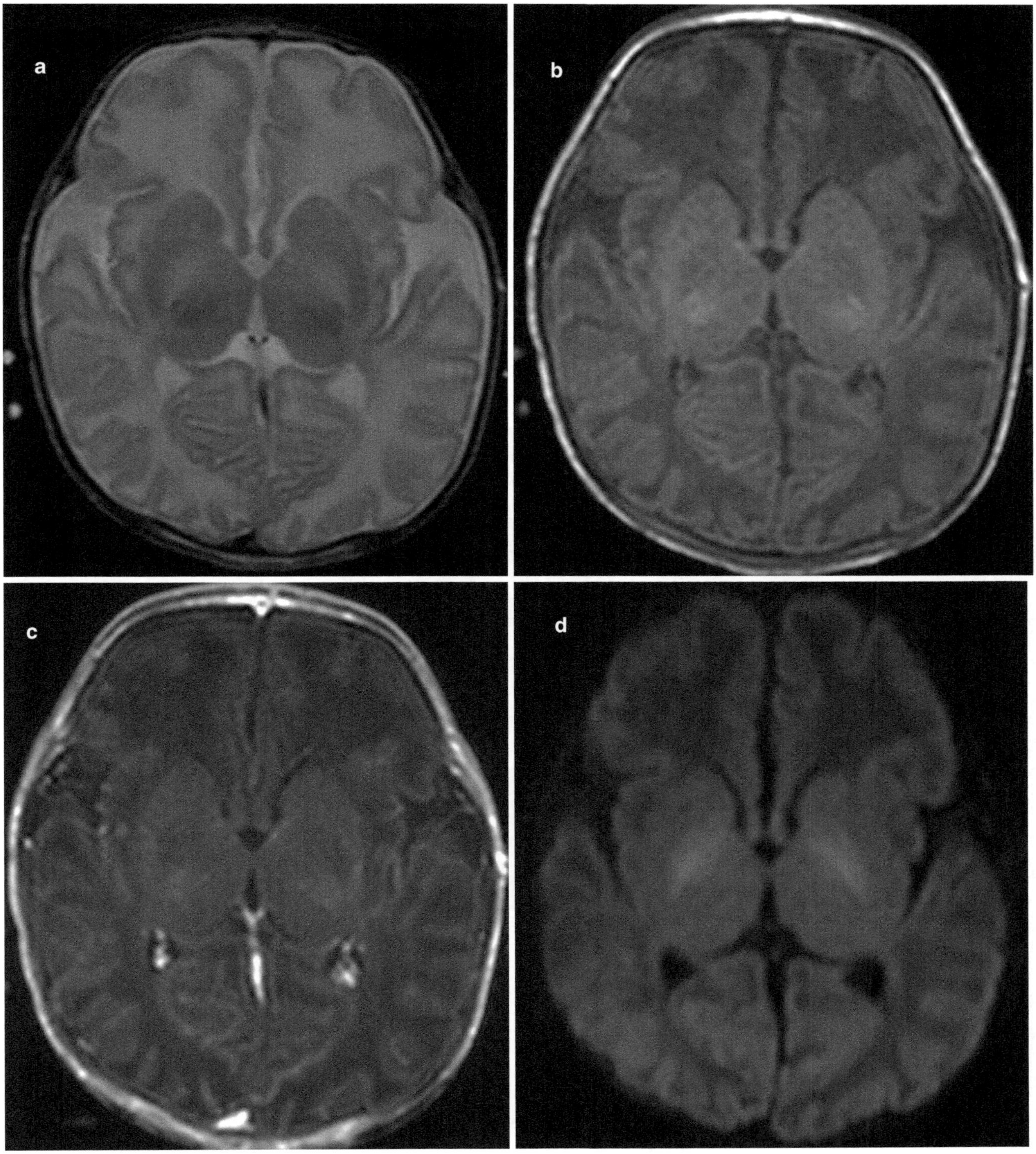

Fig. 5.19 Propionic acidemia

inal distension can be the first signs in neonatal forms [45]. Then, it deteriorates rapidly without appropriate treatment. They have a more variable presentation in late-onset forms, including psychomotor delay, failure to thrive, and vomiting. Abnormal metabolism of propionyl-CoA can lead to dysfunction of tricarboxylic acid circulation in mitochondria, and the energy of brain is insufficient. However, the metabolism of basal ganglia is vigorous and sensitive to lack of energy [47]. The basal ganglia were involved in PA [45]. Brain MRI may show abnormal signal in the globus pallidus. In general, these lesions are localized bilaterally. It shows high signal on T2WI and low signal on T1WI. The abnormal signal usually appears during acute episodes of metabolic decompensation or due to long-term poor metabolic control over time. And they were more obvious on DWI [47]. Due to the long-standing energy shortage, it remains a series of brain injuries at late disease even after dietary therapy.

Case 5.1.3.7 Glutaric Acidemia Type I

Clinical Presentation

A 6-month-old girl went into convulsions 10 days ago, with staring eyes, loss of consciousness, and no decapitation or salivation. Then, she cannot hold her head stably, and raise her hands. Increased tension of muscle. Electroencephalogram was normal. Amino acid of blood showed elevated glutaryl carnitine. Glutaric acid in urine was significantly increased.

Imaging Findings

A. Axial T2-weighted image demonstrates bilateral widened lateral fissure, atrophic temporal lobe, and high signals in bilateral lenticular and caudate nucleus (Fig. 5.20a).
B. Axial T1-weighted image demonstrates bilateral widened lateral fissure, atrophic temporal lobe, and low signals in bilateral lenticular and caudate nucleus (Fig. 5.20b).
C. Axial T2-weighted image demonstrates widened subarachnoid space of bilateral frontal tempus and parietal part (Fig. 5.20c).

Discussion

Glutaric acidemia I (GA-I) is caused by a deficiency of glutaryl-CoA dehydrogenase enzyme (GCDH), leading to

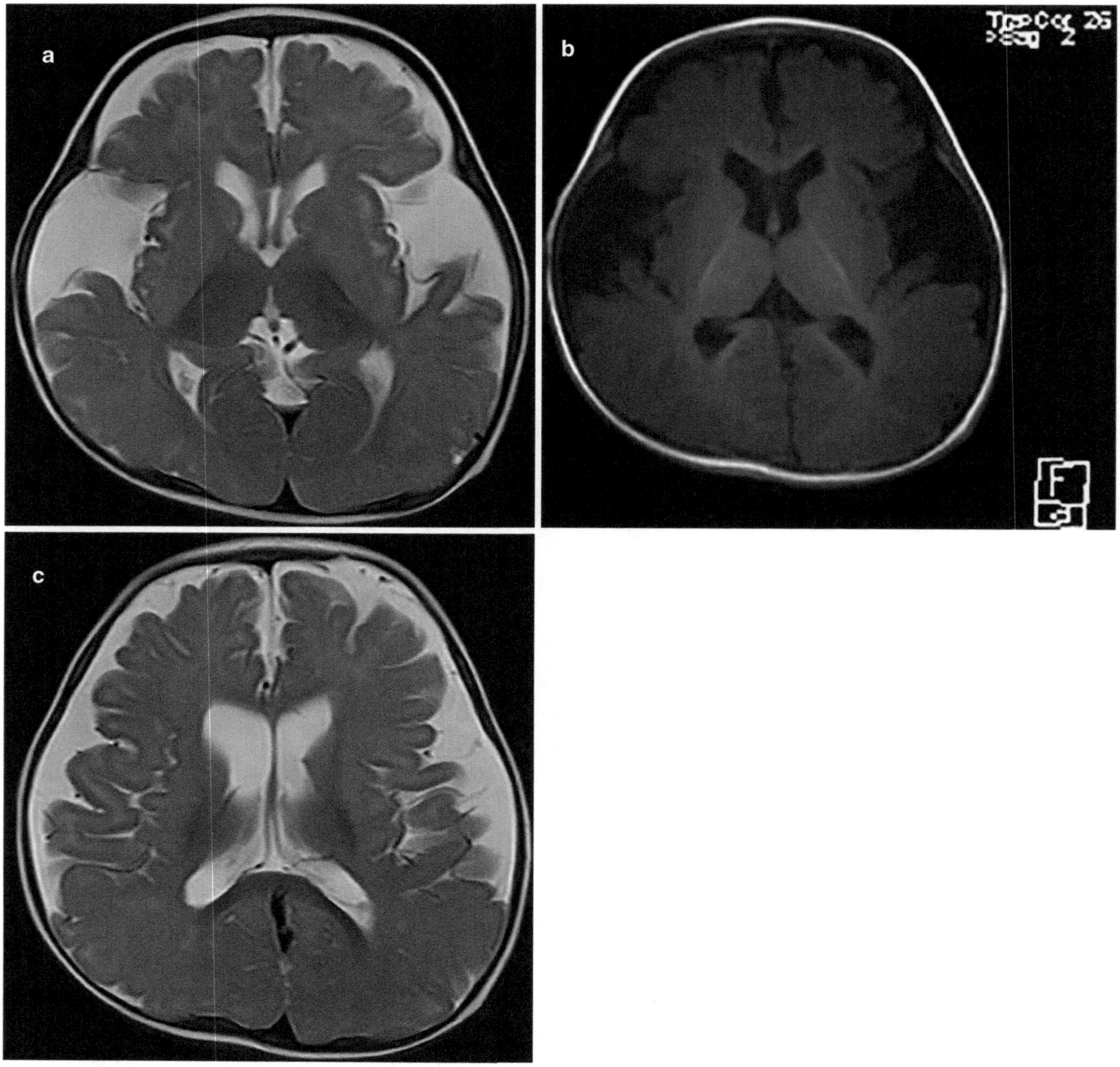

Fig. 5.20 Glutaric acidemia type I

the accumulations of several organic acids, such as glutaric acid (GA), 3-hydroxyglutaric acid (3-OH-GA), glutaconic acid, and glutarylcarnitine (C5DC), in body fluids and various organs, particularly the brain [48, 49]. And GCDH gene is located on chromosome 19p13.2, is an autosomal recessive metabolic disease [49]. Patients with GA-I are characterized by macrocephaly, frontotemporal atrophy, and acute dystonia caused by degeneration of striatum. GA-I can be manifest as acute encephalitis-like crises, induced by infection, diarrhea, immunity, and other stimuli [48, 49]. On brain MRI, the main sign is the abnormal signals on bilateral lenticular and caudate nuclei, it shows high signal on T2WI and low signal on T1WI. And the other signs include frontotemporal atrophy, widen lateral fissure pool, and outer brain space [48–50]. It has been reported that GA-I may present subdural effusion and hematoma, which may be related to frontotemporal brain atrophy and cerebrospinal fluid gap expansion, leading to mechanical injury of bridging vein.

5.1.4 Multiple Organs

Case 5.1.4.1 Mucopolysaccharidosis

Clinical Presentation

A 3-year-old boy with mental retardation for 2 years, accompanied by short stature, deformed limbs, and scoliosis.

Imaging Findings

A. The MRI horizontal axis T2WI sequence showed that bilateral white matter of the frontal lobe showed multiple cyst-like dilated perivascular spaces, bilateral lateral ventricle dilatation and abnormal signals in the parietal subcortical white matter (Fig. 5.21a).
B. The sagittal T1WI image showed multiple dilated perivascular spaces around the corpus callosum, and the odontoid soft tissue hyperplasia (arrow) and the upper cervical vertebrae stenosis (Fig. 5.21b).

Discussion

Mucopolysaccharidosis (MPS) disorders are a group of hereditary connective tissue lysosomal storage diseases. Due to the lack of lysosomal enzymes or low activity, mucopolysaccharide metabolism disorders, abnormal glycosaminoglycan (GAG) is accumulated in the lysosomes of various cells of the body. Affect the function of the tissue or organ, resulting in a series of clinical symptoms and signs such as deformed bones, hepatosplenomegaly, and mental retardation. The seven MPS types are associated with significant central nervous system (CNS) abnormalities that can manifest as impaired cognition, epilepsy, hyperactive behavior, and hydrocephalus.

MPS has characteristic neuroimaging features, and MR imaging is the best way to evaluate. Perivascular space enlargement, white matter lesions, hydrocephalus, and brain atrophy are common imaging features of MPS [51–53].

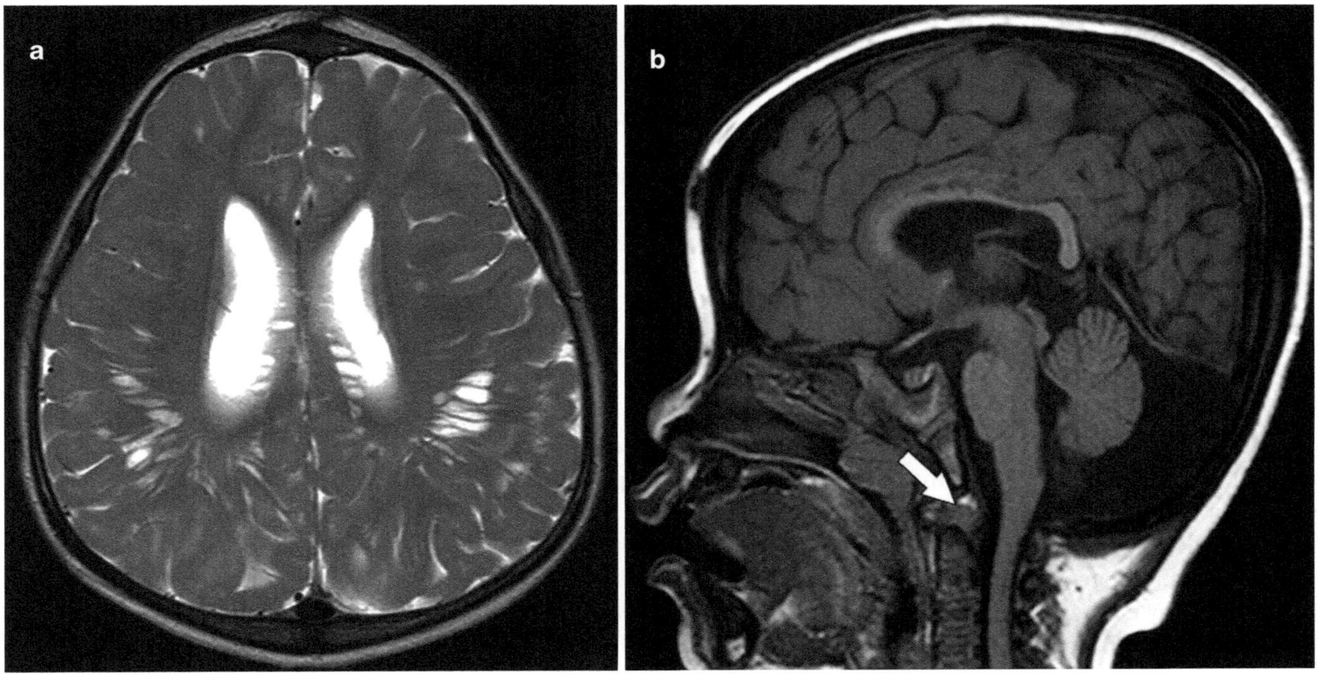

Fig. 5.21 Mucopolysaccharidosis

Enlarged perivascular space (PVS): In MR imaging, the perivascular space is similar to the CSF signal and is usually radially distributed from the subventricular zone to the cortex. The number of lesions can range from a few to a diffuse distribution, manifesting as sieving and/or fusiform cystic lesions, usually 2–8 mm in diameter. Although enlarged perivascular space can be found in the corpus callosum, basal ganglia, subcortical white matter, thalamus, or brainstem, white matter around the ventricles is the most common site of involvement. PVS expansion may be due to the deposition of GAG in the white matter that impairs the reabsorption of CSF.

White Matter Signal-Intensity Abnormalities (WMA): Changes in white matter signal abnormality are more pronounced in MPS I, II, IIIA IIIB, IIID, and VII, but less in children with MPS IV and VI. It does not become apparent until adulthood. WMA lesions can be diffuse or focal, and can occur in any area of the bilateral cerebral hemispheres, but around the ventricles are the most common sites of involvement. In MR imaging, white matter lesions are nonspecific findings, manifesting as long T1 and long T2 signal lesions. Symmetrical distribution is a common feature. White matter lesions are associated with partial degradation of GAG in neurons and oligodendrocytes in the central nervous system.

Communicating hydrocephalus: The subarachnoid space and ventricular enlargement are the main neuroradiological manifestations. The progression of ventricular enlargement is usually slow. MPS I and II typically exhibit significant ventricular enlargement, while other types of ventricular enlargement are relatively less frequent. Although the entire ventricular system is sometimes observed to expand, the involvement of the third and lateral ventricles is usually more pronounced. The subarachnoid widening occurs usually in the sella, the middle and posterior fossa, and around the optic nerve. The mechanism by which hydrocephalus is produced is that the systemic accumulation of GAG affects the function of arachnoid granules, thereby reducing the reabsorption of cerebrospinal fluid.

Brain atrophy: The main features of imaging findings are deepening of the sulci and enlargement of the cerebral fissure. It is a common neuroimaging feature of MPS development to the later stage, suggesting a poor prognosis. The deepening of the sulcus can be either symmetrical or asymmetrical, but both manifests as diffuse involvement. GAG deposition causes neuronal death and gliosis and is considered to be the main cause of the disease.

In addition to brain changes, spinal stenosis and oppressive myelopathy can occur.

Although the above imaging findings are not specific changes, it is not difficult to diagnose with typical X-ray signs of the lumbar spine, long bones of the extremities, and laboratory tests.

Normal children's brain MRI can also see the expanded Virchow-Robin spaces [51–53], the image performance is similar to MPS, but normal children do not appear white matter abnormal signals, traffic hydrocephalus, and other image changes.

Sener syndrome can also cause significant expansion of the perivascular space, but it is often accompanied by dysplasia of the corpus callosum or nodular gray matter, and has a facial deformity of the frontal dysplasia, without the cerebrospinal fluid malabsorption.

The differential diagnosis of MPS is limited, since the constellation of imaging findings is highly suggestive of the disease.

Case 5.1.4.2 Menkes Disease

Clinical Presentation

A 6-month-old boy presents with repeat convulsions for 2 months.

Imaging Findings

A. Axial T2WI showed mild cerebral atrophy in the cerebellum and cerebrum, and extensive high signal abnormalities in white matter areas (Fig. 5.22a).
B. Axial T2WI showed also abnormal high signal in bilateral thalamus and caudate nucleus (Fig. 5.22b).
C. Axial T1WI show extensive low signal abnormalities in white matter areas of cerebellum and cerebrum (Fig. 5.22c).
D. Axial T1WI showed low signal in bilateral thalamus and caudate nucleus (Fig. 5.22d).
E. MRA showing multiple contortions in bilateral anterior cerebral arteries and middle cerebral arteries (Fig. 5.22e).

Discussion

Menkes disease (MD) is a rare X chromosome-linked recessive genetic disorder, also known as curly hair syndrome, in which ATP7A gene mutation leads to abnormal copper ion absorption and metabolism in the small intestine, leading to nervous system damage. First reported by Menkes et al. [54] in 1962, the incidence was 1/(100 ~ 25 million). MD is mainly caused by male, while female is the carrier. The main cause of female disease is X chromosome one autosomal replacement or XX/XO inlay [55].

The clinical manifestations of MD are mainly epilepsy, hypotonia, lag of motor development, hair frizz, and cognitive dysfunction in early infancy, and hypochromic brittle curl is an important characteristic of the disease. The levels of serum copper and/or ceruloplasmin decreased in children with MD. Most patients die within the first 3 years of life.

The typical magnetic resonance imaging (MRI) findings of MD [56] are progressive cerebral atrophy, cerebellar atro-

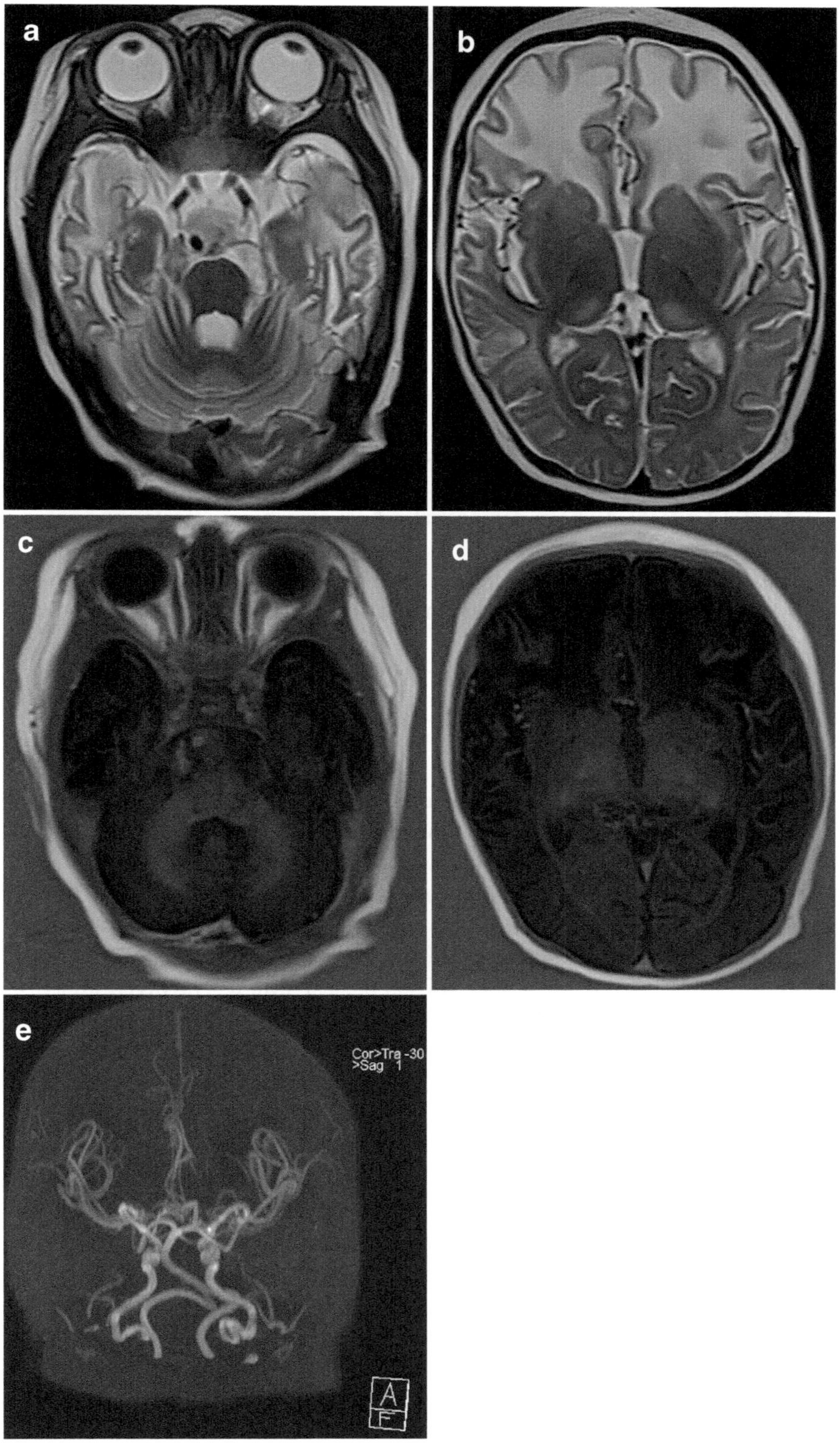

Fig. 5.22 Menkes disease

phy, subdural hematoma or effusion, and cerebrovascular wavy tortuosity. Abnormalities in white matter signaling can precede brain atrophy, usually first occurring in the temporal lobe. Abnormal signals of different degrees in bilateral cerebellar and cerebellar white matter regions, with low signal on T1WI and high signal on T2WI. The lesions may involve bilateral basal ganglia, and the lesions are symmetrical or asymmetric. As the disease progresses, softening foci appeared in the white matter area of the brain.

The main differential diagnosis of DM is encephalitis, ischemic encephalopathy, and other metabolic diseases [57]. The diagnosis of DM depends on genetic testing.

5.2 Toxic and Metabolic Encephalopathy

Case 5.2.1 Wernicke's Encephalopathy

Clinical Presentation

A 13-month-old girl, she cannot crawl, decreased tension of muscle. The ability to interact is backward and regressive. Eye movement disorder, and there are tremors in the limbs and head. Vitamin B1 was deficient.

Imaging Findings

A. Axial T2-weighted image demonstrates high signals in cerebral peduncle and periaqueductal gray (Fig. 5.23a).
B. Axial T2-weighted image demonstrates high signals in periaqueductal gray (Fig. 5.23b).
C. Axial T2-weighted image demonstrates high signals in bilateral thalamus (Fig. 5.23c).
D. Axial T2-weighted fluid-attenuated inversion recovery image demonstrates high signals in bilateral thalamus (Fig. 5.23d).
E. Axial T1-weighted image demonstrates low signals in bilateral thalamus (Fig. 5.23e).

Discussion

Wernicke's encephalopathy (WE) is an acute neuropsychiatric syndrome caused by deficiency of thiamine (vitamin B1) [58–60]. Alcoholism is the most common cause. Children's case is rarely seen at present and often misdiagnosed due to atypical clinical manifestations. If it cannot be treated in time, it can cause severe neurological sequelae and even death [58]. About one-third of WE patients present with a characteristic triad, including eye movement disorder, ataxia, mental and consciousness disorders. But the clinical symptoms of children patients are atypical, they show hypothermia and aphonia [58]. MRI is considered to be the most valuable auxiliary examination for diagnosing WE, with a specificity of 93% and sensitivity of 53%. Typical MRI showed abnormal symmetrical signals around of bilateral medial thalamus, midbrain aqueduct, papillary body, tetras, third and fourth ventricles, with low signal on T1WI, high signal on T2WI and hyperintensity on T2WI-FLAIR, no enhancement [58–60]. The early pathological changes of WE were cytotoxic edema and vasogenic edema. So, if it is identified in time and treated with vitamin B1, the symptoms can be quickly relieved and the prognosis is good [58].

Case 5.2.2 Toxic Encephalopathy

Clinical Presentation

A 7-year-old boy was detected unconscious in the shower, when used a gas water heater. Then, he was diagnosed with carbon monoxide (CO) poisoning.

Imaging Findings

A. Axial T2-weighted image demonstrates high signals in bilateral lenticular nucleus, caudate nucleus, and cerebral cortex (Fig. 5.24a).
B. Axial T2-weighted fluid-attenuated inversion recovery image demonstrates high signals in bilateral lenticular nucleus, caudate nucleus, and cerebral cortex (Fig. 5.24b).
C. Axial T1-weighted fluid-attenuated inversion recovery image demonstrates low signals in bilateral lenticular nucleus, caudate nucleus, and cerebral cortex (Fig. 5.24c).

Discussion

Toxic encephalopathy refers to a group of diseases with central nervous system damage as the main clinical manifestation caused by various toxic substances poisoning. Carbon monoxide (CO) poisoning is one of the most common causes of morbidity due to toxicity. Patients with CO poisoning present with mild symptoms such as headache and nausea and may progress to coma and death clinically. The history of CO exposure makes an important role in the diagnosis of acute CO poisoning. On brain MRI, CO poisoning usually causes ischemic lesions in the bilateral globus pallidus of the basal ganglia, various sites including corpus callosum, thalamus, hippocampus, periventricular white matter, and cerebral cortex may be involved [61–63]. It shows high signals on T2WI and T2WI-FLAIR, low signals on T1WI [61–63]. According to literature report, diffusion-weighted imaging (DWI) can play an important role to detect the involved areas [61]. Diffuse brain atrophy and cerebral white matter demyelination are delayed manifestations of CO poisoning. At present, symmetrical degeneration and necrosis of bilateral globus pallidum are considered as the characteristic imaging manifestation of CO poisoning, but it is not specific. And the globus pallidus lesions in many cases do not correlate directly to clinical status and outcome [61]. However, the presence of diffuse white matter disease is a more reliable index of both.

Case 5.2.3 Pseudohypoparathyroidism

Clinical Presentation

A 13-year-old boy presented to the hospital for motor retardation. He has no history of premature delivery and perinatal asphyxia.

Imaging Findings

A. CT shows the high density in bilateral basal ganglia regions and frontal lobe, which suggested calcification (Fig. 5.25a).

Fig. 5.23 Wernicke's encephalopathy

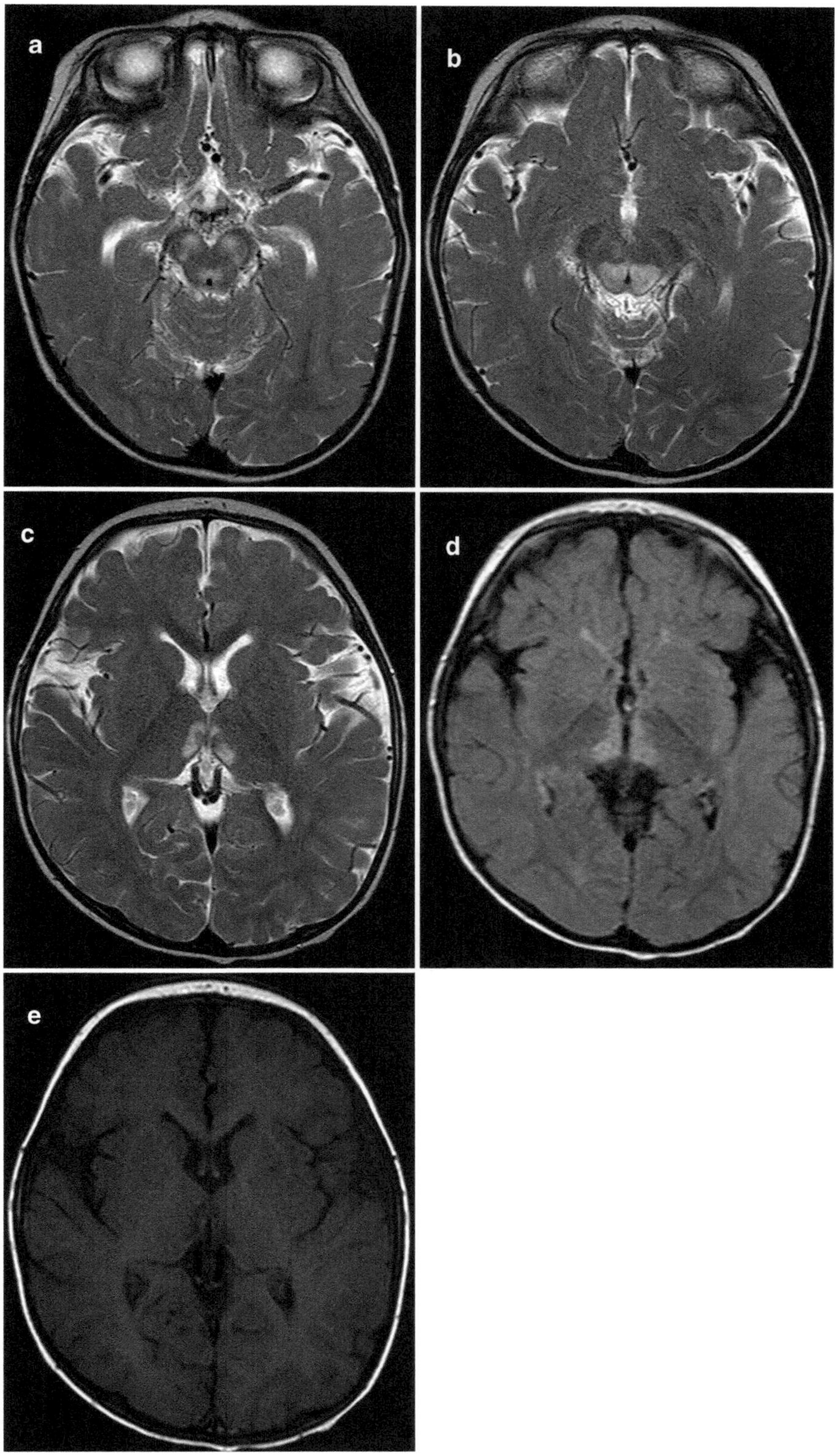

B. CT shows the high density in bilateral basal ganglia regions and frontal lobe, which suggested calcification (Fig. 5.25b).
C. T1WI shows mild swelling and abnormal high signal in bilateral basal ganglia regions (Fig. 5.25c).
D. CE-T1WI sequence shows no enhancement in bilateral basal ganglia regions (Fig. 5.25d).
E. T1WI shows mild swelling and abnormal high signal in bilateral basal ganglia regions (Fig. 5.25e).

Discussion

Pseudohypoparathyroidism (PHP) is not a true parathyroid deficiency, but the effector organs such as kidneys, bones, and digestive organs, do not respond to parathyroid hormone

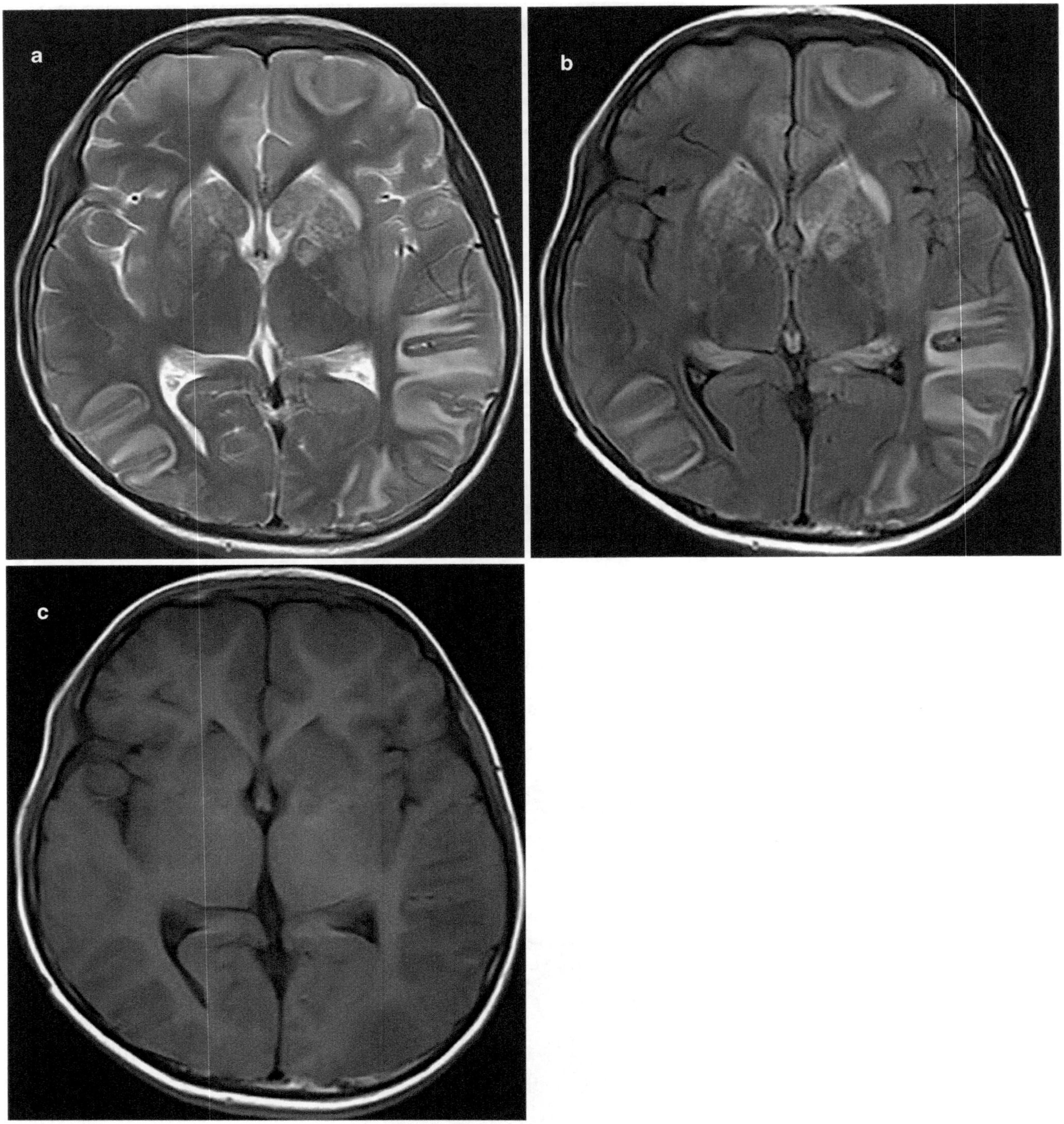

Fig. 5.24 Toxic encephalopathy

or are anti-parathyroid hormones [64]. Genetic disease is caused by mutations in the GNASI gene. It is characterized by low serum calcium, high serum phosphorus, and not low parathyroid hormone. It also is a rare neurodegenerative disease of autosomal inheritance.

The 69% of Albright hereditary osteodystrophy (AHO) in PHP I show the growth hormone (GH) deficiency, which is also the cause of AHO of short stature and obesity. The PHP is more common in women, the average age of onset is 8.5 years.

The PHP is characterized by frequent convulsions, extrapyramidal symptom damage, hypophrenia, dwarf, and obesity. The clinical classification of Pseudohypoparathyroidism can be divided into PHP I and PHP II. The PHP I is due to the PTH receptor defects on the cell membrane of the target organs (bone and kidney), the nephrogenic cAMP, and urine phosphate unresponsive after exogenous PTH stimulation. The PHP II does not have a definite genetic and family foundation.

Fig. 5.25 Pseudohypoparathyroidism

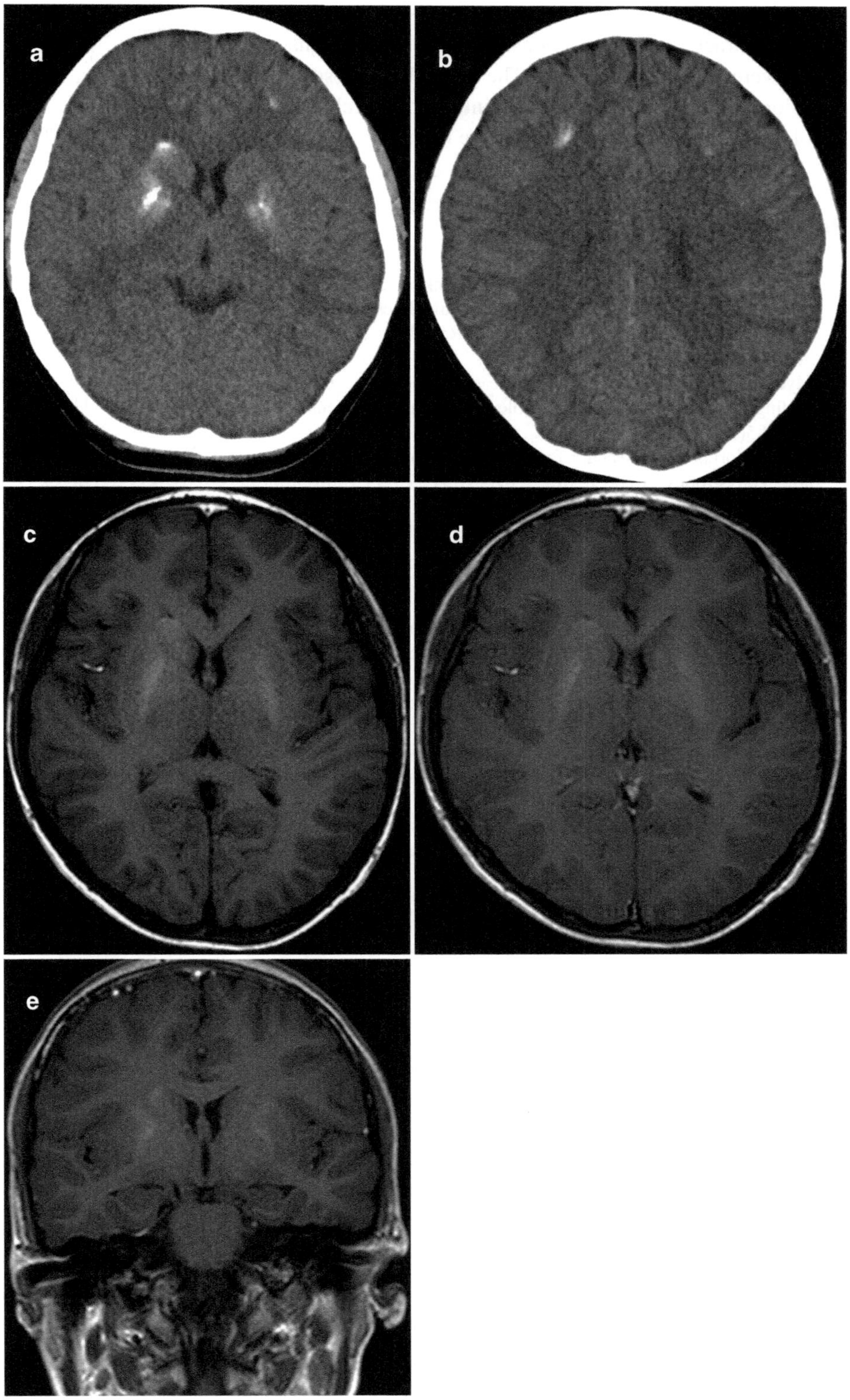

CT shows the high density in bilateral basal ganglia regions, subcortical white matter, and cerebellum, which suggested calcification. The basal ganglia region's calcification is inverted V sign. T1WI sequence shows high signal, T2WI and T2WI-FLAIR sequences show isointense signal in bilateral basal ganglia regions, and no enhancement after administration of contrast. The X-ray showed that the fourth metacarpal bone and the first metacarpal bone in the left hand were relatively short and without bone destruction.

The disease needs to be differentiated from Fahr Disease and tuberous sclerosis. The Fahr Disease shows normal serum calcium and serum phosphorus and without Albright hereditary osteodystrophy. Tuberous sclerosis also showed multiple intracranial calcifications, but the shape and distribution were irregular on the CT. The clinical manifestations were cortical adenoma, epilepsy and intellectual decline, and the blood calcium and phosphorus were normal.

References

1. Engelen M, Kemp S, Visser MD, et al. X-linked adrenoleukodystrophy (X-ALD): clinical presentation and guidelines for diagnosis, follow-up and management. Orphanet J Rare Dis. 2012;7(1):51. https://doi.org/10.1186/1750-1172-7-51.
2. Myers KA, Rho JM, Wei X-C. Teaching neuroimages: MRI findings in X-linked adrenoleukodystrophy. Neurology. 2015;85(17):e132–3.
3. Zhu J, Florian E, Alessandra B, et al. The changing face of adrenoleukodystrophy. Endocr Rev. 2020;41(4):577–93. https://doi.org/10.1210/endrev/bnaa013.
4. Liberato AP, Mallack EJ, Aziz-Bose R, et al. MRI brain lesions in asymptomatic boys with X-linkedadrenoleukodystrophy. Neurology. 2019;92:e1–e11. https://doi.org/10.1212/WNL.0000000000007294.
5. Biffi A, Lucchini G, Rovelli A, Sessa M. Metachromatic leukodystrophy: an overview of current and prospective treatments. Bone Marrow Transplant. 2008;42:S2–6.
6. Sener RN, Metachromatic leukodystrophy. Diffusion MR imaging and proton MR spectroscopy. Acta Radiol. 2003;44:440–3.
7. Seidl Z, Vaneckova M, Vitak T. Metachromatic leukodystrophy: magnetic resonance imaging (diffusion weighted image—DWI). Neuroendocrinol Lett. 2008;29:428.
8. Messing A. Chapter 44—Alexander's disease. In: Geschwind DH, Paulson HL, Klein C, editors. Handbook of clinical neurology. Elsevier; 2018. p. 693–700.
9. Leone P, et al. Long-term follow-up after gene therapy for canavan disease. Sci Transl Med. 2012;4(165):165ra163.
10. Wolfgang KH. Leukodystrophies with late disease onset: an update. Curr Opin Neurol. 2010;23(3):234–41.
11. Muthusamy K, Sudhakar SV, Thomas M, et al. Revisiting magnetic resonance imaging pattern of Krabbe disease—lessons from an Indian cohort. J Clin Imaging Sci. 2019;9:25.
12. Hwang M, Zuccoli G, Panigrahy A, Rodriguez D, Poe MD, Escolar ML. Thickening of the cauda equina roots: a common finding in Krabbe disease. Eur Radiol. 2016;26:3377–82.
13. Li H, et al. Gene suppressing therapy for Pelizaeus-Merzbacher disease using artificial microRNA. JCI Insight. 2019;4(10):e125052.
14. Barness LA. The metabolic and molecular bases of inherited disease, 7th ed.C.R. Scriver, A.L. Beaudet, W.S. Sly, D. Valle, Vol. 3, McGraw Hill, New York, 1995, pp. 4605. Am J Med Genet. 1996;66(1):87.
15. Leegwater P, et al. Identification of novel mutations in MLC1 responsible for megalencephalic leukoencephalopathy with subcortical cysts. Hum Genet. 2002;111(1):114.
16. Bu S, Zhu Y, Xiao J, et al. MRI features of phenylketonuria in brain. Chin J Med Imag Technol. 2017;33(12):1802–5. https://doi.org/10.13929/j.1003-3289.201703118.
17. Writing Group For Practice Guidelines For Diagnosis And Treatment Of Genetic Diseases Medical Genetics Branch Of Chinese Medical Association, Huang S, Song F. [Clinical practice guidelines for phenylketonuria]. Zhonghua Yi Xue Yi Chuan Xue Za Zhi. 2020:37(3):226–34. https://doi.org/10.3760/cma.j.issn.1003-9406.2020.03.002.
18. Karimzadeh P, Ahmadabadi F, Jafari N, et al. Study on MRI changes in phenylketonuria in patients referred to mofid hospital/Iran. Iran J Child Neurol. 2014;8(2):53–6.
19. Sadek AA, Hassan MH, Mohammed NA. Clinical and neuropsychological outcomes for children with phenylketonuria in upper Egypt; a single-center study over 5 years. Neuropsychiatr Dis Treat. 2018;14:2551–61. https://doi.org/10.2147/NDT.S176198.
20. Wang X, Yu YQ, Qian YF, et al. Diagnostic value of conventional MRI and ~1H-MRS in brain lesions caused by PKU in children. J Clin Radiol. 2011;10:1515–8. https://doi.org/10.1111/j.1600-0714.2011.01024.x.
21. Pavlakis SG, Phillips PC, Dimauro S, et al. Mitochondrial myopathy, encephalopathy, lactic acidosis, and strokelike episodes: a distinctive clinical syndrome. Ann Neurol. 1984;16(4):481–8.
22. Iizuka T, Sakai F. Pathogenesis of stroke-like episodes in MELAS: analysis of neurovascular cellular mechanisms. Curr Neurovasc Res. 2005;2(1):29–45.
23. Malhotra K, Liebeskind DS. Imaging of MELAS. Curr Pain Headache Rep. 2016;20(9):54.
24. Wang XY, Noguchi K, Takashima S, et al. Serial diffusion-weighted imaging in a patient with MELAS and presumed cytotoxic oedema. Neuroradiology. 2003;45(9):640–3.
25. Barkovich AJ, Good WV, Koch TK, et al. Mitochondrial disorders: analysis of their clinical and imaging characteristics. Am J Neuroradiol. 1993;14(5):1119.
26. Yuwu J, Yihui H, Jiong Q, et al. Clinical, neuropathological and molecular genetics research of Leigh syndrome in children. Chin J Pediatr. 2001;06:13–7.
27. Xiaolu T, Yanqiu L, Xiaojuan T, et al. Brain MRI imaging features and diagnosis of Leigh syndrome in children. J Med Imag. 2019;29(02):178–83.
28. Frydman M, et al. Assignment of the gene for Wilson disease to chromosome 13: linkage to the esterase D locus. Proc Natl Acad Sci U S A. 1985;82(6):1819–21.
29. Bowcock AM, et al. Refining the position of Wilson disease by linkage disequilibrium with polymorphic microsatellites. Am J Hum Genet. 1994;54(1):79–87.
30. Batla A, et al. Deconstructing Fahr's disease/syndrome of brain calcification in the era of new genes. Parkinsonism Relat Disord. 2017;37:1–10.
31. Gordon N. Pantothenate kinase-associated neurodegeneration (Hallervorden–Spatz syndrome). European Journal of Paediatric Neurology Ejpn Official Journal of the European Paediatric Neurology Society. 2002;6(5):243–7.
32. Hayflick SJ, et al. Genetic, clinical, and radiographic delineation of Hallervorden-Spatz syndrome. N Engl J Med. 2003;348(1):33–40.
33. Laugel V, et al. Mutation update for the CSB/ERCC6 and CSA/ERCC8 genes involved in Cockayne syndrome. Hum Mutat. 2010;31(2):113–26.
34. Brunetti-Pierri N, Scaglia F. GM1 gangliosidosis: review of clinical, molecular, and therapeutic aspects. Mol Genet Metab. 2008;94:391–6.
35. Chen CY, Zimmerman RA, Lee CC, Chen FH, Yuh YS, Hsiao HS. Neuroimaging findings in late infantile GM1 gangliosidosis. AJNR Am J Neuroradiol. 1998;19:1628–30.
36. De Grandis E, Di Rocco M, Pessagno A, Veneselli E, Rossi A. MR imaging findings in 2 cases of late infantile GM1 gangliosidosis. AJNR Am J Neuroradiol. 2009;30:1325–7.
37. Autti T, Joensuu R, Aberg L. Decreased T2 signal in the thalami may be a sign of lysosomal storage disease. Neuroradiology. 2007;49:571–8.
38. Jain A, Jagdeesh K, Mane R, et al. Imaging in classic form of maple syrup urine disease: a rare metabolic central nervous system. J Clin Neonatol. 2013;2(2):98–100.

39. Shah T, Purohit S, Raval M. Imaging in maple syrup urine disease. Indian J Pediatr. 2018;85(10):927–8.
40. Ailan C, Lianshu H, Yun F, et al. MRI and clinical features of maple syrup urine disease: preliminary results in 10 cases. Diagn Interv Radiol. 2017;23(5):398–402.
41. Li Y, Liu X, Duan CF, et al. Brain magnetic resonance imaging findings and radiologic review of maple syrup urine disease: report of three cases. World J Clin Cases. 2021;9(8):1844–52. https://doi.org/10.12998/wjcc.v9.i8.1844.
42. Karimzadeh P, Jafari N, Ahmad AF, et al. Methylmalonic acidemia: diagnosis and neuroimaging findings of this neurometabolic disorder (an Iranian pediatric case series). Iran J Child Neurol. 2013;7(3):63–6.
43. Baker EH, Sloan JL, Hauser NS, et al. MRI characteristics of globus pallidus infarcts in isolated methylmalonic acidemia. AJNR Am J Neuroradiol. 2015;36(1):194–201.
44. Baumgartner MR, Hörster F, Dionisi-Vici C, et al. Proposed guidelines for the diagnosis and management of methylmalonic and propionic acidemia. Orphanet J Rare Dis. 2014;9(1):130.
45. Pfeifer CM, Van Tassel DC, Miller JH. Unique neuroradiological findings in propionic acidemia. Radiol Case Rep. 2018;13(6):1207–11.
46. Kandel A, Amatya SK, Yeh EA. Reversible diffusion weighted imaging changes in propionic acidemia. J Child Neurol. 2013;28(1):128–31.
47. Leonard JV. Propionic acidemia. Berlin: Springer; 2009.
48. Zayed H, El Khayat H, Tomoum H, et al. Clinical, biochemical, neuroradiological and molecular characterization of Egyptian patients with glutaric acidemia type 1. Metab Brain Dis. 2019;34(4):1231–41. https://doi.org/10.1007/s11011-019-00422-3.
49. Chen YC, Huang CY, Lee YT, et al. Audiological and otologic manifestations of glutaric aciduria type I. Orphanet J Rare Dis. 2020;15(1):337. https://doi.org/10.1186/s13023-020-01571-w.
50. Tsai FC, Lee HJ, Wang AG, et al. Experiences during newborn screening for glutaric aciduria type 1: diagnosis, treatment, genotype, phenotype, and outcomes. J Chin Med Assoc. 2017;80(4):253–61. https://doi.org/10.1016/j.jcma.2016.07.006.
51. Matheus MG, Castillo M, Smith JK, Armao D, Towle D, Muenzer J. Brain MRI findings in patients with mucopolysaccharidosis types I and II and mild clinical presentation. Neuroradiology. 2004;46:666–72.
52. Rasalkar DD, Chu WCW, Hui J, Chu C, Paunipagar BK, Li C. Pictorial review of mucopolysaccharidosis with emphasis on MRI features of brain and spine. Br J Radiol. 2011;84:469–77.
53. Zafeiriou DI, Batzios SP. Brain and spinal MR imaging findings in mucopolysaccharidoses: a review. AJNR Am J Neuroradiol. 2013;34:5–13.
54. Menkes JH, Alter M, Steigleder GK, et al. A sex-linked recessive disorder with retardation of growth, peculiar hair, and focal cerebral and cerebellar degeneration. Pediatrics. 1962;29:764–79.
55. Moore CM, Howell RR. Ectodermal manifestations in Menkes disease. Clin Genet. 1985;28:532–40.
56. Tayal A, Elwadhi A, Sharma S, et al. An unusual presentation of menkes disease masquerading as a leukodystrophy with macrocephaly. J Pediatr Neurosci. 2020;15(1):57–9.
57. Wei Z, Wei Z, Ming Y, et al. Comparative analysis of intracranial MRI findings and genetic mutation types in Menkes disease. Radiol Pract. 2020;35(12):1595–8.
58. Song Y, Zhang Y, Guo PB, et al. Clinical features, diagnosis and treatment of children's Wernicke's encephalopathy. Neuro Quantol. 2018;16(5):35–8.
59. Jan K. Wernicke encephalopathy: (MRI) picture worth a thousand words. Oxf Med Case Reports. 2018;5:147–9.
60. Patel S, Topiwala K, Hudson L. Wernicke's encephalopathy. Cureus. 2018;10(8):e3187. https://doi.org/10.7759/cureus.3187.
61. Khanal A, Thapa S, Chhetri PK. Conventional brain MRI in carbon monoxide poisoning. JNMA J Nepal Med Assoc. 2015;53(199):197–9.
62. Kim DM, Lee IH, Park JY, et al. Acute carbon monoxide poisoning: MR imaging findings with clinical correlation. Diagn Interv Imaging. 2016:S2211568416302649.
63. Yasmin D, Bita D, Reza A, et al. Structural findings in the brain MRI of patients with acute carbon monoxide poisoning. Asia Pac J Med Toxicol. 2014;3(3):124–9.
64. Mantovani G, et al. Diagnosis and management of pseudohypoparathyroidism and related disorders: first international consensus statement. Nat Rev Endocrinol. 2018;497:1.

Craniocerebral Trauma

6

Hong Yu and Jingshi Wang

Craniocerebral Trauma are the most common cause of morbidity and mortality in children. Head trauma alone, or in combination with injuries to other organs, is responsible for 50% of deaths in children from the ages of 1–14 years. In infants younger than 2 years, the most common causes of head trauma are the infant being dropped, and nonaccidental trauma (NAT) (e.g., Shaken Baby Syndrome and Infant Abuse Syndrome). NAT accounts for more than 80% of deaths from head trauma in this group. Skull fractures, subdural hematomas, cerebral edema, and parenchymal contusions are common injuries before the age of 2 years. In children older than 3 years of age, falls, sporting activities and motor vehicle accidents are the most common causes of head trauma. Fractures, parenchymal contusions diffuse axonal injury (DAI) are the most common injuries in this group [1].

Case 6.1 Neonatal Craniocerebral Trauma

Clinical Presentation

A female infant, 3 days old, was delivered with the help of forceps due to prolonged second stage of labor. Fetal distress and neonatal asphyxia occurred during the delivery.

Imaging Findings

A. Axial T1-weighted image demonstrates left frontal-parietal subdural hematoma (high signal) (Fig. 6.1a).
B. Axial T2-weighted image demonstrates the hematoma was hypointense (Fig. 6.1b).
C. Axial Susceptibility-weighted image a small amount of subarachnoid hemorrhage in sagittal sinus and tentorium cerebellum (Fig. 6.1c).
D. Axial T1-weighted image demonstrates scalp hematoma (Fig. 6.1d).

H. Yu · J. Wang (✉)
Department of Medical Imaging, Dalian Women and Children's Medical Center (Group), Dalian, Liaoning, China

Discussion

Neonatal craniocerebral trauma is often caused by birth injury, and it refers to the brain injury caused by mechanical factors to the fetus or newborn during the delivery. The incidence rate is 0.1–0.7%. Since the newborn still has immature development in the central nervous system and adjacent skulls during childbirth, the pathological and imaging findings of this type of craniocerebral trauma are unique.

Extracranial Trauma

Extracranial trauma includes three types: scalp hematoma, subarachnoid hematoma, and head hematoma. Scalp hematoma often occurs after vaginal delivery, and it is soft textured and superficial; it can span across the cranial suture, and gradually disappear within a few days after birth. The subarachnoid hematoma occurs below the occipital or frontal muscles. The subaponeurotic hematoma is hard textured, with a fluctuation sensation, and the lesions gradually disappear after 2–3 weeks. The aforementioned two types generally do not require imaging examination. The head hematoma is a post-traumatic subperiosteal hematoma, which is often caused by the delivery with obstetric forceps. It is located below the outer layer of the periosteum, does not span across the cranial suture, and occurs mostly in the parietal, occipital, and tibial bones. The ossification process of the subperiosteal hematoma of the skull is: no visible calcification, peripheral calcification, shell-like calcification, all calcification, and ossification. Pathological evolution and CT findings: 1 week ago, the CT shows the sickle- or bump-like soft tissue density shadows, attached to the outer plate of the skull, at a slightly higher density, with clear demarcation between the outer border of hematoma and the scalp. One week thereafter, multiple bone resorption areas are seen in the skull below the hematoma, and the thickness of the skull is approximately normal. Three weeks thereafter, the hematoma became harder. The hematoma pseudocapsule and the lifted cranial periosteum became calcified. The CT findings presented an arc-like shape and shell-like high-density shadows. Two months thereafter, the pseudocapsule and perios-

H. Liu, X. Zhang (eds.), *Pediatric Neuroimaging*, https://doi.org/10.1007/978-981-16-7928-5_6

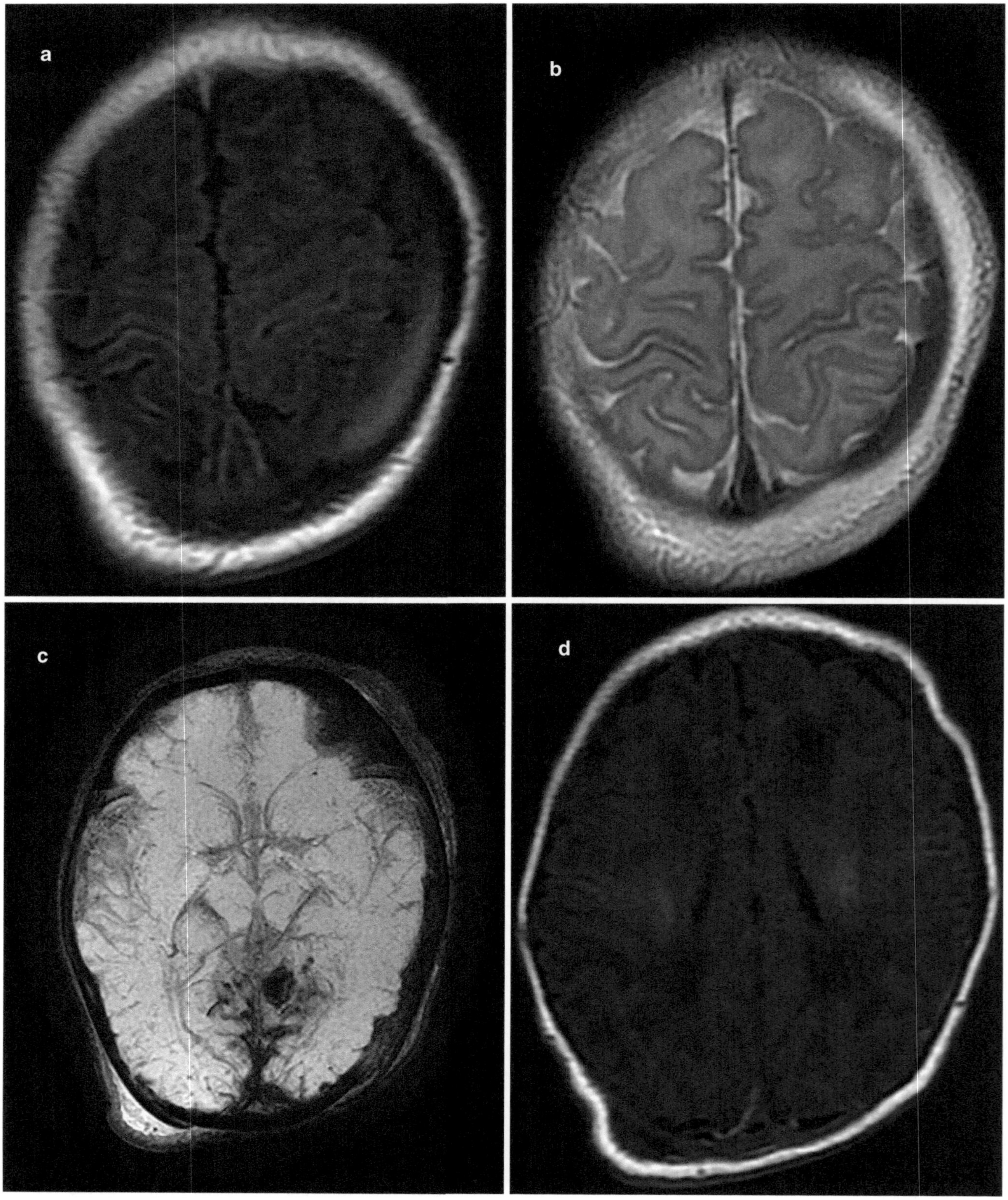

Fig. 6.1 Neonatal craniocerebral trauma

teal calcifications are more obvious. Four months thereafter, the hematoma capsules are completely calcified and ossified. The CT shows the inner border of the calcified foci (cranium) and the outer border (calcified lifted periosteum), which show the convex lens-like or sandwich biscuit-like double-layer structure.

Skull Fractures
Neonatal skull fractures are often linear and depressed fractures. Linear fractures often occur in the parietal or frontal bone, and if there is no displacement, the fracture can heal itself without any treatment. Depressed fractures are often caused by the compression of the fetal head and pelvis during labor or the use of forceps. CT can accurately determine the degree of displacement of the depressed fracture. Skull fractures occasionally have a concomitant dural tear, and the meningeal and cerebral tissue break into the fracture fissures, making it impossible for osteoblasts to span across the fracture and prevent fracture from healing.

Intracranial Hemorrhage
Mechanical injury during childbirth usually leads to subdural hematoma, epidural hematoma, subarachnoid hemorrhage, and intraventricular hemorrhage. Subdural hemorrhage is common and induced by subdural laceration due to head deformation during childbirth. Subdural hemorrhage is divided into four categories: cerebellar tear, occipital separation, cerebral falx tear, and bridging venous tear on the surface of brain. Both cerebellar tentorium tear and occipital separation can lead to subdural hemorrhage in the posterior cranial fossa. A severe cerebellar tear causes a rupture of the Galen vein, the straight sinus, or the transverse sinus, which eventually causes a large amount of subdural hemorrhage. CT shows increased density and thickening of the affected cerebellum, with the high-density shadows extending downward, and it is located at the posterior region of the cerebellar hemisphere. The lesion shows a better display at the coronal and sagittal planes, and the hematoma is located under the cerebellum. Since the cerebral falx tear and the superficial venous rupture of the brain often lead to subdural hematoma on the cerebellar tentorium. CT and MRI coronal images are helpful in assessing the actual size and involvement extent of subdural hematoma.

Case 6.2 Infant Brain Trauma

Clinical Presentation
A baby boy, 10 months old. Four days earlier, the infant fell accidentally from his bed at home and hit his head to bedside with occiput. After injury, the infant developed apathy, limb jerking, and vomiting. Investigation: brudzinski (−) Kernig (−), Babinski (−); Right sided muscle strength was slightly reduced (grade 4).

Imaging Findings
A. CT showed uneven highdensity shadow (Fig. 6.2a).
B. Axial T1-weighted image demonstrates high signal (Fig. 6.2b).
C. Axial T1-weighted image demonstrates low signal (Fig. 6.2c).
D. Diffusion weighted image demonstrates a large area of patchy hyperintense shadow in the left occipital lobe along the course of the cerebral white matter, (Fig. 6.2d).
E. Axial Susceptibility-weighted image demonstrates left parietal frontal sulcus is blurred Subarachnoid hemorrhage (Fig. 6.2e)
F. Axial T1-weighted enhanced scan demonstrates showed no obvious abnormalities (Fig. 6.2f).

Discussion
Cerebral traumas of infants are similar to that of adults, but their causes between them are very different, which include occasional and non-occasional ones, with their proportion being 1:10–15. The severe occasional traumas are common in the elder, and rare in babyhood [2, 3].

Skull fractures, according to shapes of fractures, can be divided into several kinds including parting from the cranial sutures (normal cranial suture reaches 2 mm), linear fracture (rupture of internal and external plates of the skull), denting fracture (denting fracture of the skull plate, which needs to measure the denting degree), comminuted fracture (there often are shifting of fractured pieces and intracranial injuries and fracture of skull base).

In intracranial hematomas, epidural hematomas result mainly from rupture of emissary veins, venous sinus, and diploic veins. By CT examination, shuttle-like high-density shadows with sharp edges can be found. And in the hematomas, low-density areas can sometimes be seen, which hints that there exists bleeding or oriented bleeding. Subdural hematomas result from injuries of cortical pontine veins, which occur in the convex surface of the brain, most emerge in the top of the forehead, among of which 80% can harm both sides of it, which are manifested as crescent high-density areas by CT examination, and by MRI examination, which are different with duration of foci. In the phase of hematomas, signals like T1WI resulting from deoxygenated hemoglobin in red blood cells emerge, with T2WI being lower. With the deoxygenated hemoglobin being turned into methemoglobin, high signals of T1WI/T2WI emerge. At this time, because the undestroyed red blood cells are located in the lower position (signals like T1WI and low signal of T2WI), free methemoglobin floats in the upper layer of the hydrops. Thus, stratification phenomenon of the liquid emerges. Finally, because substances resulting from destruction of blood are reabsorbed, T1WI and T2WI take on signals of subdural effusion similar to that of cerebrospinal fluid. Subarachnoid hemorrhage is caused by rupture of

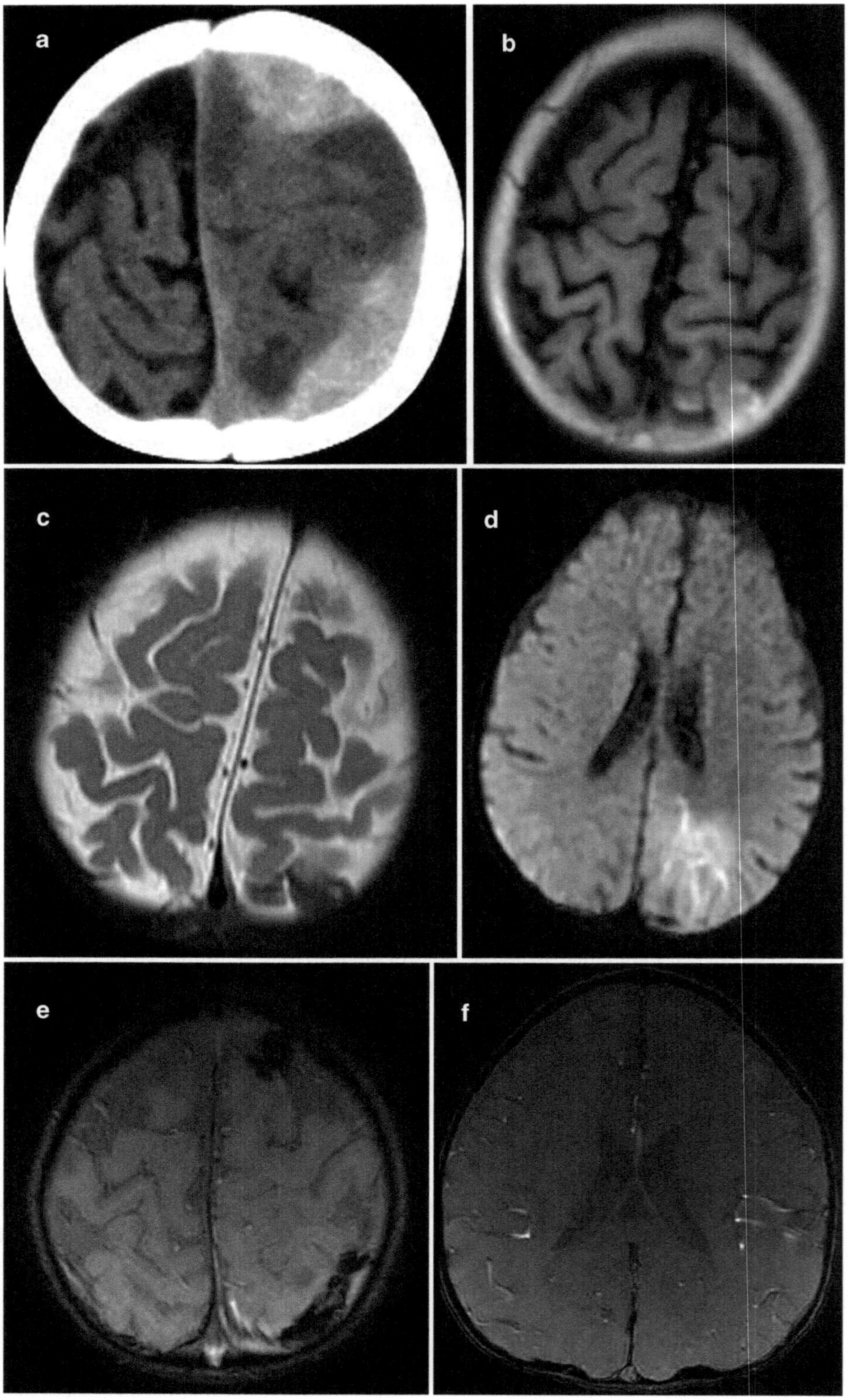

Fig. 6.2 Infant brain trauma

cortical veins or subdural hemorrhage into the cisterns, which often occurs with contusion and laceration of brain. T2-FLAIR and SWI are highly sensitive to subarachnoid hemorrhage. Intracerebral hematomas may result directly or indirectly from injuries, around which there emerge low-density areas. And within 2–3 weeks after the traumas, the hematomas become to have equal density, and after 4 weeks, become to have low density. Contusion and laceration of brain occur in the surface of the brain, and juries of the gyrus occur at the intersection of the gray and the white matters, subcortical white matter, or at the deeper position, which include two types of blast injury and hedge injury. After brain trauma in infants, it can show that brain contusion and laceration exist at the same time. Diffusive axonal injury is the most severe primary foci that are most common in craniocerebral traumas, which are irreversible injuries of diffusive axinal focus injuries caused by pulling, tearing of white matter fibers quick, linear or spiral traumas, which often harm subcortical white matters, callosum, brainstem and endocysts, and have poor manifestations prognosis. By MRI examination, they are manifested multiple foci, and might not be distributed along blood vessels. Encephaledema is more common, and when it becomes serious, it is manifested as diffusive low density by CT examination. And it is manifested as low signals of T1 and weighted high signals of T2. SWI is sensitive to hemorrhagic foci, with low signals. FLAIR is manifested as the hemorrhagic components, around which high signals mean edemas or leakage of axoplasm. In the acute phase, DWI takes on high signal, with ADC value lowering, which hints at swelling of cells and toxic edema of cells. By MRI examination, lactic acid level can be seen rising, and in the subacute phase, NAA of white matters lower, which has certain hinting effects on prognosis. Post-traumatic infarction (PTI) is secondary cerebral infarction after trauma due to abnormal coagulation function and other factors. More common in children. Most of them occurred 24 h or more after injury. PTI in children often occurs in the basal ganglia, mostly single lacunar infarction, with a diameter of less than 10 mm. Severe craniocerebral trauma is prone to large area cerebral infarction.

Case 6.3 Shaken Baby Syndrome

Clinical Presentation

A baby boy, 9 months old. The infant suffered from vigorous shaking of his father's head. The patient presented with unresponsiveness, vomiting, and apathy.

Imaging Findings

A. Axial T2-weighted image demonstrates slightly lower signal in the right frontal lobe (Fig. 6.3a).
B. Axial T1-weighted image demonstrates slightly higher signal, compression and displacement of adjacent brain parenchyma and lateral ventricle. A small amount of left frontal epidural hematoma appeared (Fig. 6.3b).

Discussion

Shaken Baby Syndrome(SBS) is a form of maltreatment that generally refers to hyperextension and hyperflexion of the infant's neck by adults through violent shaking, and then causes brain parenchymal lesions (cerebral edema, diffuse axonal injury(DAI)), subdural hematoma (SDH), and retinal hemorrhages (RH). Because the neck muscles of infants and young children have not yet fully developed, the head is relatively heavy, and the skull and brain are not mature, it is more likely to suffer inertial effects during strenuous shaking and lead to intracranial small vessel rupture, as well as collisions between the brain and skull (especially during head deceleration) to form brain injury. The US Centers for Disease Control and Prevention (CDC) statistics showed that the incidence of SBS from 2003 to 2008 was 32.3 per 100,000 [4].

Bechtel et al. reported that only 10% of cases with retinal hemorrhage manifestations were under 2 years of age without SBS, while 60% were in SBS. Due to the severe shear force and rotational forces generated by violent shaking of children can rapidly deform and recover the vitreous in an oscillatory form, produce traction forces on the retina, and congestion and rupture blood vessels, causing characteristic RH [5].

In short, the diagnosis of abusive traumatic brain injury is often delayed because the infant is not expressive, and parents or other caregivers deliberately conceal the history or do not have sufficient awareness of the behavior that causes the damage. Delayed diagnosis may lead to disease progression or continued injury. Clinicians need to deepen their understanding of such injuries and increase vigilance to avoid misdiagnosis and missed diagnosis.

Case 6.4 Infant Abuse Syndrome

Clinical Presentation

A 3-month-old male infant was abused by a house nanny. Recently, the infant often presented with poor feeding, vomiting, convulsions, and other symptoms. Clinical investigation: the infant had a poor movement of the right limbs and grade 3 muscle tone. Intracranial pressure increased to 130 mmH_2O.

Imaging Findings

A. Axial T2-weighted image demonstrates left intracranial hematoma (subacute phase), located at the junction of left frontal lobe and parietal lobe, showing isosignal or hypersignal. In addition, T2WI demonstrates bilateral frontotemporal subdural hematoma (chronic phase) (Fig. 6.4a).
B. Axial T1-weighted image demonstrates that the hematoma is high signal or low signal (Fig. 6.4b).
C. Diffusion weighted imaging demonstrates low signal and peripheral high signal (Fig. 6.4c).
D. Susceptibility weighted imaging demonstrates "low signal" (Fig. 6.4d).

Discussion

Infant Abuse Syndrome (IAS) is the leading cause of traumatic death in infants and young children, and the difference between IAS and SBS is not very clear. In recent years, the American Academy of Pediatrics has recommended that pediatricians should use the word "abusive head trauma" in diagnosis and medical communication. SHI is an infantile

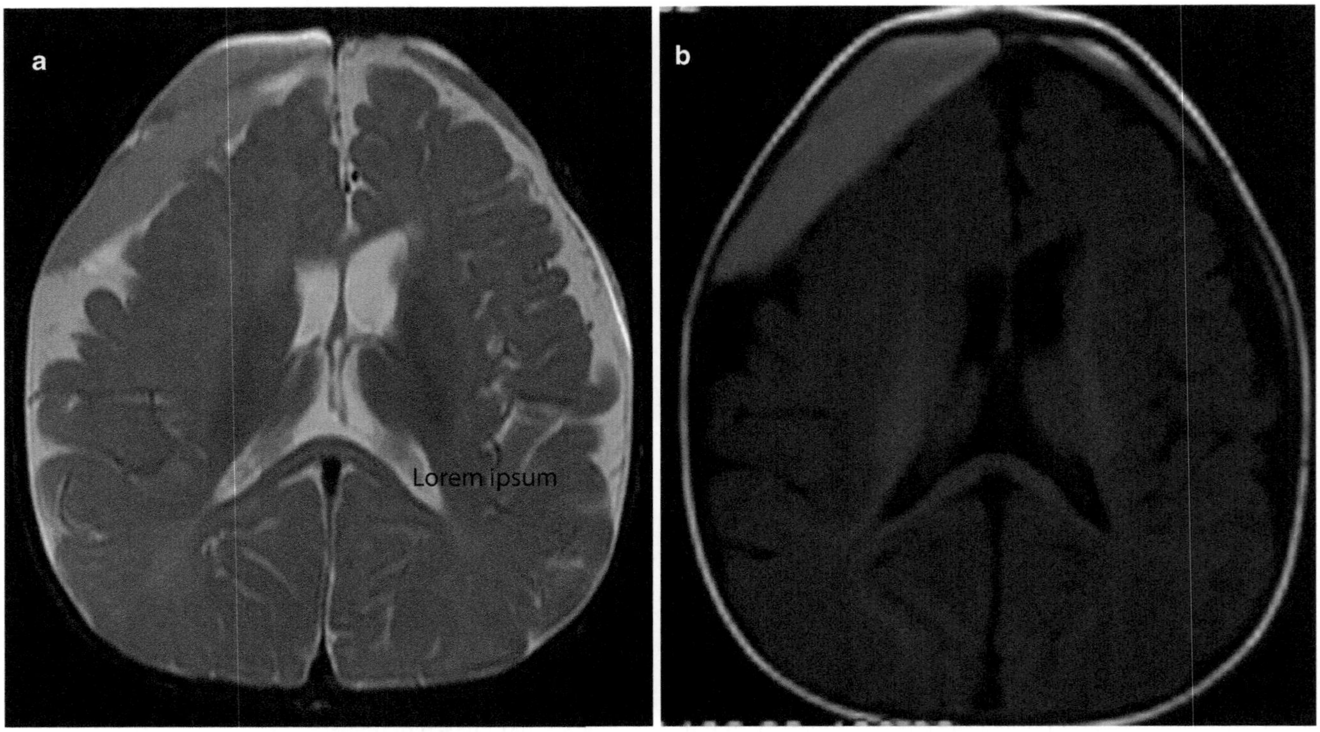

Fig. 6.3 Shaken baby syndrome

traumatic brain injury caused by human factors such as spanking, even evil, and abuse. According to statistics, approximately one in every four infant abusive head trauma events results in infant death. Data from the Centers for Disease Control and Prevention show that abusive head trauma is the leading cause of physical abuse deaths in children under 5 years of age in the United States; while abusive head trauma accounts for one-third of all child abuse deaths. Because of its special affected population, unknown pathogenesis, easy misdiagnosis, and missed diagnosis, and poor prognosis, it also involves social and legal problems and is often very difficult in clinical practice [6].

The clinical symptoms of IAS are nonspecific and often present with symptoms such as poor feeding, vomiting, crying, irritability, binocular retinal hemorrhage, epilepsy, and abnormal mental status. In severe cases, disturbance of consciousness, shock, and even death may occur. The most common clinical manifestations of IAS are subdural hematoma, cerebral contusion, retinal hemorrhage, skull fracture, etc.

IAS and SBS belong to the same kind of disease, and as for the imaging findings and differential diagnosis of IAS, please refer to SBS.

Case 6.5 Sequelae of Head Injury

Clinical Presentation

A boy, 2 years old. A severe traumatic head injury was encountered 1 year ago, and the optimal duration of treatment was missed because he did not seek medical attention in time at that time. However, patients often present with headaches, dizziness, and secondary seizures. In the activities of fingers and toes, EEG showed spikes and spikes.

Imaging Findings

A. Axial T2-weighted image demonstrates the right parietal lobe formed a brain softening focus (Fig. 6.5a).
B. Axial T2-weighted image demonstrates The bilateral lateral ventricles were slightly widened (Fig. 6.5b).
C. Axial T1-weighted image demonstrates decreased volume in the right hemisphere and mild atrophy of bilateral frontal lobes (Fig. 6.5c).
D. Axial T1-weighted image demonstrates Chronic subdural hematoma at the top of the right forehead (Fig. 6.5d).

Discussion

After the craniocerebral injury, due to different degrees of injury, treatment time, and method, a small number of patients may have organic changes, namely Sequelae of Head Injury, such as brain atrophy, encephalomalacia, porencephaly, hydrocephalus, and arachnoid cyst, are irreversible changes. Clinically, headache, dizziness, seizures, hemiplegia, aphasia, and visual impairment may occur, and a few patients have psychiatric symptoms and high intracranial pressure [3].

Encephalomalacia is common in brain contusion and intracranial hematoma and can also be seen after traumatic cerebral infarction. Encephalomalacia is close to ventriculo-

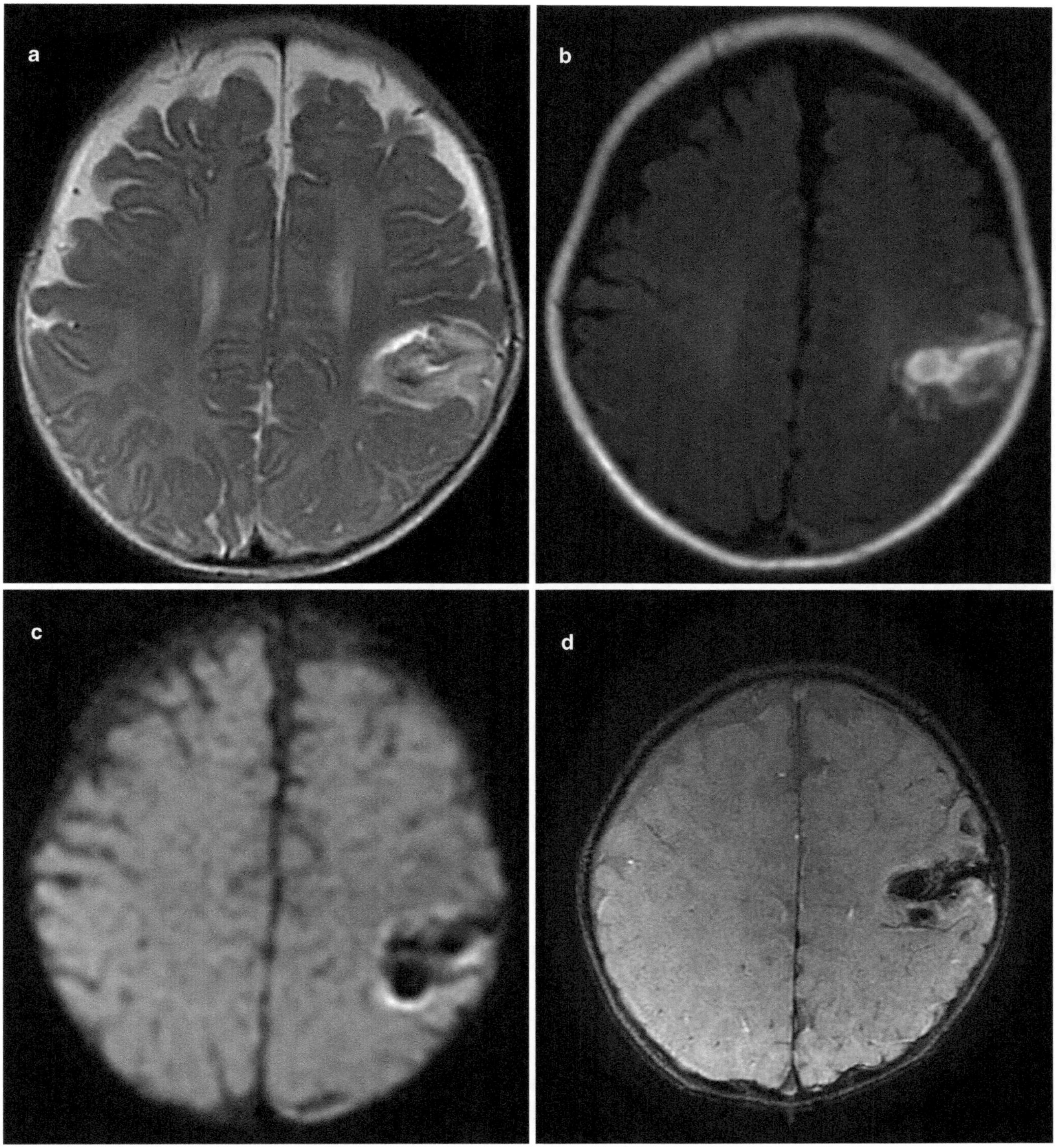

Fig. 6.4 Infant abuse syndrome

megaly and sulci deepening, which is different from other space-occupying lesions. Gliosis is one of the important causes of epilepsy after traumatic brain injury. FLAIR sequence can clearly show cord-like and lamellar hyperintense gliosis around the softening lesion without enhancement on contrast-enhanced scans. Brain atrophy can occur in 30% after severe traumatic brain injury. On MRI images, diffuse brain atrophy is characterized by enlargement of both ventricles, sulci, and cisterns. Localized brain atrophy can enlarge the sulci and ventricles in the corresponding areas. Unilateral brain atrophy only has the above changes, and the midline structure is displaced toward the affected side. Porencephalia refers to the communication with the lateral ventricle due to necrosis and softening of brain tissues after

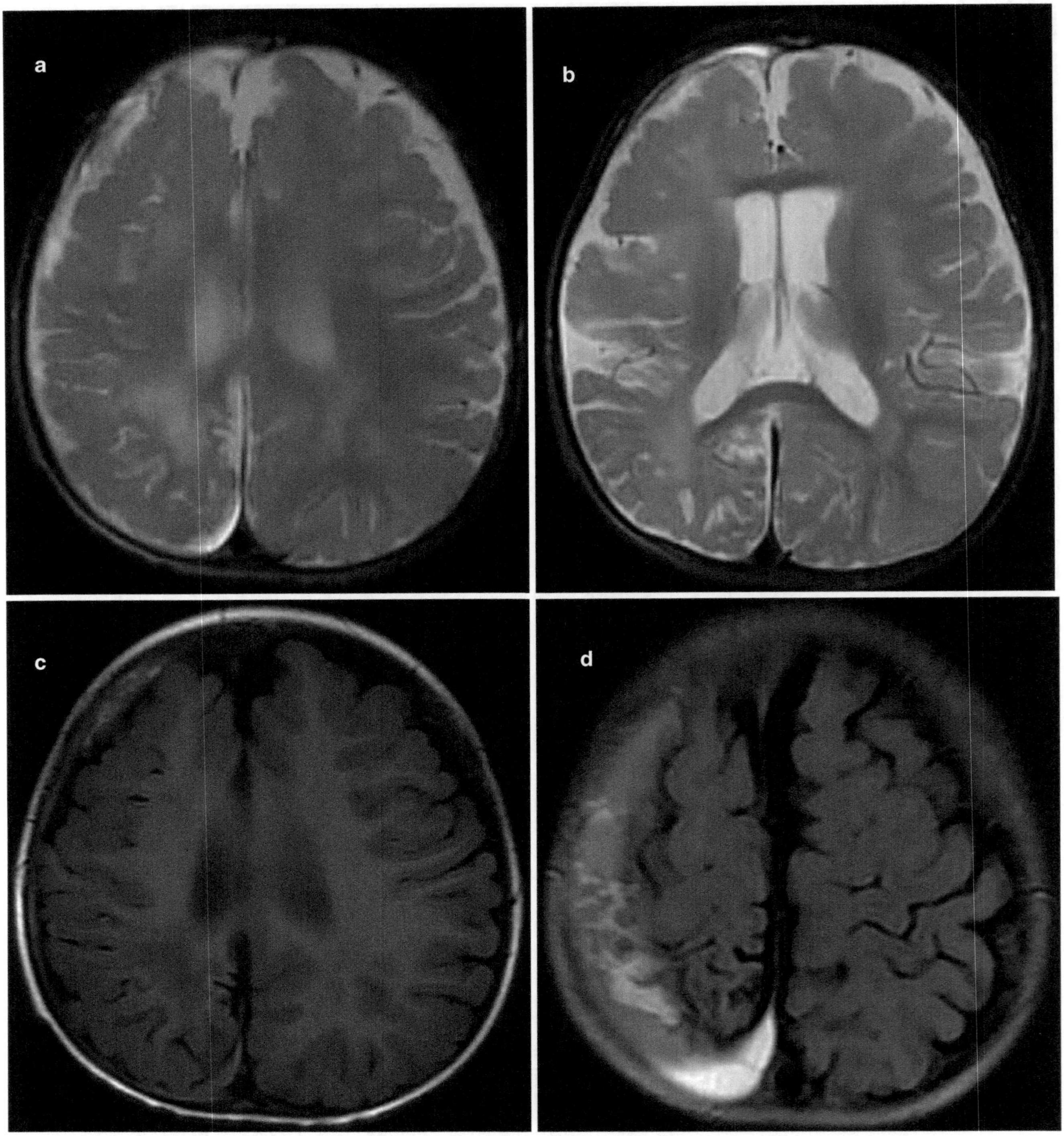

Fig. 6.5 Sequelae of head injury

intracerebral hematoma or brain contusion and laceration. CT shows a well-defined hypodense area with CT values similar to that of cerebrospinal fluid, and the corresponding ventricles are significantly enlarged and communicated with the above-softened areas. On MRI, the shape of the lesion is the same as that of CT, the signal intensity of the lesion is similar to that of cerebrospinal fluid, and MRI images are clearer than CT images.

Sequelae of Head Injury requires a full understanding of the child's history and differentiation from sequelae of intracranial infection, congenital craniocerebral lesions of the brain, and childbirth-related diseases.

References

1. Coley BD. Caffey's pediatric diagnostic imaging, 2-volume set: expert consult—online and print, 12e[M]. Saunders. 2013.
2. Figaji AA, Fieggen AG, Peter JC. Early decompressive craniotomy in children with severe traumatic brain injury. Childs Nerv Syst. 2003;19:666–73.
3. Araki T, Yokota H, Morita A. Pediatric traumatic brain injury: characteristic features, diagnosis, and management. Neurol Med Chir (Tokyo). 2017;57(2):82–93.
4. Lee Y, Lee KS, Hwang DH, et al. MR imaging of shaken baby syndrome manifested as chronic subdural hematoma. Korean J Radiol. 2001;2(3):171–4.
5. Kujiraoka Y, Sato M, Tsuruta W, et al. Shaken baby syndrome manifesting as chronic subdural hematoma: importance of single photon emission computed tomography for treatment indications—case report. Neurol Med Chir (Tokyo). 2004;44(7):359–62.
6. Orman G, Kralik SF, Meoded A, er al. MRI findings in pediatric abusive head trauma: a review. J Neuroimaging. 2020;30(1):15–27.

Brain Damage, Destructive Diseases

7

Hong Yu and Jingshi Wang

This chapter is titled head injury, devastating disease. The resulting brain damage, devastating diseases (e.g., hypoxic-ischemic encephalopathy, hypoglycemia, hyperbilirubinemia, vitamin K deficiency, etc.) covered in this chapter all result from physical factors and usually have one or two defined etiologies, and the disease course is often static. MRI is the most sophisticated modality to evaluate the head injury and devastating diseases, and with advanced imaging techniques such as diffusion-weighted imaging (DWI), functional magnetic resonance imaging (fMRI), and magnetic resonance spectroscopy (MRS), it has the advantage of providing information regarding physiology, function, and metabolism [1, 2].

7.1 Polycystic Encephalomalacia, Hydrancephaly, and Porencephaly

Case 7.1.1 Polycystic Encephalomalacia

Clinical Presentation

A male infant, 4 months old, was born in the spontaneous delivery after (41 + 2) gestation weeks, with intracranial hemorrhage and severe HIE. The baby with epilepsy has intermittent seizures. EEG showed hypsarrhythmia and diffuse abnormality.

Imaging Findings

A-B. Axial T1-weighted image demonstrates low signal intensity with clear contour of bilateral frontal lobe, which contained multiple cyst cavities inside. Bilateral lateral ventricle and third ventricle were obviously dilated with leukoaraiosis (LA). The corpus callosum became thinner obviously (Fig. 7.1a–b).

C-D. Axial T2-weighted image demonstrates high signal intensity in the cystic cavities and the subdural effusion adjacent to inner plate of skull occurred with a small amount of old hemorrhage (Fig. 7.1c–d).

Discussion

Polycystic encephalomalacia is the result of diffuse injury to the brain during the third trimester, childbirth, or after birth, forming multiple cystic spaces of varying sizes with the center separated by glial tissues. Glial cell hyperplasia is present in the white matter or gray matter, not in the periventricular region. Periventricular leukomalacia has clinical manifestations of cerebral palsy [3].

The area of polycystic encephalomalacia lesions varies depending on the specific type of injury. If a lesion is caused by thrombi or embolic infarction, the affected area is located in the distribution area of the main cerebral arteries. If a lesion is caused by mild to moderate hypotension, the affected area is distributed in the cortex and the peripheral white matter (vascular junction where blood supply happens). Severe hypotension may result in damage to the deep cranial nerve nuclei and cortices to varying extents, and the selected site for resection varies when the injury is at different periods. The injury caused by infection factors demonstrates no specificity in the site of resection [4].

The affected area is characterized by illy-demarcated T1 low signal and T2 high signal shadows, which contain multiple cystic spaces. The concomitant manifestations include the presence of some heterogeneous signals, which are composed of glial intervals of varying sizes and cerebrospinal fluid within the lesion. The glial interval is a high signal region compared to the cerebrospinal fluid space.

This disease needs to be differentiated from polycystic brain. Polycystic brain appears as mental retardation, tonic convulsion of the extremities, and no cerebral palsy. Magnetic resonance imaging (MRI) shows multiple rounds, elliptical or stratified saclike structures of varying sizes appear in both sides of the cerebral hemisphere with similar signal intensity

H. Yu · J. Wang (✉)
Department of Medical Imaging, Dalian Women and Children's Medical Center (Group), Dalian, Liaoning, China

H. Liu, X. Zhang (eds.), *Pediatric Neuroimaging*, https://doi.org/10.1007/978-981-16-7928-5_7

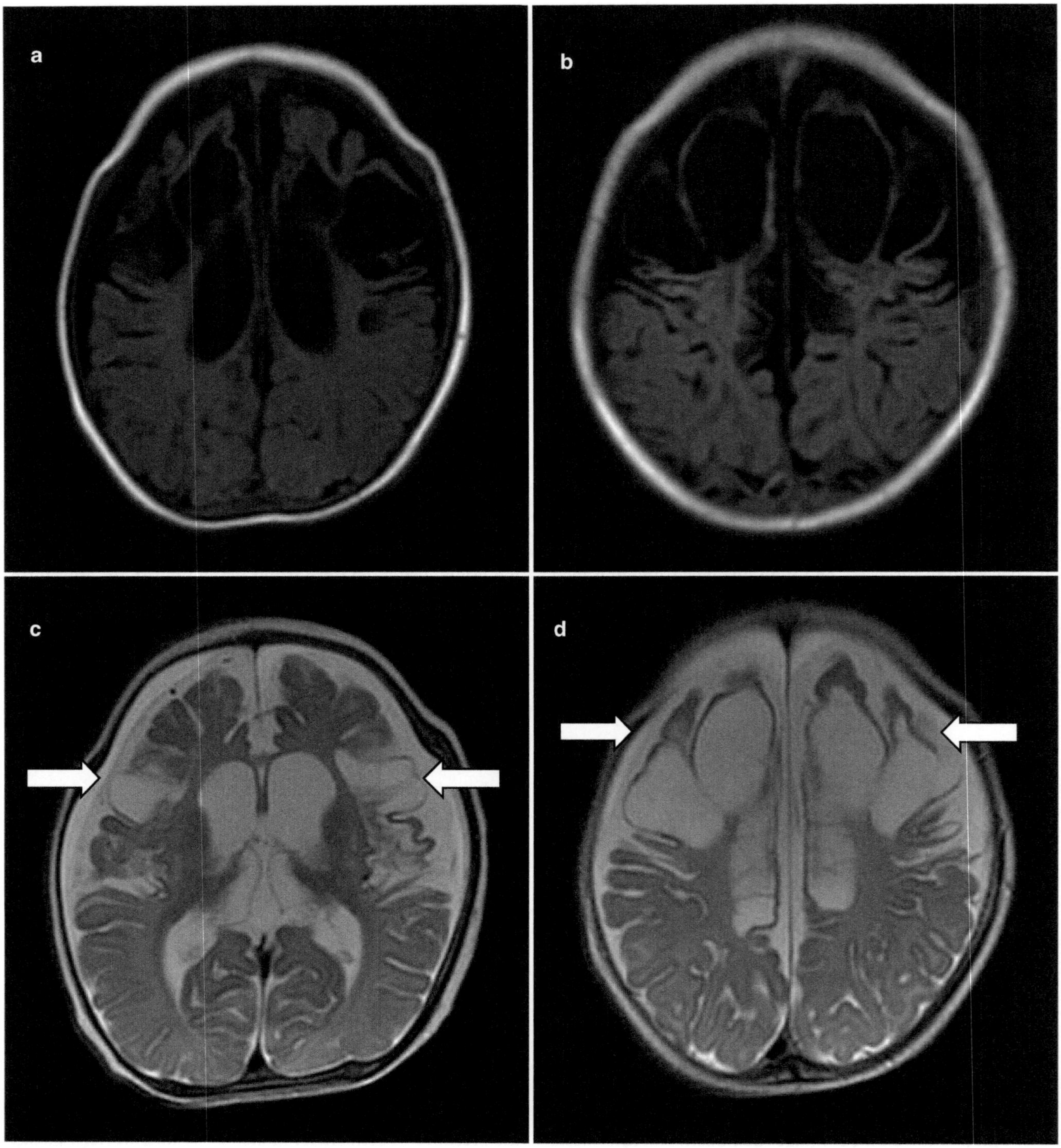

Fig. 7.1 Polycystic encephalomalacia

to that of cerebrospinal fluid, and are highly dilated perivascular spaces. In addition, the disease should be differentiated from periventricular leukomalacia (PVL), ependymal pseudocysts, and so on.

Case 7.1.2 Hydranencephaly

This case was provided by Xia Men Children's Hospital, China.

Clinical Presentation

A. Axial T2-weighted image demonstrates "cerebral cortex was absent and the midline structure was discontinuous". Thalamus and brain stem protruded into cystic cavity (Fig. 7.2a).
B. Sagittal T2-weighted image demonstrates huge supratentorial cystic lesions filled the whole cranial cavity (Fig. 7.2b).

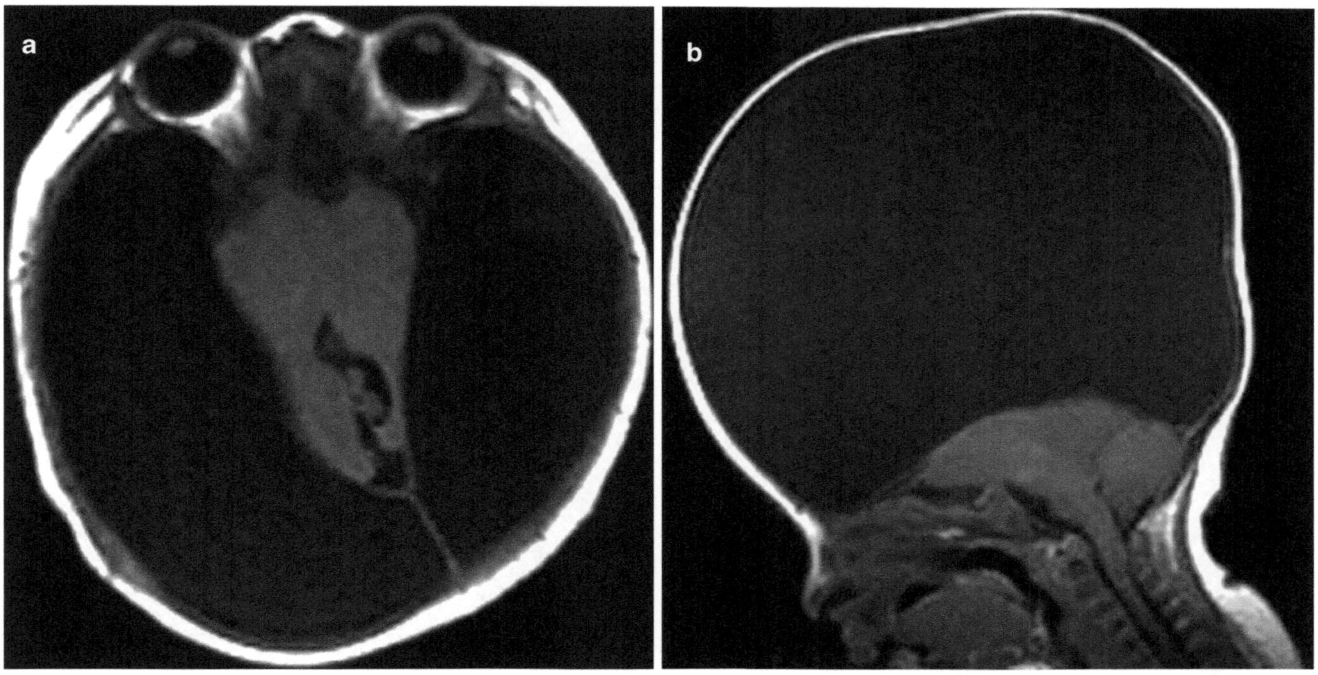

Fig. 7.2 Hydranencephaly

Imaging Findings

MRI showed huge supratentorial cystic lesions filled the whole cranial cavity, cerebral cortex was absent and the midline structure was discontinuous. Thalamus and brain stem protruded into cystic cavity.

Discussion

Hydranencephaly is a condition in which most of the brain mantle (cortical plate and hemispheric white matter) has been damaged, liquefied, and resorbed; it can be considered as porencephaly of nearly the entire cerebrum.

Hydroanencephalus is composed of hydrocephaly and anencephaly, with unknown etiology. Most scholars prefer the theory of internal jugular vein occlusion, i.e. embryonal malformation of bilateral internal carotid arteries leads to parenchymal brain underdevelopment or nondevelopment in arteria cerebri anterior and area where the arteries supply blood in the brain. Because of cerebrospinal fluid circulation disorder, the cerebral hemispheres are replaced by large amounts of cerebrospinal fluids, therefore there always are parts of the brain line. The developments of posterior cerebral artery and basilar artery blood supplying area (cerebellum, occipital lobe, and some basal ganglia areas) are normal. And parts of the cases are caused by congenital infection (toxoplasmosis and cytomegalovirus infection) [5]. The characteristic of clinical manifestations is significant. Generally, the newborn baby has no special signs and symptoms, but later there will be progressive cranial enlargement, fontanelle enlargement, and mental development gradually going low. Corresponding symptoms include crying, increased intracranial pressure, underdeveloped or undeveloped brain.

Imaging studies of patients with hydranencephaly show that the cerebral hemispheres are nearly completely replaced by CSF. The thalami are usually preserved. The inferior medial aspects of the frontal lobes and the inferior medial aspects of the temporal and occipital lobes may also be preserved. The brainstem is usually atrophic; the cerebellum is almost always normal.

The disease needs to be differentiated from hydrocephalus and alobar holoprosencehaly. The thalami of children with alobar holoprosencehaly are fused, and their frontal lobes present a pancake-like fusion. The thalami of children with hydroanencephalus are not fused, and they lack fused cortical tissue. The cortical margin can be seen in children with hydrocephalus.

Case 7.1.3 Porencephaly

Clinical Presentation

A baby boy, 2 years old, was born with birth injuries, has occasional epileptic attacks currently with limb weakness.

Imaging Findings

A-B. Axial T1-weighted image demonstrates cystic lesions were seen in the body of the right lateral ventricle, taking on T1WI low signal (arrow). The boundary was clear and could be interlinked with the adjacent right lateral ventricle, with local ventricular dilatation, and the cyst wall had no gray matter lining (Fig. 7.3a–b).

C-D. Axial T2-weighted image demonstrates that the cystic focus was high signal intensity (arrow) (Fig. 7.3c–d).

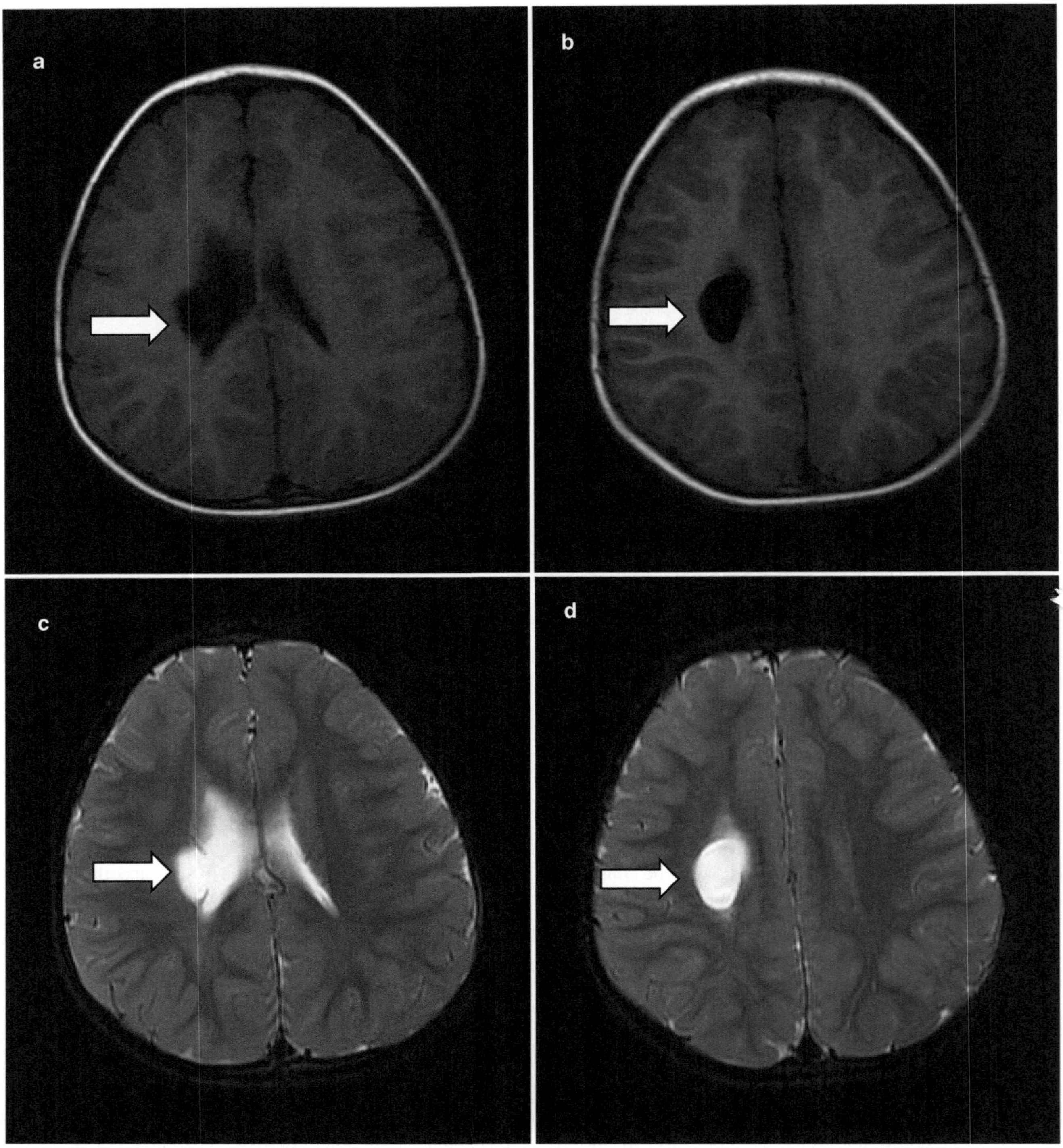

Fig. 7.3 Porencephaly

Discussion

Porencephaly means non-neoplastic fluid lumen in the brain caused by congenital or acquired reasons. In most cases, it is connected to the subarachnoid space in the encephalocoele. Both multicystic encephalomalacia and hydroanencephaly are tissue reactivity changes after end-stage injury which is specific to the brain.

Porencephaly is classified into congenital and acquired types. Congenital porencephaly is caused by dysplasia, cerebral infarction, and other destructive diseases. Border of hypogenetic ectocinerea can be found around the porencephaly caused by dysplasia, as well as cortical dysplasia, such as cerebellar gyrus malformation. The porencephaly caused by cerebral infarction, after 24 weeks of gestation, generally is cortical arteriotic porencephaly caused by arterial ischemic stroke; Germinal stromal hemorrhage before 34 weeks of gestation cause compression on medullary veins, leading focal white matter venous infarction around the encephalocoele which is limited in the medullary veins area, thereby cystic degeneration will appear before the formation of porencephaly. The acquired generative necrotic porencephaly is caused by hypoxia, bleeding, cerebrovascular disease, infection, trauma, etc. [5].

The CT of porencephaly presents cystic low-density foci, with irregular shapes and no enhancement after strengthening. MRI shows that cyst presents a shape of T1WI low signal, T2WI high signal, clear border, single or multiple features, unilateral or bilateral distribution. Cystic diseases may be connected to adjacent encephalocoele and (or) subarachnoid space, with corresponding limited expansion of encephalocoele and subarachnoid space. There is no gray matter lining on the cyst wall. Diseased lateral brain tissue may have the symptom of localized atrophy and softening lesions.

The disease needs to be differentiated from the cerebromalacia lesion, the intracerebral cystic space, and separate fissure. The cerebromalacia lesion and the intracerebral cystic space do not communicate with the ventricle or the subarachnoid space. Separate fissure mostly belongs to bilateral lesions with poor prognosis, which traverse the cerebral hemisphere fissure and reach the ventricle from the brain surface, where the cortical gray matter folds inward along both edges of the fissure and reaches the ventricular wall.

7.2 Hypoxic-Ischemic Encephalopathy

Case 7.2 Hypoxic-Ischemic Encephalopathy

Clinical Presentation

A female infant, 7 days old, full-term infant, was delivered with the help of obstetric forceps due to fetal distress, with a history of severe asphyxia, low muscle tension, and no spontaneous breathing during delivery. Apgar score was respectively 2 in 1 min, 4 in 5 min after resuscitation, and 7 in 10 min.

Imaging Findings

A-B. Axial T1-weighted image demonstrates patchy hyperintensity in bilateral basal ganglia and thalamus; High signal intensity disappeared in the hind limbs of bilateral internal capsule (Fig. 7.4a–b).

C. T2-FLAIR demonstrates brain swelling and edema, and the boundary between gray matter and white matter is unclear (Fig. 7.4c).

D. Axial T1-weighted image demonstrates that patchy slightly high signals in bilateral basal ganglia and thalamus (Fig. 7.4d).

Discussion

Hypoxic-ischemic encephalopathy (HIE) refers to fetal or brain damage caused by partial or complete hypoxia, reduced or suspended cerebral blood flow. As one of the most common causes of cerebral palsy and other severe neurologic deficits in children, HIE occurs in two to nine of every 1000 live births. The decrease of blood flow and oxygen content in blood will cause the loss of brain autoregulation function, resulting in different degrees of brain injury. Therefore, how to make early diagnosis and predict the prognosis of HIE is very important [6].

The pathological changes of neonatal hypoxic-ischemic encephalopathy (HIE) were significantly correlated with gestational age, degree, and nature of cerebral injury. The main pathological changes include neuronal necrosis, brain damage in the parasagittal region, paraventricular white matter damage, apoptosis, cerebral edema, intracranial hemorrhage, etc. [7].

Cranial Computed Tomography (CT) scanning helps to determine lesion range and prognosis. CT diagnosis for HIE can be divided into four levels: Level I (normal), Level II (regional local density is reduced, and lesions are spotted), Level III (regional density for more than two lesions is reduced), Level IV (the general density of the cerebral hemisphere decreases, the difference between the gray matter and white matter disappears, and the lateral ventricle narrows [8]. Conventional MRI is diverse in their performance and often presents as coexistence of multiple signs. Mild HIE usually presents as a lesion in the subcortical region of the parasagittal region on MRI, while basal ganglia or thalamic lesions usually appear in moderate or severe HIE. The disappearance of high signal for posterior limb of internal capsule on the T1WI sequence is one of the important signs predicting the poor prognosis of neonatal HIE. The pathological changes of HIE images are more obvious on T1WI than on T2WI. On T1WI, they can present as: Brain swelling, cerebral edema (unclear boundaries between gray matter and white matter, cortical, subcortical white matter and spotted deep white matter, curved strip high signal, spotted high signal in basal ganglia and thalamus); selective neuronal necrosis in the cerebral cortex, brainstem, and cerebellum (present as low T1WI signal); softened leukoventricular white matter (the white matter around the ventricles presents as a small cystic low T1WI signal); brain injury in parasagittal region; intracranial hemorrhage

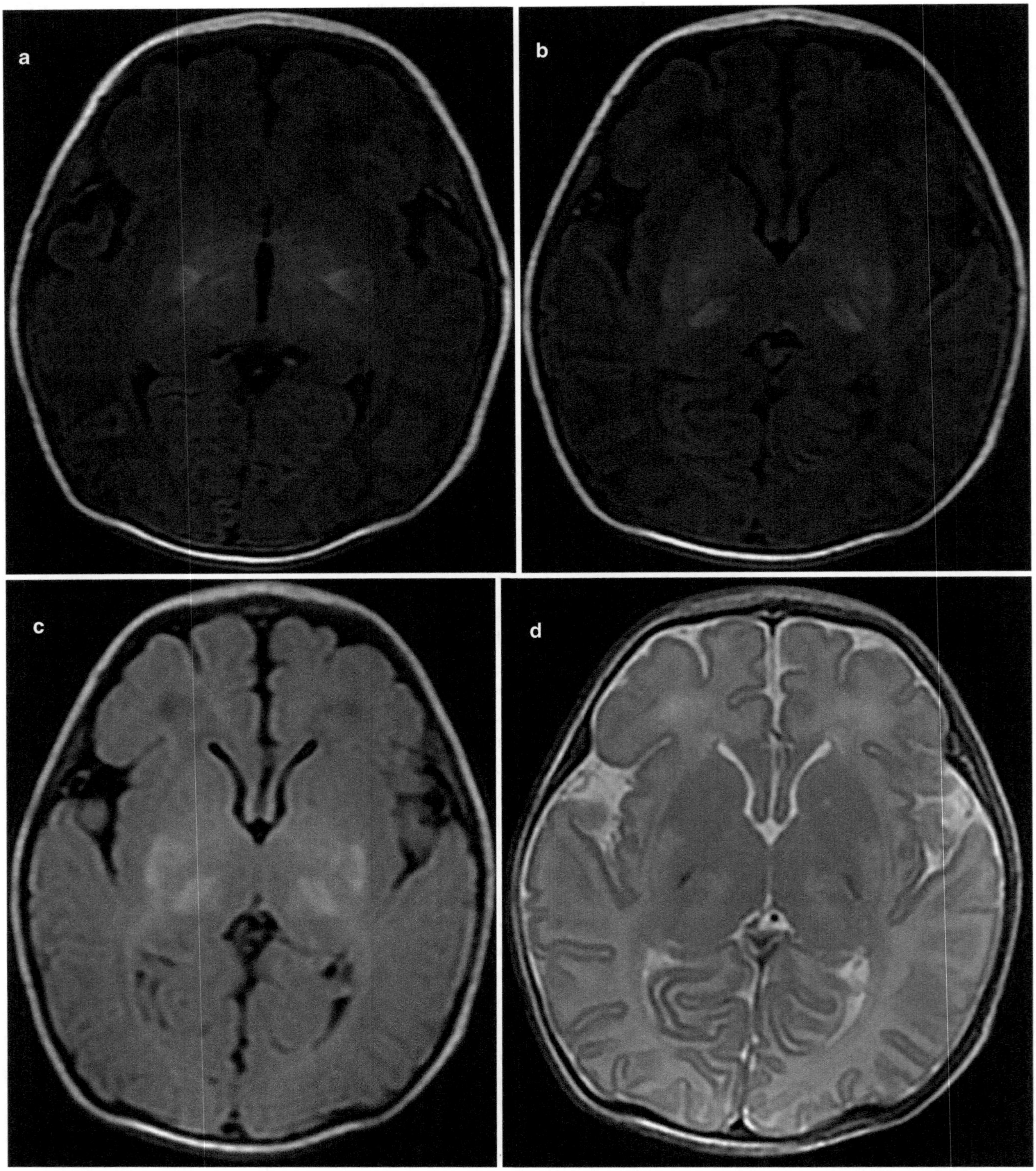

Fig. 7.4 Hypoxic-ischemic encephalopathy

(including subdural hemorrhage, subarachnoid hemorrhage, and parenchymal hemorrhage); there may be venous sinus embolism as well. In addition, diffusion-weighted imaging (DWI) can reflect early diffusion limitation caused by neonatal HIE cytotoxic edema. Susceptibility weighted imaging (SWI) is most sensitive to the detection of intracranial hemorrhage, especially to early and micro hemorrhage. Micro hemorrhage refers to hemorrhagic focus of less than 5 mm in the basal ganglia, thalamus, cortex, brainstem, and so on. The combined analysis for multiple modalities of MRI has higher sensitivity and specificity, which makes the judgment of prognosis get more accurate [9].

7.3 Premature Infant Hypoxic-Ischemic Encephalopathy

Case 7.3.1 Hair Layer and Intraventricular Hemorrhage

Clinical Presentation

A baby girl, 7 days old, was born prematurely due to premature rupture of membranes after 33 gestation weeks. The weight is 1600 g.

Imaging Findings

A-B. Axial T1-weighted image demonstrates the left Hair Layer hemorrhage, subependymal hemorrhage, and hemorrhage of cistern of great cerebral vein (subacute phase)(arrow) (Fig. 7.5a–b).

C. Sagittal T1-weighted image demonstrates lateral ventricular hemorrhage with high signal intensity (arrow) (Fig. 7.5c).

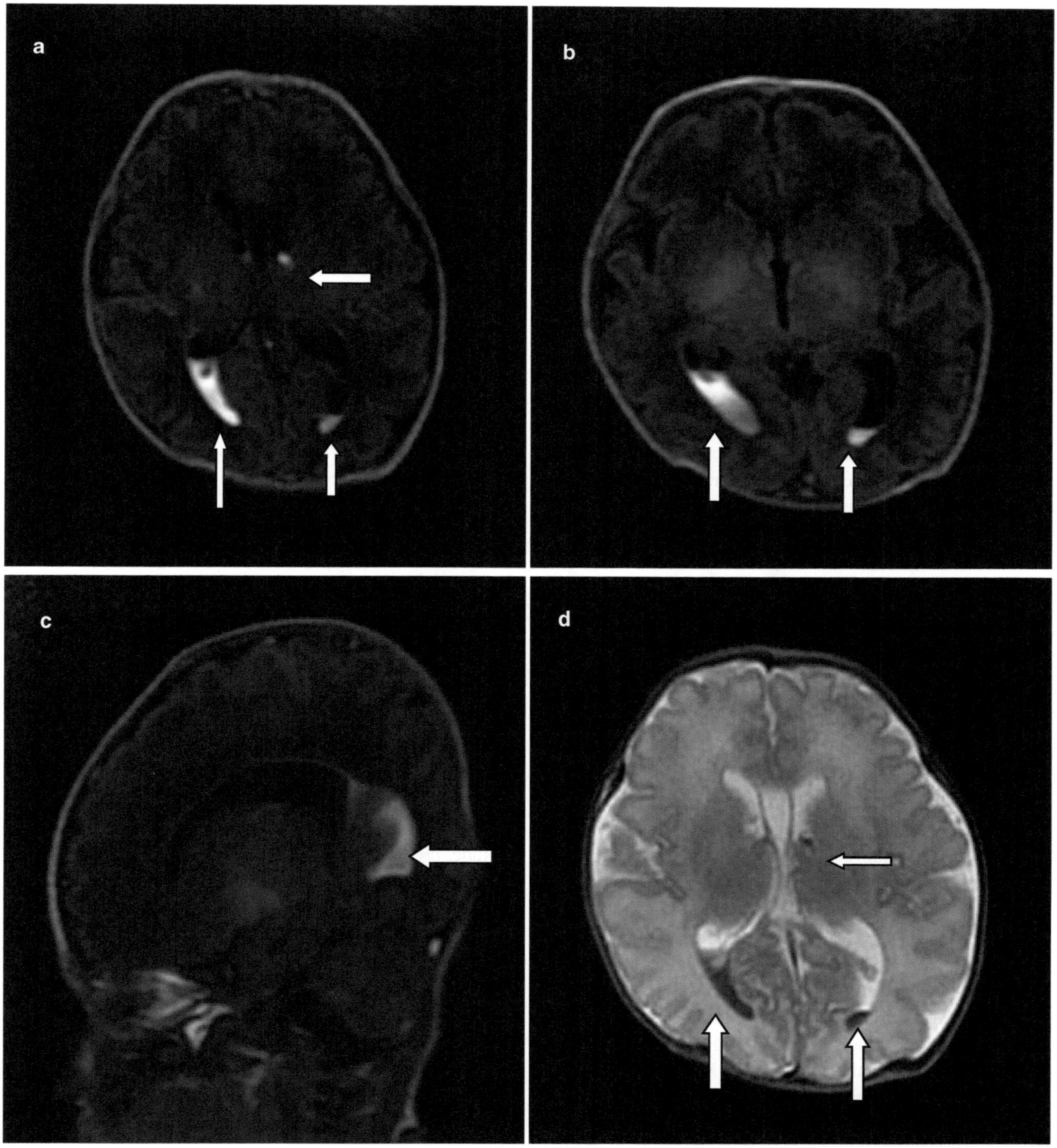

Fig. 7.5 Hair layer and intraventricular hemorrhage

D. Axial T2-weighted image demonstrates low signal shadow in the bilateral lateral ventricle and subependymal (arrow) (Fig. 7.5d).

Discussion
Common cerebral injury in premature infants is mainly hair layer and intraventricular hemorrhage and periventricular leukomalacia (PVL), which are closely related to developmental immaturity in the anatomy and physiology and neurobiology of the central nervous system of premature infants. The former is a hemorrhagic lesion and often leads to serious complications such as hydrocephalus and periventricular hemorrhagic medullary vein infarction after intraventricular hemorrhage [10]. The latter is an ischemic lesion, is also associated with intrauterine infections, and is the main cause of early death, cerebral palsy, visual disturbance, hearing disorder, and cognitive impairments in premature infants [11].

Hair layer and intraventricular hemorrhage is the most common type of intracranial hemorrhage in premature infants and mostly originates from the germinal matrix under the ventrolateral subependymal membrane of the lateral ventricle. The vascular structure and distribution of the germinal matrix of premature infants lack the specificity of supporting tissues, which determines that the germinal matrix is highly sensitive to hypoxia, hypercapnia, and acidosis and is prone to necrosis and disintegration to result in subependymal hemorrhage. Periventricular-intraventricular hemorrhage is mainly related to the intravascular and extracellular factors of the germinal matrix and the factors of the blood vessel itself [12].

Classification of germinal layer and intravenous hemorrhage: Level I. Bleeding is limited to the subependymal zone/germinal matrix, without involving the lateral ventricle. MRI presents as a small spotted high T1WI signal and a low T2WI signal in the subependymal/germinal matrix. Level II. Subependymal/germinal matrix hemorrhage entering the lateral ventricle or intravenous hemorrhage without ventricular dilatation. MRI presents as high T1WI signal shadow in the lateral ventricle. Level III. intravenous hemorrhage with ventricular dilatation. Intravenous hemorrhage causes secondary subarachnoid hemorrhage by entering the subarachnoid space along the cerebration fluid pathway and may cause cerebration fluid circulation pathway obstruction, leading to hydrocephalus. MRI presents as high T1WI signal shadow in the lateral ventricle accompanied with lateral ventricular dilatation. Level IV. Periventricular hemorrhage involves adjacent ventricular hemorrhagic infarction. Subventricular germinal matrix hemorrhage can also block the terminal veins to cause a hemorrhagic infarction of medullary veins that drain the white matter. MRI presents as high and low mixed signals of T1WI and uneven high signal of T2WI around the ventricles. The display rate of T1-FLAIR for lateral paraventricular white matter lesions in premature infants is the highest. In addition, SWI displays subependymal germinal matrix and intravenous hemorrhage significantly better than conventional sequences do, and SWI shows a distinctly low signal because most of the products in the blood such as deoxyhemoglobin, methemoglobin, and hemosiderin are paramagnetic.

Case 7.3.2 Periventricular Leukomalacia

Clinical Presentation
A male infant, 19 days old, was born prematurely after 32 gestation weeks, with neonatal respiratory distress syndrome (NRDS). The baby was hyporesponsive, with poor sucking and hypotonia. EEG showed central area sharp wave discharges.

Imaging Findings
A. Axial T1-weighted image demonstrates small multiple irregular cystic lesions were seen around bilateral lateral ventricle and in the white matter of centrum semiovale (low signal). The Hemorrhagic focus was seen around the posterior horn of bilateral lateral ventricles and in optic radiation area (patchy high signal shadow) (arrow) (Fig. 7.6a).
B. AX-T2 FLAIR demonstrates delay of myelination (arrow) (Fig. 7.6b).
C-D. Axial T1-weighted image demonstrates high signal in the lesion area.The wall of ventricle is unsmooth and the virchow-robin space was slightly enlarged (arrow) (Fig. 7.6c–d).

Discussion
The dural cortical arterial anastomotic branches of premature infants are abundant, and the blood supply of the gray matter is almost all from the centripetal blood flow of the brain surface. Therefore, it usually causes ischemic edema and necrosis of the white matter around the cerebral ventricle called PVL. PVL can cause pediatric neurological sequelae such as cerebral palsy, visual and auditory dysfunction, and cognitive impairment. Vascular developmental characteristics and susceptibility of oligodendrocyte precursors to ischemia are the basis of PVL formation. The causes of PVL include premature birth (especially less than 32 weeks), brain tissue ischemia in unhealthy status, infection, white matter lesion and so on [13].

White matter damage has different pathological changes at different stages: (1) Edema period (6–12 h after ischemia to several days after damage): Edema can be localized focally besides the ventricles or around the ventricles, and can even cause white matter to be widely affected (2). Formative period for softening lesion: Common sites include the parts near the anterior horn of the lateral ventricle, near the central part of the lateral ventricle, and near the posterior horn of the

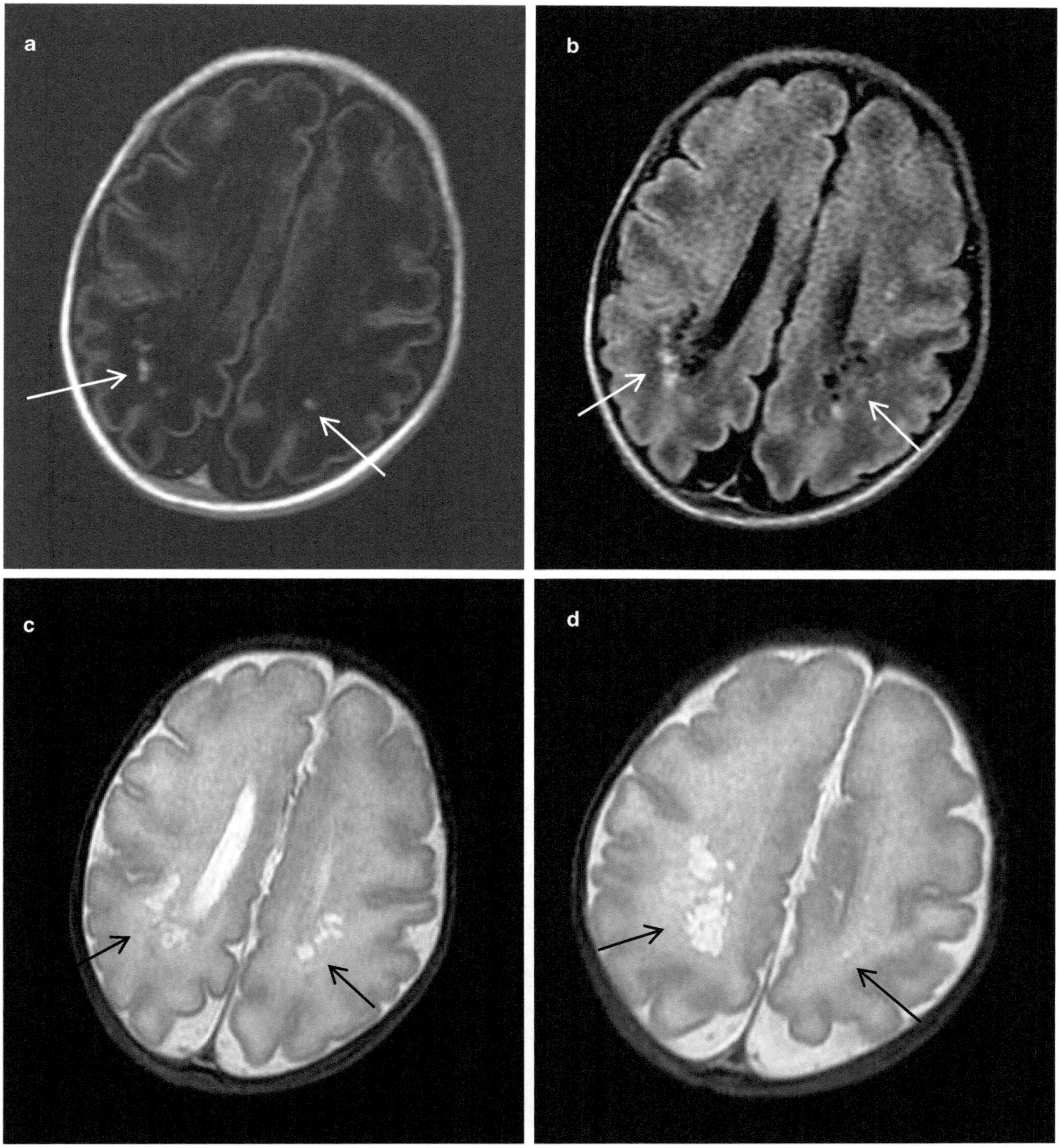

Fig. 7.6 Periventricular leukomalacia

lateral ventricle as well as extensive white matter softening lesion (3). The late stage of softening lesion formation: Microglia repair and calcification and atrophy of white matter can be seen [6].

PVL most commonly occurs in the white matter of the lateral margin of the triangle area of the bilateral lateral ventricle and in the white matter adjacent to the interventricular foramen area. The watershed damage usually appears as coagulation necrosis, and complete cystic change needs 2–6 weeks. CT shows the ventricle is enlarged, paraventricular white matter density and the white matter density in semioval center decreases, and it is obvious around the triangle area; the higher white matter density is similar to cerebrospinal fluid. It is a high-density shadow when hemorrhage occurs simultaneously. MRI can better show the above lesions, and the abnormalities seen were associated with neurological dysfunction in child patients. Spotted or strip low T1 signal and high T2 signal for the white matter around the lateral ventricle can be seen in 2–3 days after hypoxia, and T2 signal decreases during 6–7 days. Thereafter, cystic changes and unsmooth ventricular wall occur gradually due to necrosis and softening of the white matter, and the perivascular space is enlarged. A few MRI images show high T1 signals due to hemorrhage, paramagnetic deposition, and cerebral cortical necrosis. Fluid attenuated inversion recovery (FLAIR) can show the delay of myelination, and SAG-T1WI shows that the corpus callosum gets thinner, which is most obvious in its posterior and splenium parts, and sometimes visual radiation and visual cortex can be involved. In addition, diffusion-weighted imaging (DWI) is more sensitive than conventional MRI in lesion detection, showing a high signal, which is caused by cytotoxic edema. MR spectroscopy (MRS) shows lactic acid (Lac) increases and N-acetyl aspartate (NAA) decreases in paraventricular white matter.

This disease needs to be differentiated from the diseases such as late development of myelin sheath in normal term infants, congenital leukoencephalopathy, and abnormal neuronal migration. The myelination of the white matter over the posterior triangle area in the normal term infants is rather late, showing a high T2 signal, but the medullary type of the white matter is normal and there is no diffusion limitation. White matter disease is often bilaterally symmetrical, and laboratory tests are helpful for its identification. There is no abnormal neuronal migration such as multiple micro-cerebral gyrus, signal and density abnormalities, white matter thinning, and abnormal ventricular wall morphology.

Case 7.4 Perinatal Asphyxia in Term Infants

Clinical Presentation

A 37 week neonate, delivered by cesarean section for "fetal distress."Birth weight 2500 g, amniotic fluid clear, umbilical cord coiled around neck 1 week, twist 20 weeks. After birth, the child had no spontaneous breathing, pale complexion, flaccid extremities, and occasional convulsions, Apgar score of 3 for 5 min, and metabolic acidosis (umbilical vein blood pH: 6.76. The clinical diagnosis was perinatal asphyxia in term infants.

Imaging Findings

A. Axial T1-weighted image demonstrates bilateral periventricular focal cerebral white matter lesions. A small patchy shadow was seen around bilateral lateral ventricles (arrow) (Fig. 7.7a).
B. Diffusion Weighted Imaging demonstrates high signal (arrow) (Fig. 7.7b).

Discussion

Perinatal Asphyxia in term infants refers to a pathophysiological condition in which the newborn cannot normally breathe after birth for various reasons in the process of delivery, causing oxygen deficiency and acidosis. In severe cases,

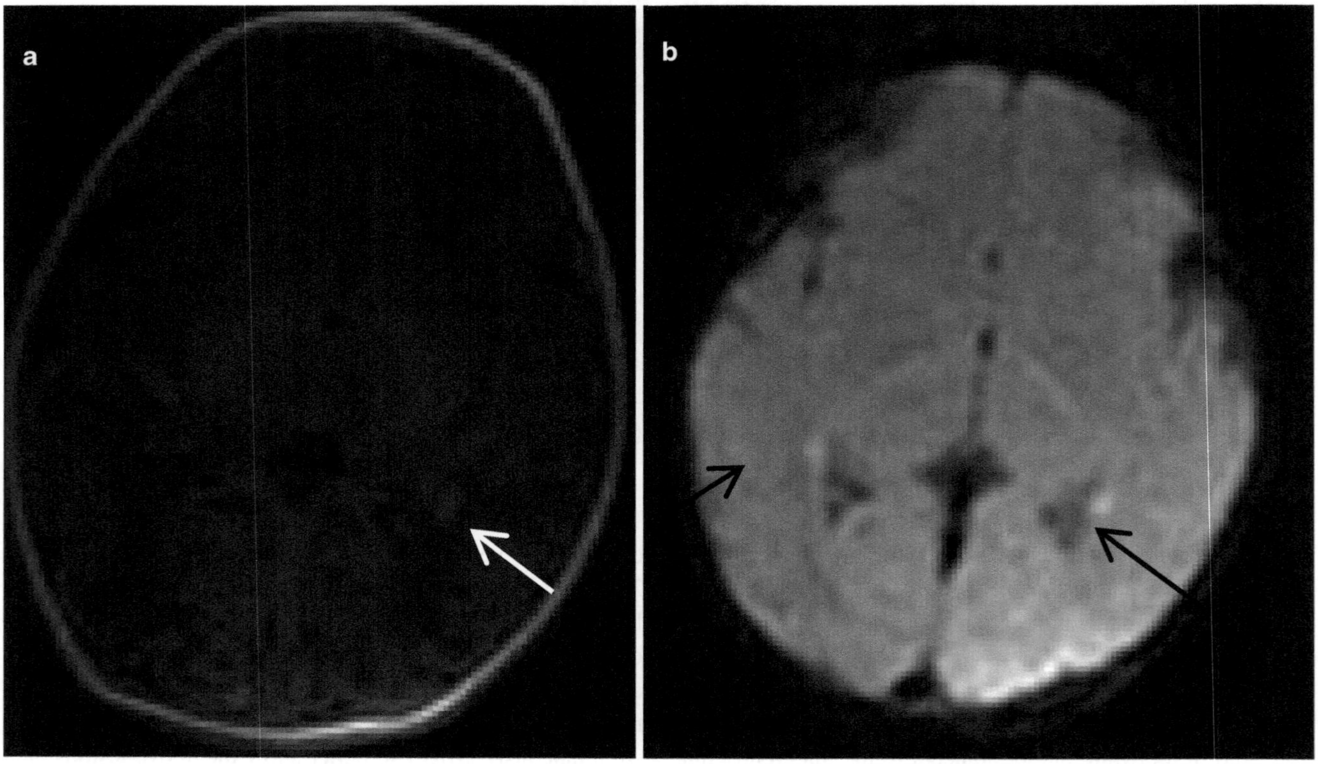

Fig. 7.7 Perinatal Asphyxia in term infants

multiple organ damage of the whole body may be caused. It is the main reason for the death and disability of newborns in the perinatal stage. Neonatal asphyxia often causes cerebral injury of different degrees. In severe cases, it may cause hypoxic-ischemic encephalopathy (HIE). At present, in the field of imaging, HIE is often studied. There are few studies on the cerebral injury caused only by asphyxia of full-term infants in the perinatal stage [14].

The pathological changes causing cerebral injury after Perinatal Asphyxia in term infants mainly include cerebral edema, neuronal death, decreased number of nerve cells, and damage of neuroglia network. And then, there is the reactive gliosis [15]. Although they are not diagnosed with HIE, newborns with asphyxia have a cerebral injury of a certain degree. MRI mainly showed subarachnoid hemorrhage, punctate white matter lesions (PWML), subcutaneous hematoma, and Subcutaneous hematoma. PWML appear as puncta in the centrum semiovale, periventricular white matter, and some of them can fuse into threads or clusters. It is hyperintense on T1WI, hypointense, or isointense on T2WI and ADC maps, and its diameter is mostly less than 5 mm. Besides, DTI and other special imaging sequences also have diagnostic significance for the cerebral injury of the newborn after asphyxia. The study of Dawn Gano et al. showed that in the first hours after the occurrence of the ischemic and anoxic event, the DTI sequence could display the cerebral injury. Therefore, they were not diagnosed with HIE, the newborns with asphyxia had cerebral injury of a certain degree, which should be paid attention to by clinicians. Early intervention and treatment should be made.

Case 7.5 Kernicterus

Clinical Presentation

A male infant, 4 days old. The baby was found to have xanthochromia at 50 h after birth, with a total bilirubin of 335 mmol/L and direct bilirubin of 18.6 mmol/L.

Imaging Findings

A-C. Axial T1-weighted image demonstrates MRI showed symmetrical high signal on bilateral globus pallidus (Fig. 7.8a–c).

D. There was no obvious abnormality in Axial T2-weighted image (Fig. 7.8d).

Discussion

Kernicterus is the persistent or severe hyperbilirubinemia that happened in the neonatal period. Free bilirubin in the serum becomes deposition in the cerebrospinal fluid and the brain tissue through incomplete blood–brain barrier, causing damage to neuron and astrocyte. The damage in the pallidum is the most obvious, but the shell core is not affected. Bilirubin encephalopathy may present with abnormal clinical and subclinical manifestations of the nervous system, which is one of the most important factors affecting neonatal survival rate and its quality [16].

Erythrocytic hemolysis is the most common cause of neonatal bilirubin encephalopathy, for example, the blood types of the mother and the baby do not match, or there is a lack of G-6PD. The bilirubin encephalopathy has three stages: reversible damage, recoverable damage, and irreversible damage (i.e., kernicterus) to the brain tissue by bilirubin. Kernicterus can be avoided if it is diagnosed and treated early in the first two stages. The current clinical approach is to assess the risk of bilirubin encephalopathy by monitoring total bilirubin of serum and level of uncombined bilirubin. The concentration of serum bilirubin within 1 week after the birth of baby will raise, with term infant greater than 220 μmol/L, and a premature infant less than 255 μmol/L. The serum direct bilirubin is greater than 26 μmol/L, lasting for 2–4 weeks. Currently, there is no golden standard for the diagnosis of bilirubin encephalopathy, which should be carried out combining with clinical manifestation, laboratory examination, and imageological examination [17].

MRI is an important supplementary means for diagnosis of bilirubin encephalopathy. T1WI of severe hyperbilirubinemia presenting globus pallidus symmetry high signal is the important performance of ABE of the newborn baby, which is closely related to the severity of hyperbilirubinemia [16]. When it is severe, there may be T2WI symmetry high signal. And the T2WI symmetry high signal of globus pallidus in the infants and young children period is the important feature of chronic bilirubin encephalopathy. But because the myelination of the newborn baby develops early, the regular MRI diagnosis has a false positive rate. 1H-MRS shows that the NAA is going low, but there is no lactate peak. In the chronic phase, T2 time extension and atrophy occur in globus pallidus, subthalamic nucleus, and hippocampal [18, 19].

The disease should be identified with other lesions that happened in the basal ganglia region. HIE involved basal ganglia: globus pallidus, putamen, or dorsal thalamus of the newborn baby present T1WI high signal. The globus pallidus may be involved, but the putamen will be involved the most. Cortex and subcortical and deep white matter may be involved too, causing diffuse cerebral edema and intracranial hemorrhage, which present high signal in DWI. Hepatolenticular degeneration is a kind of disease caused by autosomal recessive hereditary copper metabolism disorder. Most of the lesions present T1 low signal and T2 high signal. The lesions form presents "butterfly's spreading wings," which are liable to occur in the shell nucleus and caudate nucleus, followed by thalamus and globus pallidus. Hypoglycemia brain injury generally presents T1 low signal and T2 high signal. The occipital lobe is involved, and the DWI presents a limited spreading signal.

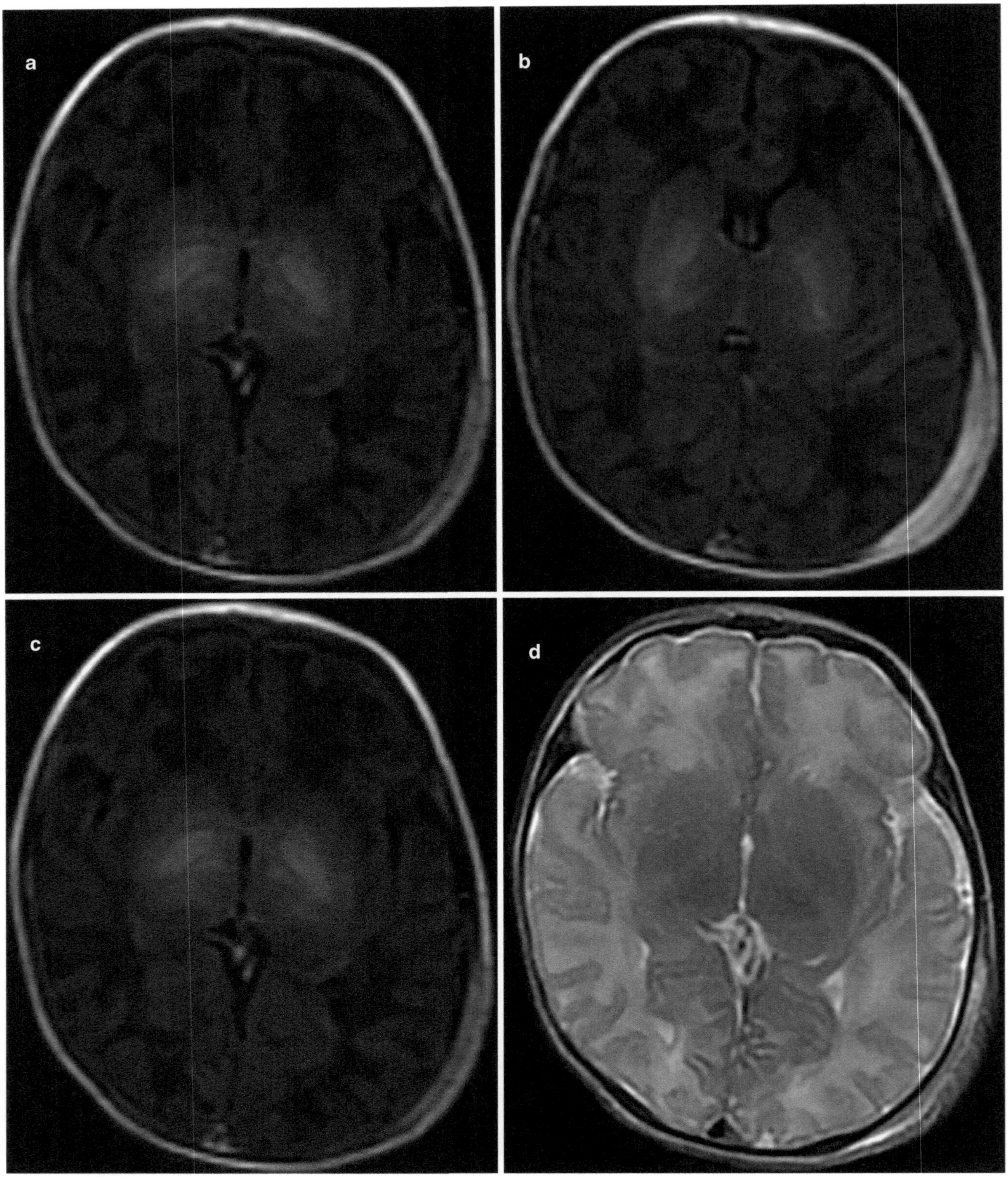

Fig. 7.8 Kernicterus

Case 7.6 Neonatal Hypoglycemia

Clinical Presentation

A male infant, 6 days old, with birth weight of 4000 g. The baby has poor feeding with shortness of breath. The mother had gestational hyperglycemia with blood sugar of 1.3 mmol/L, OGTT: 5.2–8.3–7.1 mmol/L.

Imaging Findings

A-C. Diffusion Weighted Imaging demonstrates bilateral occipital lobe and parietal lobe injure with high signal intensity, and the splenium of corpus callosum and posterior limb of internal capsule as well as corticospinal tract were involved (Fig. 7.9a–c).

D. There was no obvious abnormality in Axial T2-weighted image (Fig. 7.9d).

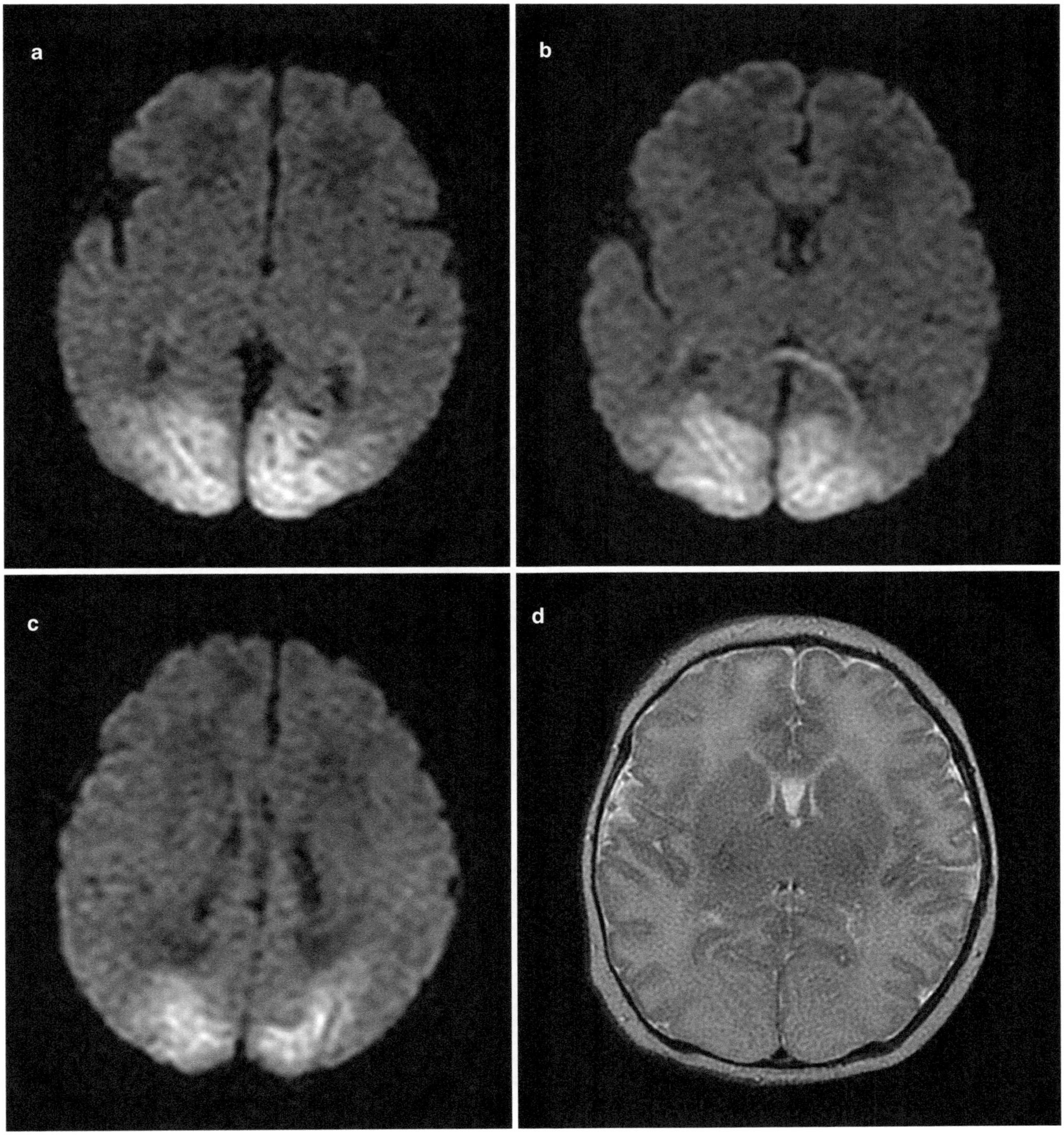

Fig. 7.9 Neonatal hypoglycemia

Discussion

Hypoglycemia is a common metabolic disease in early neonatal period. Glucose, as a necessary substance for brain energy metabolism, is the only energy source for the metabolism of neonatal brain tissue. In neonatal period, severe and persistent hypoglycemia can cause brain damage, further leading to acute and long-term neurological impairment, cerebral palsy, developmental disorder, visual impairment, and other sequelae [20].

The brain injury resulting from neonatal hypoglycemia may also cause lethargy, low muscle tension, easy to panic, screaming, shaking, restlessness, coma and seizures, and other neurological dysfunction [20]. The threshold for hypoglycemia is not yet well defined. The most common areas suffering from brain injury are posterior parietal-occipital lobe on both sides, splenium of corpus callosum, posterior limb of internal capsule, corticospinal tract, often characterized by symmetry, and the least-affected areas are brain stem, cerebellum and basal ganglia. Recent studies have shown that the parietal-occipital lobe is not the most affected area, but its injury is more diverse than previously reported, including white matter injury, hemorrhage and middle cerebral artery infarction [21]. There are some causes for cortex injury of parietal-occipital lobe from neonatal hypoglycemia. First, compared with other areas of the cerebral cortex, there are signs of four layers of visual cortex evidently thickening, more neurons and synapses, a significant increasing need for glucose during the formation of axon and synapse in occipital lobe. Second, metabolic disturbance and damage to oxygen-free radical are the main causes of cell edema. Third, excitatory amino acids increase the activation of the NMDA receptor, and then the ion channels are open, resulting in cytotoxic edema [22, 23].

The mechanism of causing injury to splenium of corpus callosum is not yet to be clearly identified. However, the high signal on DWI and lower ADC in hypoglycemic brain injury indicate the possible mechanism of cytotoxic edema: lack of glucose causing insufficient metabolic energy in the brain, and therefore leading to a decrease in the activity of ion pump in cell membrane, and then extracellular intercellular transport of water molecules, which finally contributes to cytotoxic edema [24]. The MRI findings of hypoglycemic brain injury revealed a low signal on T1WI, normal or higher signal on T2WI after 5 days of hypoglycemia. Early MRI of brain injury showed that the damage of corticospinal tract is linked to impaired movement and cognitive development after 1 year old. Severe hypoglycemia, acute phase metabolic disorder, energy failure may lead to edema or necrosis of nerve cells, and further cause limited movement of water molecules in cells. In the chronic phase, it may contribute to encephalomalacia, encephalatrophy, ventricular enlargement. DWI was particularly sensitive to the movement of water molecules in cells after tissue injury, showing high signal, which could make the lesions detected earlier (within 24 h). At this time, T1WI and T2WI were not obviously examined on MRI. MRS can reflect the early stage of brain injury by measuring the levels of phosphocreatine and lactic acid, which form high-energy phosphate bonds in the brain [25, 26].

This disease needs to be differentiated from HIE, cerebral infarction, and other diseases. HIE often occurs in the watershed area, and premature infant is mainly caused by white matter injury, term infants mainly caused by gray matter injury, severe injury caused by both of the injury, often accompanied with different degrees of cerebral hemorrhage. The severity of hypoglycemia brain injury is related to the duration of hypoglycemia, and the distribution of lesion does not match that of cerebral vessels, and cerebral hemorrhage is unlikely to occur.

Case 7.7 Intracranial Hemorrhage Due to Vitamin K Deficiency

Clinical Presentation

A male infant was admitted to hospital for crying and vomiting on the 43rd day after birth; PT:100 s and APTT:190 s.

Imaging Findings

CT demonstrates cerebral hemorrhage of right frontal-parietal lobe, with adjacent parenchyma slightly compressed; A small amount of subarachnoid hemorrhage occurred (arrow) (Fig. 7.10a).

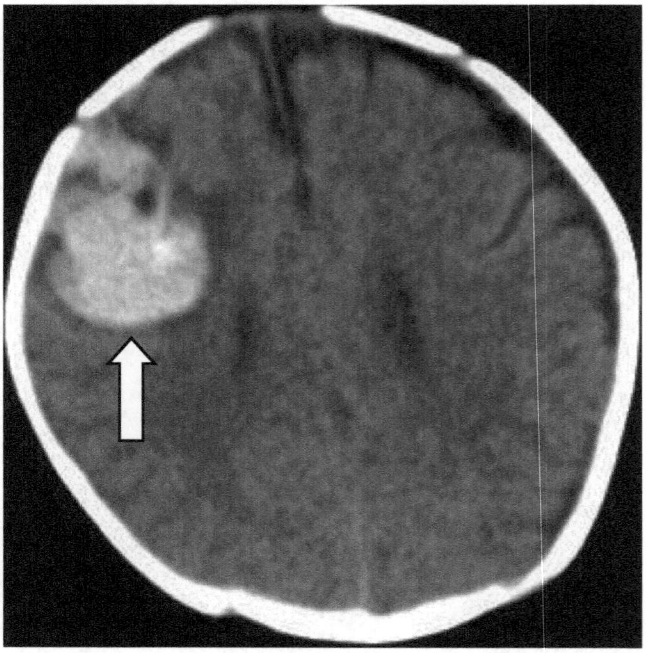

Fig. 7.10 Intracranial hemorrhage due to Vitamin K deficiency

Discussion

Vitamin K deficiency bleeding (VKDB) is a hemorrhagic syndrome caused by a severe lack of vitamin K in infants who are breastfed after birth. VKDB can be classified into three categories by age of onset: Early VKDB (<24 h after birth), classic VKDB (2–14 days), and late VKDB (2–12 weeks). About 50% of VKDB patients may suffer from intracranial hemorrhage. In accordance with European and Asian reports, the incidence of intracranial hemorrhage is (4.4 ~ 7.2)/100,000 [27]. Late VKDB can suddenly lead to the onset of intracranial hemorrhage, which progresses rapidly, has the disability rate to the nervous system as high as 33~50%, and cause great suffering to society and families. The bleeding site and hematoma characteristics of this disease are not specific, and its diagnosis needs to be combined with medical history [28].

Vitamin K deficiency is caused by that vitamin K cannot be fully utilized to synthesize prothrombin (coagulation factors II, VII, IX, X, etc.) due to insufficient intake and absorption of vitamin K or liver dysfunction. In general, if the level of prothrombin is reduced by 30%, bleeding may be caused; if its level is as low as 20% or less, spontaneous bleeding may occur. It has been reported that hemostatic effects can be achieved within 6 h after the application of vitamin K1 [29].

Computed tomography (CT) shows: Intracranial hemorrhage can occur in the brain parenchyma, subarachnoid space, subdural space, ventricular system, and other parts, and it is more common in the supratentorial brain parenchyma and subarachnoid space. In general, cerebral hematoma is larger, and has crumby homogeneous high density and mixed density; a blood-liquid level may occur in subacute hemorrhage. It can also be expressed as scattered patchy high-density shadows of varying sizes, which can involve several lobes. Hypoxic-ischemic encephalopathy (HIE) and large cerebral infarction can be accompanied: For the patients with large hematomas, especially those with a large area of cerebral infarction, there are often changes in cerebromalacia lesion and other sequelae. In addition, cerebral palsy can occur in 25% of cases, causing deformation, stenosis, displacement, or occlusion of the cistern around the suprasellar cistern and brainstem. The affected ventricle is compressed to get narrow due to hemorrhage and edema, and moves to the uninjured side together with the midline structure, causing expansion of the lateral ventricle. Magnetic Resonance (MR) has obvious advantages in judging bleeding time, and it is also the best way to observe white matter damage.

The disease needs to be differentiated from hemorrhage caused by cerebral vascular malformation, hypoxic ischemia, and obstetric injury. The hemorrhage site and hematoma characteristics of the disease are not specific, so the diagnosis needs to be combined with the medical history of the disease [30, 31].

Case 7.8 Hydrocephalus

Clinical Presentation

A baby boy, 17 months old, had enlargement of skull and anterior fontanelle, increased intracranial pressure, and delayed motor development with Babinski (+).

Imaging Findings

A. Axial T2-weighted image demonstrates "significant enlargement of supratentorial ventricular system"; (Fig. 7.11a).

B-C. The vein in the fornix and the brain were displaced downward, the diaterma was protruded into enlarged sella turcica, and the interstitial edema was evident around the ventricular horn; (Fig. 7.11b–c).

D. Sagittal T1-weighted image demonstrates "aqueductal stenosis and The corpus callosum thinned and stretched upward" (Fig. 7.11d).

Discussion

Hydrocephalus is a complicated neurologic condition with numerous causes and treatment approaches. In basic terms, it implies fluid (CSF) volume and concomitant increase in ventricular size [32].

At present, the core problem of basic research on hydrocephalus is the exploration of pathogenesis thereof. It is well known that the pathogenesis of hydrocephalus includes excessive secretion (choroidal papilloma), circulatory obstruction (congenital malformation, tumor and hematoma compression of the aqueduct, blockment of interventricular pores, etc.), and malabsorption (traffic hydrocephalus). The pathogenesis of the first two cases is relatively clear, and the cause of cerebrospinal fluid malabsorption has become a key issue in the research of hydrocephalus pathogenesis. The circulatory dynamics of cerebrospinal fluid is an extremely complex process. In the past, it was thought that the decrease in brain tissue compliance led to an increase in intraventricular pressure due to an increase in the pressure of intracranial arterial pulsations. Thereafter, the enlargement of the ventricles and the reduction of the subarachnoid space occur. The occurrence of hydrocephalus is actually the redistribution of cerebrospinal fluid in the brain, and the capillaries participate in the absorption of cerebrospinal fluid. In 2004, Greitz believed that arachnoid granules were not the only way to absorb cerebrospinal fluid, mainly because it was absorbed through the surface of the central nervous system. In 2011, Klarica et al. proposed a new hypothesis on cerebrospinal fluid dynamics: not formed mainly by the choroid plexuses, CSF does not then circulate to finally be absorbed. However, it appears and disappears throughout the entire CSF system, depending on the hydrostatic and osmotic forces between the CSF, interstitial fluid (ISF), and blood capillaries [33, 34].

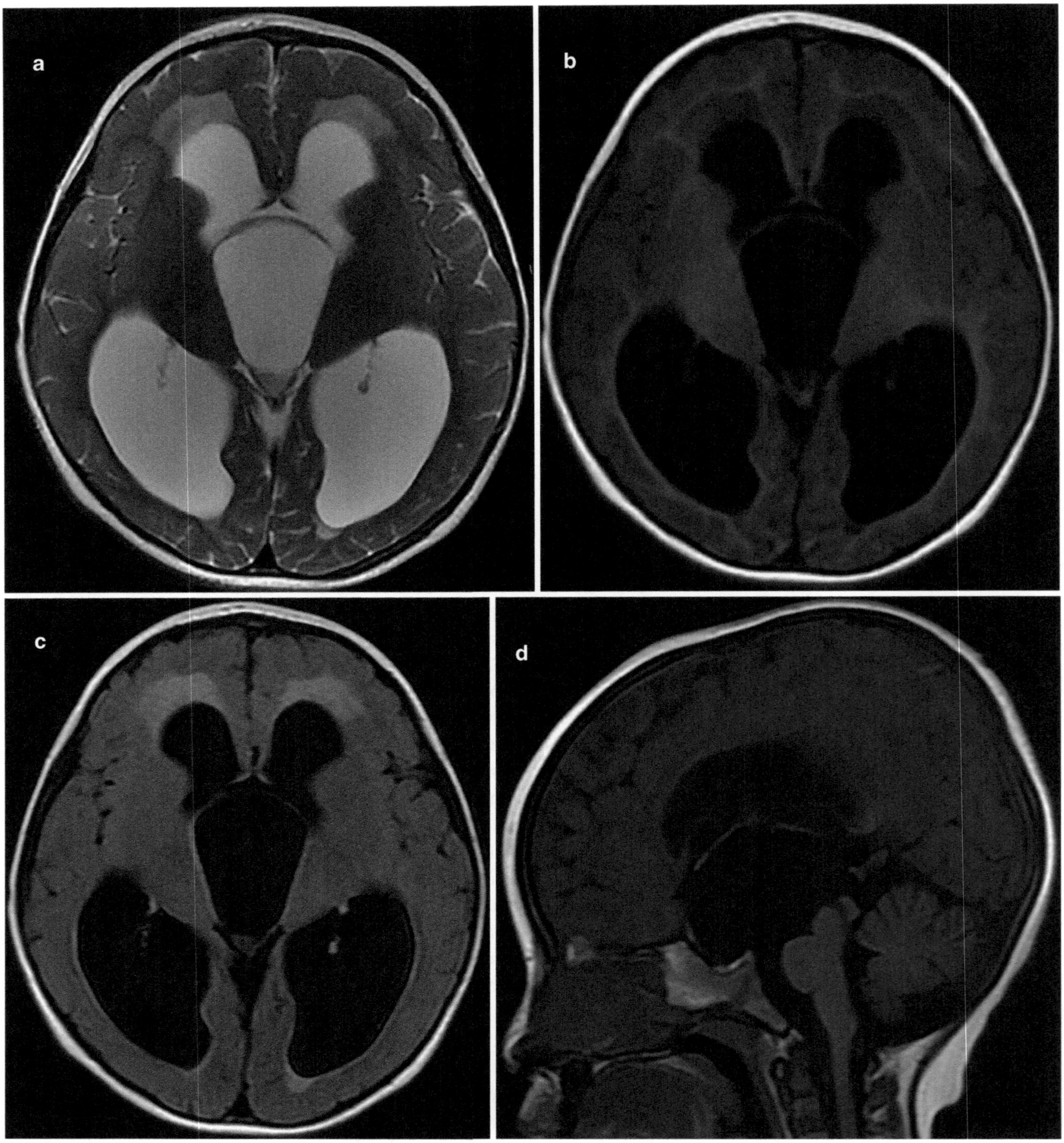

Fig. 7.11 Hydrocephalus

Severe hydrocephalus can cause brain tissue deformation around the ventricles, brain herniation, ventricular diverticulum, and secondary midbrain aqueduct stenosis. The most common brain herniation is the anterior recess hemia of the third ventricle and the upper recess hemia in the third ventricle. The anterior recess hemia is caused by the optic chiasm and the funnel crypt extending downwards, deep into the upper saddle pool, and compressing the funnel to cause hypothalamic-pituitary dysfunction. The anterior recess hemia of the third ventricle in the pineal gland is due to the expansion of the recess into the gap of the tentorial incisure and the pineal gland down, and even the Galen vein elevation is visible. When the upper recess hemia is further enlarged, the cover can be pressed back, causing the cover to be thinned and the midbrain aqueduct to be narrow. The ventricular diverticulum is due to the infiltration of the ventricular wall into the upper cerebellar and quadrant pools, which may indicate that the lateral ventricle triangle is connected to the diverticulum. If the hydrocephalus is combined with the absence of the corpus callosum, the ventricular diverticulum can enter the cerebral hemisphere intervertebral fissure, which is a type I hemispheric cyst, which may be associated with skull defect or meningeal bulging. Severe hydrocephalus can compress the midbrain back, the quadrilateral pool, and the midbrain aqueduct, and then the primary traffic hydrocephalus combined with the secondary midbrain aqueduct stenosis [33].

Hydrocephalus is caused by cerebrospinal fluid circulation disorder (channel blocking), cerebrospinal fluid malabsorption, excessive cerebrospinal fluid secretion, brain parenchyma atrophy, and other reasons. In clinical application, obstructive pathogenesis is the most common, such as blocking of different parts of the ventricular system (interventricular foramen, aqueduct, median aperture), space-occupying lesion compression of adjacent parts of the ventricular system and congenital malformation of the central nervous system. This nomenclature divides hydrocephalus as communicating (with or without obstruction to CSF absorption) or noncommunicating and forms the basis for our article. Recently, members of the International Society for hydrocephalus and CSF Research suggested a simple "point of obstruction" model. Members of the Hydrocephalus Classification study group including Rekate proposed a simple scheme where they suggested that all hydrocephalus is obstructive and nomenclature is based on the site of obstruction to the CSF circuit. The point of obstruction could be the foramen of Monroe, aqueduct of sylvius, fourth ventricle, basal cisterns, arachnoid granulations, or venous outflow.

Communicating hydrocephalus is hydrocephalus caused by blocking below the exit level of the fourth ventricle. CT and MRI show that the ventricular system is generally enlarged and the sulci are flattened or disappear. If the tentorium cerebelli hiatus is blocked, all the ventricles are enlarged with the enlargement of cisterna magna and pontine cistern. When the basilar cistern expands and cerebral convex sulci do not change, the horizontal blocking of cisterna chiasmatica is often suggested. The blocking of arachnoid granulations on the surface of the brain should be considered when the upper sulci are generally widened to the level of the sagittal sinus.

Non-communicating hydrocephalus refers to the blocking above the exit of the fourth ventricle, expansion of the ventricular system above the blocking level to varying degrees, and normal or shrinking distal ventricle. Monro blocking on one or both sides can lead to unilateral or bilateral ventricular enlargement. Midbrain aqueduct stenosis (<1 mm, anteroposterior diameter of proximal aqueduct is greater than 4 mm) is characterized by the enlargement of bilateral ventricles and the third ventricle. The fourth ventricle is normal or becomes smaller. It is common in congenital diseases, inflammatory and tumorous lesions. Sagittal MRI can show the morphology of midbrain aqueduct, ventricular hernia, and other local pathological signs. Ventricle enlargement can result in thinning, compression, and upward movement of callosum. Hydrocephalus can cause intracranial blood stasis in pia mater, and T1WI can be significantly enhanced. The aqueduct emptying phenomenon often disappears in non-communicating hydrocephalus. The 3D-CISS sequence can highlight the signals of CSF with the effect of heavy T2WI, reduce the flow artifact of CSF, and display the edge of ventricle clearly. Phase-contrast cine MRI can display and measure changes in flow rate, flow and direction of cerebrospinal fluid flowing through the aqueduct. In case of communicating hydrocephalus, flow rate and flow of cerebrospinal fluid increase; and in non-communicating hydrocephalus, flow rate and flow of cerebrospinal fluid decrease [34].

Hydrocephalus should be distinguished from cerebral atrophy, hydroanencephalus, and other diseases. In case of brain atrophy, sulci and cistern are obviously widened, the ventricle enlargement is often obvious in the frontal angle, and the enlargement of the third ventricle is rare. In case of hydroanencephalus, no normal frontal lobe, temporal lobe or parietal lobe can be seen, and no lateral ventricle structure can be found. Even in case of severe hydrocephalus, the anterior horn of bilateral ventricle and brain parenchyma of the occipital lobe are compressed and thinned.

Case 7.9 Osmotic Demyelination Syndrome

This case was provided by Guangzhou Women and Children's Medical Center, China.

Clinical Presentation

A boy, 7 years old, was admitted to hospital for vomiting, aphasia, and limb weakness, with the blood sodium of 105 mmol/L at admission. The boy was given symptomatic treatment such as correcting electrolyte disturbance. After 2 days, the blood sodium of the boy returned to normal, but his condition did not improve significantly.

Imaging Findings

A-C. Axial T2-weighted image demonstrates that bilateral basal ganglia, semioval center and pons had symmetrical high signals (Fig. 7.12a–c).

D. Axial T2-weighted image demonstrates low signal corresponding to T2WI, (Fig. 7.12d).

E-F. It was significantly enhanced after enhanced scanning (Fig. 7.12e–f).

Discussion

Osmotic demyelination syndrome (ODS) is a rare acute non-inflammatory demyelinating central nervous system disease. Depending on diseased parts, it can be divided into central

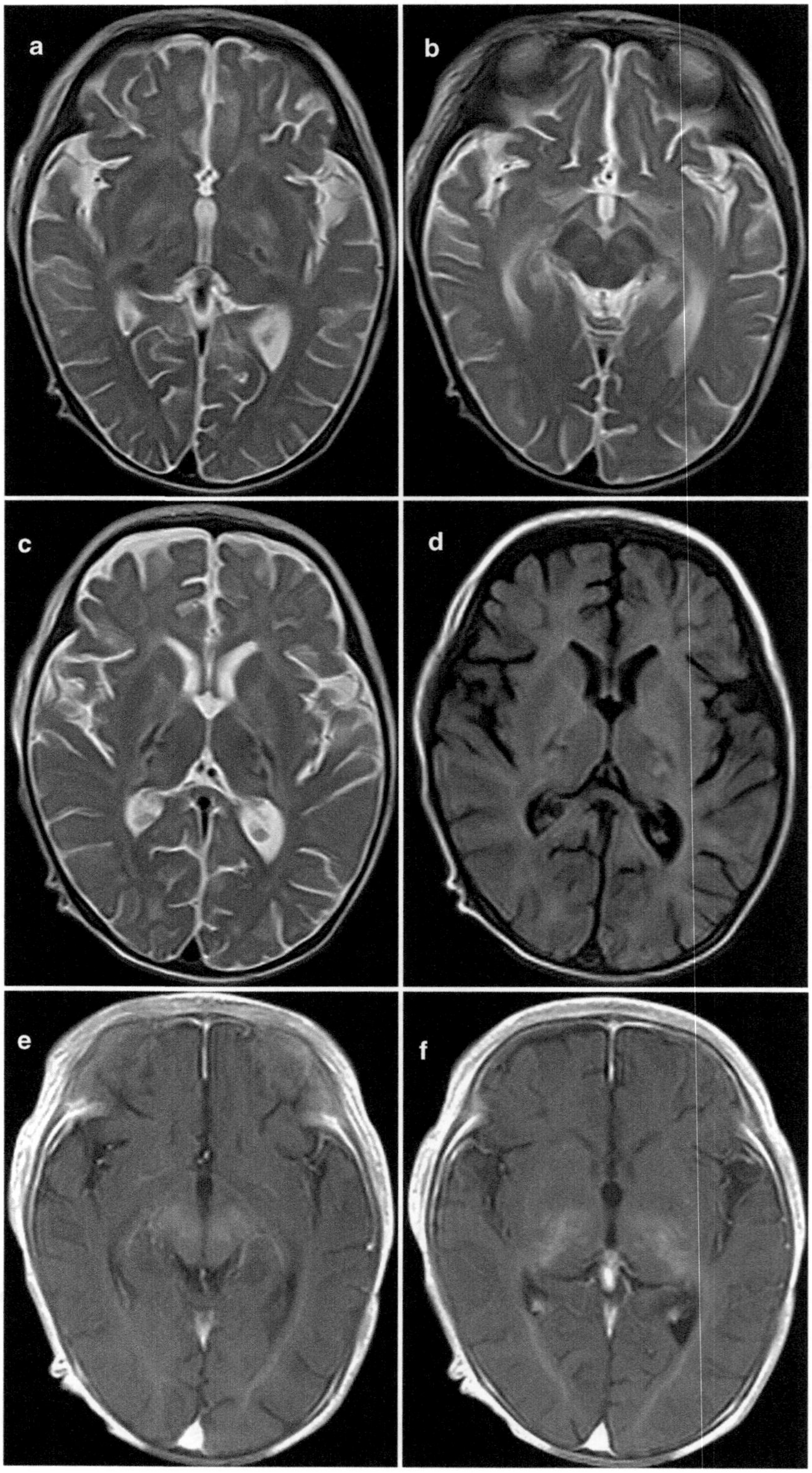

Fig. 7.12 Osmotic demyelination syndrome

pontine myelinolysis (CPM) (involving pons) and extrapontine myelinolysis (EPM) (involving basal ganglia, thalamus, hippocampus, cerebellum, etc.), which can exist separately or simultaneously [35].

Etiology and pathogenesis of ODS are still unclear. Hyponatremia is the main risk factor, and some ODS patients are associated with the rapid correction of hyperosmolar status. Clinical manifestations of ODS are diversified. It usually occurs 5–7 days after hypertonic injury, but occurs 2 weeks or more later. Typical cases of CPM appear as bipolar clinical passage: It appears as a convulsion of limbs or encephalopathy in the early stage. With the correction and improvement of hyponatremia, symptoms become worse in the process of treatment. The pseudobulbar palsy, central quadriparesis, different levels of disturbance of consciousness and other symptoms appear. In severe cases, the patients are silent or have complete/incomplete locked-in syndrome. This is due to the damage of corticobulbar tract, corticospinal tract, and ascending reticular activating system near the midline of the basal part of the pons [36, 37].

The magnetic resonance manifestations of ODS are characteristic, and the lesions located at the base of pons are butterfly-shaped, appearing as symmetric low signal of T1WI and high signal of T2WI. After enhancement, most patients have no enhancement, while some patients have mild to moderate enhancement, which is not consistent with the direction and distribution of vessels. There is no obvious occupying effect. The typical manifestations of EPM are symmetrical low signal of T1WI and high signal of T2WI in the brain [36]. Lesions are most common in cerebellar hemisphere, lateral geniculate body, basal ganglia region, etc. Cortex involvement is rare. The time of abnormal signals on ODS MRI may be significantly later than the time when symptoms appear. The time difference is about 1–2 weeks. Therefore, no abnormality is found by MRI examination at the early stage of the disease.

The disease needs to be differentiated from Wernicke encephalopathy, cerebral infarction, and Hepatolenticular degeneration. Wernicke encephalopathy: The disorder of glucose metabolism caused by vitamin B1 deficiency, often appears as symmetrical low T1WI signal and high T2WI signal in the gray matter and other areas around the thalamus, mamillary body and aqueduct, mainly in the mamillary body. Cerebral infarction often has risk factors and is consistent with vascular distribution. Hepatolenticular degeneration: It is a recessive hereditary disease caused by a copper metabolism defect on the autosome. It presents as symmetrical long low T1 signal and high T2 signal in the basal ganglia, thalamus, brainstem, and cerebellum [38]. It has no obvious space-occupying effect and edema effect, mostly accompanied by brain atrophy, but it will not be strengthened after enhancement. Its pathogenic site is mainly on the basal ganglia.

References

1. James B, Charles R. Pediatric neuroimaging (Pediatric Neuroimaging (Barkovich)) [M]. Lippincott Williams & Wilkins. 2011.
2. Coley BD Caffey's pediatric diagnostic imaging, 2-volume set: Expert consult—online and print, 12e[M]. Saunders. 2013.
3. Tatsuharu S, Mitsuhiro K, Kaoru M, et al. A case of tubulinopathy presenting with porencephaly caused by a novel missense mutation in the TUBA1A gene. Brain Dev. 2018;40(9):819–23.
4. Naomi HF, Noriko T, Ritsuko T, et al. Neuroepidemiology of porencephaly, schizencephaly, and hydranencephaly in miyagi prefecture, Japan. Pediatr Neurol. 2016;54:39–42.
5. Harada T, Uegaki T, Arata K, et al. Schizencephaly and porencephaly due to fetal intracranial hemorrhage: a report of two cases. Yonago Acta Med. 2017;60(4):241–5.
6. Chao CP, Zaleski CG, Patton AC. Neonatal hypoxic-ischemic encephalopathy: multimodality imaging findings. Radiographics. 2006;26(Suppl 1):S159–72. https://doi.org/10.1148/rg.26si065504.
7. Back SA. Perinatal while matter injury: the changing spectrum of pathology and emerging insights into pathogenetic mechanisms. Ment Retard Dev Disabil Res Rev. 2006;12(2):129–140.
8. Chao CP, Zaleski CG, Patton AC, et al. Neonatal hypoxic-ischemic encephalopathy: multimodality imaging findings. Radiographics. 2006;26(Special):S159–72.
9. Krishnan P, Shroff M. Neuroimaging in neonatal hypoxic ischemic encephalopathy. Indian J Pediatr. 2016;83(9):995–1002.
10. D'Alton ME, Hankins GD, Berkowitz RI, et al. Neonatal encephalopathy and neurologic outcome: report of the American College of Obstetricians and Gynecologists' Task force on Neonatal Encephalopathy. Pediatrics. 2014;133:e1482–8.
11. Ballabh P. Intraventricular hemorrhage in premature infants: mechanism of disease. Pediatr Res. 2010;67(1):1–8.
12. Kuperman AA, Kenet G, Papadakis E, et al. Intraventricular hemorrhage in preterm infants: coagulation perspectives. Semin Thromb Hemost. 2011;37(7):730–6.
13. Huang BY, Castillo M. Hypoxic-ischemic brain injury: imaging findings from birth to adulthood. Radiographics. 2008;28:417–39.
14. Groenendaal F, de Vries LS. Fifty years of brain imaging in neonatal encephalopathy following perinatal asphyxia. Pediatr Res. 2017;81(1–2):150–5. https://doi.org/10.1038/pr.2016.195.
15. Barkovich AJ, Westmark KD, Bedi HS, et al. Proton spectroscopy and diffusion imaging on the first day of life after perinatal asphyxia: preliminary report. AJNR Am J Neuroradiol. 2001;22:1786–94.
16. Okumura A, Kidokoro H, Shoji H, et al. Kernicterus in preterm infants. Pediatrics. 2009;123(6):e1052–8.
17. Wang XY, Wu WL, Hou BL, et al. Studying neonatal bilirubin encephalopathy with conventional MRI, MRS, and DWI. Neuroradiology. 2008;50(10):885–93.
18. Coskun A, Yikilmaz A, Kumandas S, et al. Hyperintense globus Pallidus on T1-weighted MR imaging in acute Kernicterus: is it common or rare? Eur Radiol. 2005;15:1263–7.
19. Watanabe H, Fukatsu H, Katsuno M, et al. Multiple regional 1H-MR spectroscopy in multiple system atrophy: NAA/Cr reduction in pontine base as a valuable diagnostic marker. BMJ. 2004;75:103–9.
20. Wong DS, Poskitt KJ, Chau V, et al. Brain injury patterns in hypoglycemia in neonatal encephalopathy. AJNR Am J Neuroradiol. 2013;34:1456–61.
21. Yalnizoglu D, Haliloglu G, Turanli G, et al. Neurologic outcome in patients with MRI pattern of damage typical for neonatal hypoglycemia. Brain Dev. 2007;29(5):285–92.
22. Parvaneh K, Sepideh T, Mohammad G. Hypoglycemia-occipital syndrome: a specific neurologic syndrome following neonatal hypoglycemia? J Child Neurol. 2011;26(2):152–9.
23. Thompson BA, Havranek T. Neonatal hypoglycemia. Pediatr Rev. 2017;38(4):147–57.
24. Adamkin DH. Neonatal hypoglycemia. Curr Opin Pediatr. 2016;28(2):150–5.
25. Burns CM, Rutherford MA, Boardmall JP, et al. Patterns of cerebral injury and neurodevelopmental outeorrles after symptomatic neonatal hypoglycemia. Pediatrics. 2008;122(1):65–74.
26. Arya VB, Senniappan S, Guemes M, et al. Neonatal hypoglycemia. Curr Opin Endocrinol Diabetes Obes. 2014;8l(1):58–65.
27. American Academy of Pediatrics Committee on fetus and Newborn. Controversies concerning vitamin K and the newborn. Pediatrics. 2003;112(1 Part1):191–2.
28. Von KR, Hachmeister A, Gobel U. Oral mixed micellar vitamin K for prevention of late vitamin K deficiency bleeding. Arch Dis Child Fetal Neonatal Ed. 2003;2:F109–12.

29. Sutor AH, Dagres N, Niederhoff H. Late form of vitamin K deficiency bleeding in Germany. Klin Padiatr. 1995;207(3):89–97.
30. Anita J, Petra P, Ana P, et al. Neonatal prophylaxis: prevention of vitamin K deficiency haemorrhage and neonatal ophthalmia. Zdr Varst. 2015;54(3):184–93.
31. Schulte R, Jordan LC, Morad A, et al. Rise in late onset vitamin k deficiency bleeding in young infants because of omission or refusal of prophylaxis at birth. Pediatr Neurol. 2014;50(6):564–8.
32. Huff N, Naik S. Hydranencephaly in monochorionic-diamniotic twins. Pediatr Neurol. 2017;67:107–8.
33. Kahle KT, Kulkarni AV, Limbrick DD, et al. Hydrocephalus in children. Lancet. 2016;387(10020):788–99.
34. Amit A, Girish B, Sangam K. Imaging of communicating hydrocephalus. Semin Ultrasound CT MRI. 2016;37(2):100–8.
35. Shah B, Tobias J. Osmotic demyelination and hypertonic dehydration in a 9-year-old girl: changes in cerebrospinal fluid myelin basic protein. J Intensive Care Med. 2006;21(6):372–6.
36. Turnbull J, Lumsden D, Siddiqui A, et al. Osmotic demyelination syndrome associated with hypophosphataemia: 2 cases and a review of literature. Acta Paediatr. 2013;102(4):e164–8.
37. Lalit RB, Timothy Z. Osmotic demyelination syndrome in children. Pediatr Neurol. 2019;97:12–7.
38. Yo-ichi T, Chiho A, Shu-ichi I. Osmotic demyelination Syndrome: reversible MRI findings in bilateral cortical lesions. Intern Med. 2003;42(9):867–70.

Neurodegenerative Diseases

8

Honglei Shang, Xin Zhao, and Xiaoan Zhang

Neurodegenerative diseases are characterized by the gradual loss of selectively vulnerable neuronal populations, in contrast to selected static neuronal loss due to metabolic or toxic diseases. Neurodegenerative diseases can be classified according to major clinical features (such as dementia, Parkinson's disease, or motor neuron diseases), anatomical distribution of neurodegenerative diseases (such as anterior temporal lobe degeneration, extrapyramidal disease, or spinocerebellar degeneration), or major molecular abnormalities. The common neurodegenerative diseases in adults such as Alzheimer's disease, frontotemporal lobe degeneration, Parkinson's disease, and multiple system atrophy are really rare in children. The childhood neurogenerative diseases of as yet unclear pathophysiology are sometimes categorized based on whether they affect the brain homogenously (diffuse encephalopathies) or preferentially affecting the cerebral cortex (poliodystrophies), the cerebral white matter (leukodystrophies), the basal ganglia (corencephalopathies), or the cerebellum, brainstem, and spinal cord (spinocerebellar diseases). In this chapter, we only introduce two relatively common neurodegenerative diseases in children and hope to contribute to a more comprehensive and detailed study of childhood neurogenerative diseases in the future.

Case 8.1 Olivopontocerebellar Atrophy

Clinical Presentation

A 9-month-old girl presented to unresponsiveness, weakness in the limbs, and limbs irregular shaking. There was no history of genetic, infectious, or similar cerebral palsy in the family.

H. Shang
Department of Radiology, The Third Affiliated Hospital of Zhengzhou University, Zhengzhou, Henan, China

X. Zhao · X. Zhang (✉)
Department of Radiology, The Third Affiliated Hospital of Zhengzhou University, Institute of Neuroscience, Zhengzhou University, Zhengzhou, Henan, China
e-mail: zdsfyzx@zzu.edu.cn; zxa@zzu.edu.cn

Imaging Findings

A. Axial T2-weighted image passing through mid-pons demonstrates the "hot cross bun" sign typically (arrow) (Fig. 8.1a).
B. Midline sagittal Ti-weighted image shows moderate atrophy in the cerebellum and in the pons, with flattening of its inferior part. The atrophy is severe and involves the whole pons (arrow) (Fig. 8.1b).
C-D. Axial T1-weighted and T2-FLAIR images show the "hot cross bun" sign atypically (arrow). Note the atrophy in the cerebellum (Fig. 8.1c–d).

Discussion

The term "olivopontocerebellar atrophy" was introduced by Dejerine and Thomas [1] in 1900 to designate the pathological presentation in a patient with sporadic adult-onset progressive cerebellar ataxia, and it has survived the test of time and enjoys widespread recognition in either the full expression or its acronym OPCA [2]. In general, OPCA is a slowly progressive neurodegenerative disease of unknown cause, which can be divided into genetic and sporadic types. In genetic OPCA group, the onset age was early. Cerebellar sign was obvious, and it was the most common first symptom, accompanied by dementia, extraocular muscle paralysis, pyramidal fascicle sign, and bulbar paralysis. In sporadic type, frequent urination, urination urgency, and unstable standing were seen in the early stage, followed by common relief disorder, dysarthria, and so on. A small number of patients can also be complicated with bilateral vertebral tract signs, limb muscle atrophy, nystagmus or extraocular muscle paralysis, and other symptoms.

The pathological changes of OPCA were cerebellum, pons, olivary nucleus atrophy, neuronal loss with glial hyperplasia, and also involved red nucleus, nigra, basal ganglia, and cerebral cortex. At present, the pathogenesis of the disease is not clear, which may be related to heredity, immunity, virus infection, free radical damage, biochemical abnormalities, and so on. Up to now, there is no effective therapeutic method. Therefore, early detection and timely treatment can delay the

H. Liu, X. Zhang (eds.), *Pediatric Neuroimaging*, https://doi.org/10.1007/978-981-16-7928-5_8

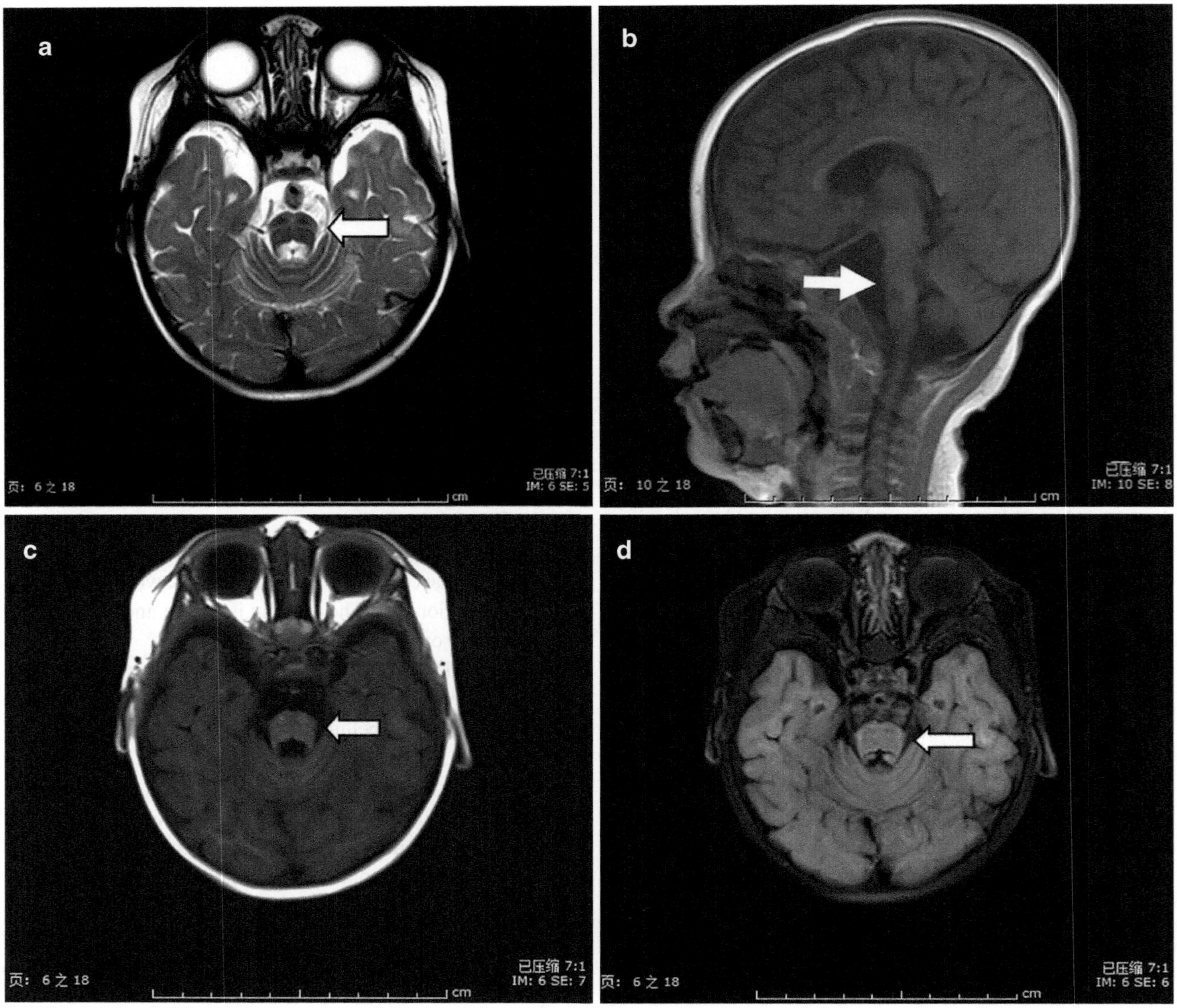

Fig. 8.1 Olivopontocerebellar atrophy (OPCA)

development of the disease, and also improve the clinical symptoms and improve the quality of life of the patients.

CT or MRI examination is a necessary technique to characterize the brain stem and cerebellar atrophy of OPCA in clinical practice [3]. MRI is crucial for the diagnosis of OPCA. The morphological characteristics of MRI in patients with OPCA were atrophy and thinning of brain stem, narrowing of anteroposterior diameter of pons, symmetrical or asymmetrical changes of cerebellar volume, widening and deepening of cerebellar sulcus, enlargement of cistern and ventricle, mild atrophy of frontal and parietal lobe. And the brain parenchyma generally has no abnormal signal. If cerebellopontine foot atrophy occurs, the transverse and longitudinal fibers of pontine are involved, T2WI shows high signal intensity and pons "cross sign," which is of great value in the diagnosis of OPCA. The more serious pons atrophy are, the more obvious the "cross sign" of OPCA are. However, not all OPCA patients were positive for MRI, especially the MRI signs of OPCA patients in the early stage of onset were not canonical. And DWI made up for it in this respect. DWI can quantitatively analyze the early neurodegeneration of OPCA patients by ADC value, and it is not necessary to wait until the late morphological manifestation of the lesion is abnormal. In addition, PET scans of OPCA patients showed significant decreases in local cerebral metabolic rates of lumbrical, cerebellar, and brain stem glucose (LCMRgluc), as compared with those of normal control subjects [4].

On the basis of the classification of genetic and sporadic types, some authors have further classified according to genetic, clinical, biochemical, and pathological characteristics [5]. The numerous and complex manifestations of OPCA not only lead to confusion in classification, but also bring difficulties to clinical work. A growing number of researchers believe that OPCA may be one of the pathological features of other diseases, such as multiple system atrophy (MSA), mitochondrial encephalopathy, hexosamine deficiency, adrenal leukodystrophy, or spongiform encephalopathy [6]. In addition, familial OPCA is often misdiagnosed as familial prion disorder (Gerstmann-scheinker Syndrome) or familial insomnia. Therefore, in addition to relying on the typical MRI manifestations ("cross sign"), the differential diagnosis of OPCA should be based on the characteristic clinical symptoms.

In summary, OPCA is a pathological marker that is often associated with lesions at all levels of the central nervous system, essentially presenting as a variable progressive cerebellar-plus syndrome.

Case 8.2 Wallerian Degeneration

Clinical Presentation

A 3-year-old girl had a cerebral hemorrhage in the right frontal temporal-parietal lobe 2 years ago. She was delivered naturally at term and had asphyxia history. Her past surgical and family histories were negative.

Imaging Findings

A. Axial T2-weighted image demonstrates a large area of high signal in the right frontal parietal lobe (arrow), which was the formation of softening focus (Fig. 8.2a).

B-C. The volume of the right pons was smaller than that of the contralateral, while he signal had no significant change (arrow) (Fig. 8.2b–c).

Discussion

Animal experiments and neuroimaging studies had ever shown that there was secondary degeneration in fiber pathways in addition to the primary focus [7, 8], which was called Wallerian degeneration (WD). It means that retrograde and anterograde axonal degeneration secondary damage would occur in distal axon and myelin sheath after neuronal cell or proximal axonal injury [9], and this phenomenon existed widely in the whole nervous system. However, it is most common in the pyramidal tract. In contrast to the WD of the peripheral nerves, the central nervous system develops more slowly.

Combining with pathological and MRI manifestations, Kuhn et al. [10] used the appearance of primary lesions as the starting points and classified WD into the following stages: (1) Within 4 weeks, the axons of the affected nerve fibers begin to degenerate, but the biochemical changes are slight; (2) At 4–10 weeks, the myelin protein of nerve fibers is destroyed, but the lipid in myelin is relatively intact. And the hydrophilicity of degenerated tissues begins to increase; (3) At 10–14 weeks, the myelin lipids of the nerve fibers are destroyed and glial hyperplasia occurs. Then, the hydrophilicity of the degenerated tissue is significantly increased; (4) After several months to several years, the nerve fiber bundle completely disintegrates, the destruction, the local atrophy is obvious.

In terms of different imaging methods, WD presents different image features. CT has hysteresis for MRI examination

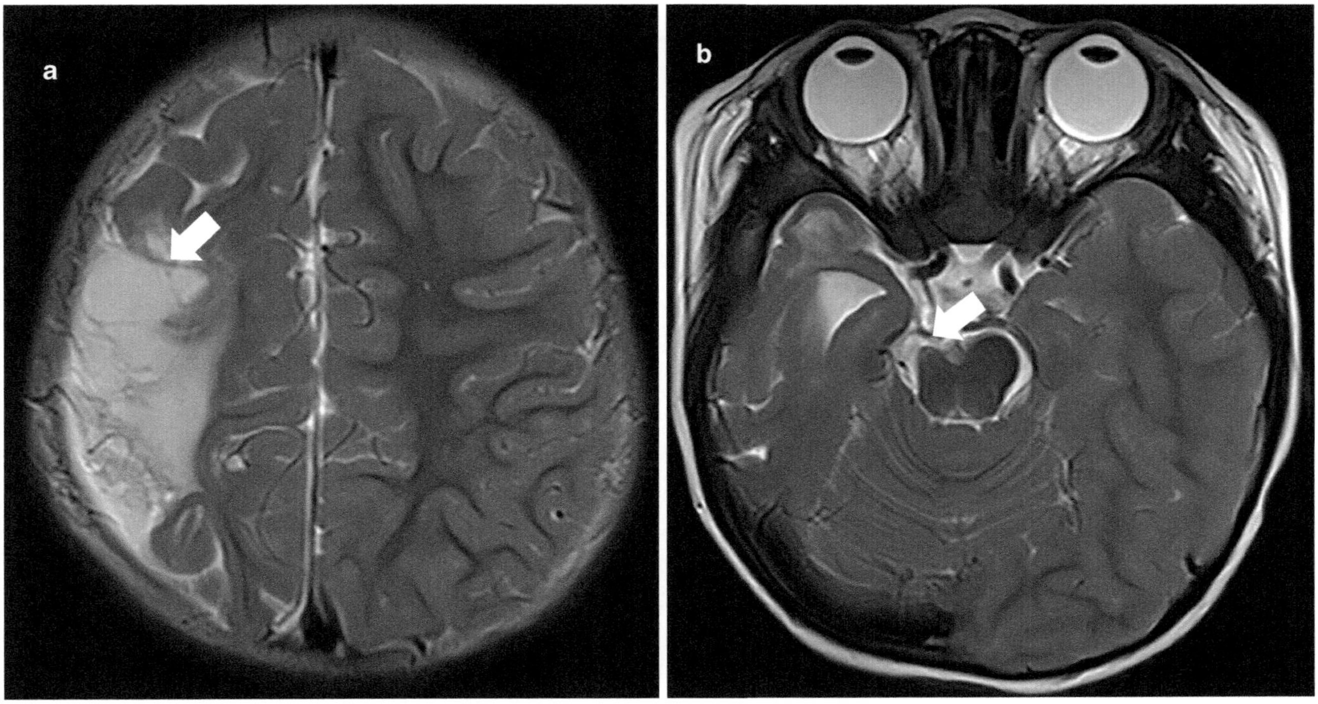

Fig. 8.2 Wallerian degeneration

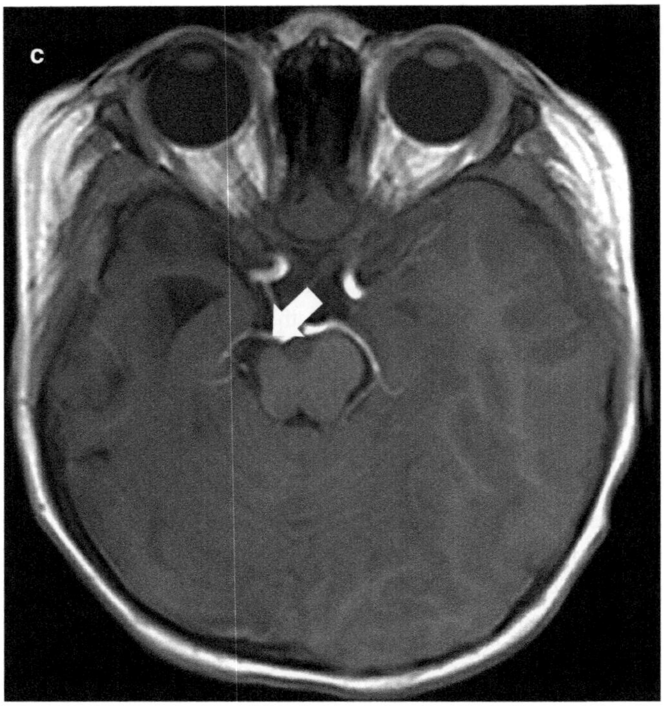

Fig. 8.2 (continued)

and can only detect brain tissue atrophy at the later stage of WD. MRI can initially detect the high signal of WD region in T1WI and low signal of T2WI in the fourth week after brain injury.

References

1. Dejerine J, Thomas A. L'atrophieolivo-ponto-cèrèbelleuse. NouvIconogr Salpêtrière. 1900;13:330–70.
2. Duvoisin RC. An apology and an introduction to the olivopontocerebellar atrophies. In: Duvoisin RC, Plaitakis A, editors. Olivopontocerebellar atrophies. New York: Raven Press; 1984. p. 13–38.
3. Jiang J, Wang J, Lin M, et al. Bilateral middle cerebellar peduncle lesions: neuroimaging features and differential diagnoses. Brain Behav. 2020;10(10):e01778.
4. Gilman S, Koeppe RA, Junck L, et al. Patterns of cerebral glucose metabolism detected with positron emission tomography differ in multiple system atrophy and olivopontocerebellar atrophy. Ann Neurol. 2010;36(2):166–75.
5. Cagnoli C, Mariotti C, Taroni F, et al. SCA28, a novel form of autosomal dominant cerebellar ataxia on chromosome 18p11.22-q22. Brain. 2006;129:235–42.
6. Bower PG. Multiple system atrophy: building a global community—30years of advocacy efforts. Auton Neurosci. 2017;211:39–42.
7. Loos M, Dihné M, Block F. Tumor necrosis factor-alpha expression in areas of remote degeneration following middle cerebral artery occlusion of the rat. Neuroscience. 2003;122(2):373–80.
8. Yu C, Zhu C, Zhang Y, Chen H, Qin W, Wang M, Li K. A longitudinal diffusion tensor imaging study on Wallerian degeneration of corticospinal tract after motor pathway stroke. NeuroImage. 2009;47:451–8.
9. Conforti L, Gilley J, Coleman MP. Wallerian degeneration: an emerging axon death pathway linking injury and disease. Nat Rev Neurosci. 2014;15(6):394–409.
10. Kuhn MJ, Mikulis DJ, Ayoub DM, Kosofsky BE, Davis KR, Taveras JM. Wallerian degeneration after cerebral infarction: evaluation with sequential MR imaging. Radiology. 1989;172(1):179–82.

Other Brain Diseases

9

Honglei Shang, Jing Chen, Guifen Zheng, Xin Zhao, Xiaoan Zhang, and Xin Li

This chapter includes some various disorders of the pediatric central nervous system other than the common diseases. Some are primary or secondary diseases during the infancy and childhood, such as trauma, infection, and so on. Others are some congenital lesions that are often with no typical symptoms and discovered incidentally. We introduced these diseases from their clinical symptoms, pathological manifestations, CT and MRI findings including advanced MR imaging methods such as arterial spin labeling(ASL) and magnetic resonance spectroscopy(MRS) to help clinicians make prompt diagnosis and treatment.

Case 9.1 Hippocampus Sclerosis

Clinical Presentation

A 11-year-old boy was admitted to hospital with intermittent convulsions for more than 3 months as the chief complaint. He first developed nausea symptoms, followed by convulsions, which were manifested as: not responding to calls, straight eyes, perioral salivation, cyanosis of the mouth, movement stopped, no obvious convulsions of the limbs, spontaneous remission lasting about 10 s, remission as usual, and no recollection after the attack.

Imaging Findings

A, B, D. Axial T2-weighted flair, axial T2-weighted and coronal T2-weighted flair images demonstrate signal intensity in the left hippocampus was increased compared with that in the contralateral, the internal structure was blurred, and the adjacent choroid fissure in the left side was slightly widened (Fig. 9.1a, b, d).

C. DWI demonstrates no obvious diffusion limitation was observed (Fig. 9.1c).

E. Arterial spin labeling demonstrates the perfusion in the left hippocampus and temporal lobe was significantly reduced compared with that in the contralateral, and the cerebral blood flow (CBF) in the left frontal and parietal cortex was slightly reduced compared with that in the contralateral (Fig. 9.1e).

F. Sagittal T2-weighted demonstrates hippocampus volume reduction (Fig. 9.1f).

Discussion

Hippocampus sclerosis (HS), a term often used interchangeably with mesial temporal lobe sclerosis (MTLS), is the most common pathological finding in temporal lobe epilepsy (TLE) and involves neuronal loss mainly within the hippocampus and also the amygdala and entorhinal cortex. It is a syndrome with a characteristic history and seizure semiology [1].

The MRI findings of hippocampus sclerosis are as follows: Hippocampus atrophy; Hippocampus volume reduction (coronal view is better); The abnormal T2WI signal increased in the hippocampus (obvious FLAIR sequence); The superficial sulcus of hippocampus head disappeared; white matter atrophy on the affected side; lateral temporal lobe atrophy; The affected side of the brain ventriculo

H. Shang
Department of Radiology, The Third Affiliated Hospital of Zhengzhou University, Zhengzhou, Henan, China

J. Chen
Department of Medical Imaging, Tianjin Children's Hospital (Children's Hospital of Tianjin University), Tianjin, P.R. China

G. Zheng
Department of Radiology, Tianjin Children's Hospital (Children's Hospital of Tianjin University), Tianjin, P.R. China

X. Zhao (✉) · X. Zhang
Department of Radiology, The Third Affiliated Hospital of Zhengzhou University, Institute of Neuroscience, Zhengzhou University, Zhengzhou, Henan, China
e-mail: zdsfyzx@zzu.edu.cn; zxa@zzu.edu.cn

X. Li
Tianjin Second People's Hospital (Tianjin Institute of Hepatology), Tianjin, P.R. China

H. Liu, X. Zhang (eds.), *Pediatric Neuroimaging*, https://doi.org/10.1007/978-981-16-7928-5_9

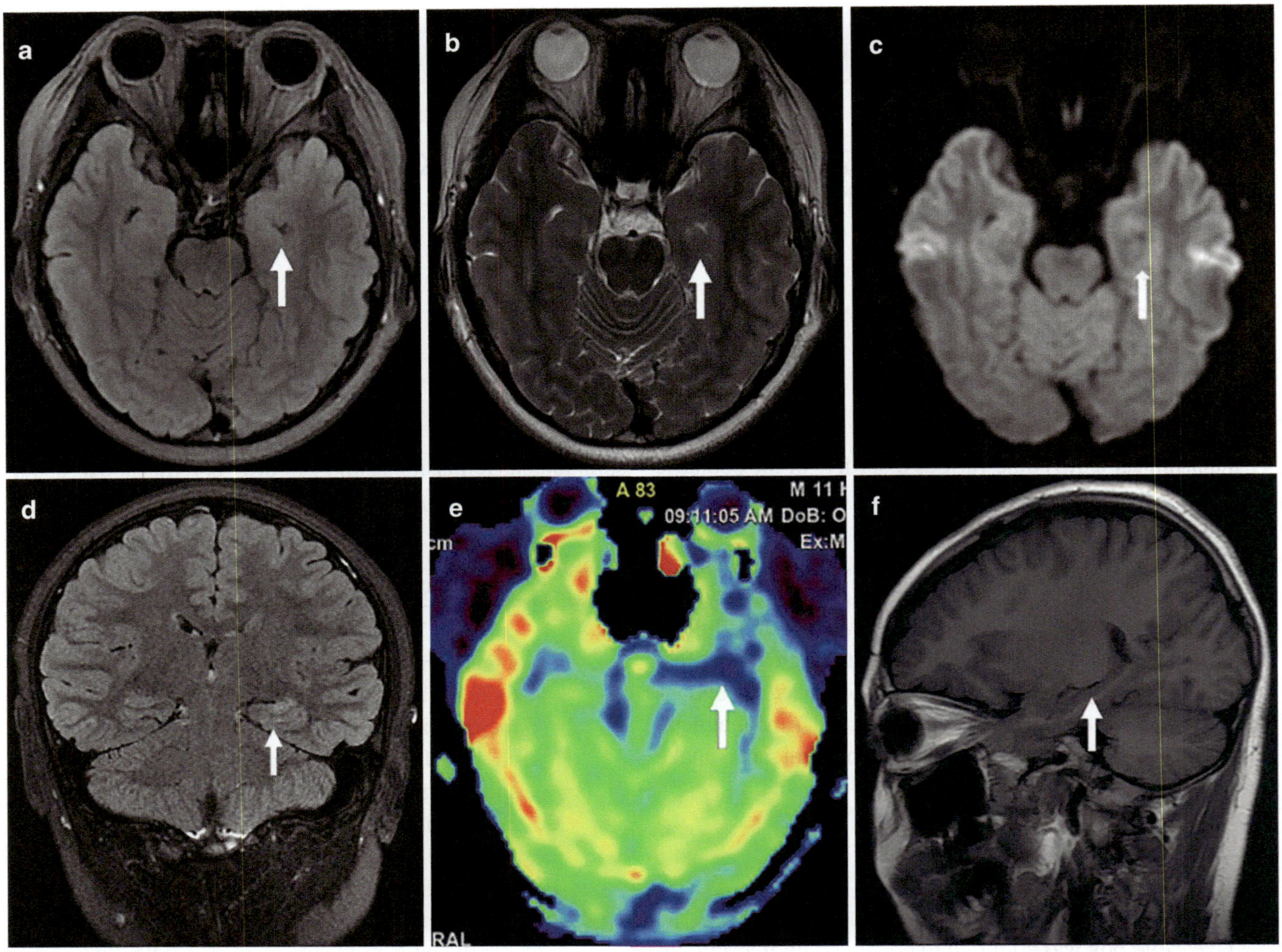

Fig. 9.1 Hippocampus sclerosis

temporal horn dilated. ASL was used to detect the absolute value of CBF in patients with epilepsy, and the CBF value of the affected hippocampus was significantly reduced in patients with unilateral hippocampus sclerosis. The MRI measure T2-signal intensity, which likely reflects gliosis of the neuropil, was not related to the histopathological findings [2].

Hippocampal mono spin magnetic resonance spectroscopy (1H-MRS) showed that the NAA peak in the affected side of the hippocampus decreased significantly. The study showed that the lowest value of normal N-acetyl aspartic acid (NAA)/creatine (CR) + choline (CHO) was 0.72. And the value lower than 0.05 suggests hippocampal sclerosis [3].

Diffusion tensor imaging (DTI) is an imaging method to study the white matter fiber bundles in the brain, which can reflect the fiber density between the fibers and network nodes in different brain regions. Patients with temporal lobe epilepsy with or without hippocampal sclerosis may have white matter tract abnormalities on DTI [3].

Blood oxygen level dependent functional MRI (BOLD-fMRI) can synchronously record electroencephalogram (EEG) in the interphase or during seizures of epileptic activity can be helpful in determining targets for surgical treatment [4].

Most patients with temporal lobe epilepsy have hippocampal sclerosis, which has high chances of postoperative seizure freedom after surgery [5]. Sometimes, HS occurs with a second lesion, either in the temporal lobe or extratemporal, most often happen on the same side to the HS [1].

Helmstaedter and Elger reported the results of a cross sectional design, it demonstrated how people who developed epilepsy in childhood expressed a block in their development of verbal memory skills with a slower progression compared to healthy controls [6].

The histopathologic diagnosis of HS is usually straightforward, it concludes granule cell dispersion, mossy fiber sprouting, and neuronal loss and chronic fibrillary gliosis centered on the pyramidal cell layer [1]. It defined by neuronal loss in the subfields CA1–CA4 in neuropathologically and gliosis of the adjacent neuropil [2]. HS type 1 involves neuronal loss in the CA1, CA3, and CA4 region, type 2 involves CA1 neuronal loss only, and type 3 describes neuronal loss restricted to CA4. While Hippocampal specimens showing reactive gliosis with little/no neuronal loss are classified as "no-HS."

Case 9.2 Reversible Compression of Corpus Callosum

Clinical Presentation

An 11-year-old boy presented with acute high fever for several hours and hyperspasmia once. His past medical, surgical, and family histories were negative. Blood routine and cerebrospinal fluid tests were negative.

Imaging Findings

A. Axial T1-weighted image demonstrates small patchy low signal lesion in the splenium of corpus Callosum (Fig. 9.2a).
B. Axial T2-weighted image demonstrates mild hyperintensity of the lesion in the splenium of corpus Callosum (Fig. 9.2b).
C. Axial T2WI-FLAIR image demonstrates moderate hyperintensity of the lesion in the splenium of corpus Callosum (Fig. 9.2c).
D. Axial DWI image demonstrates obvious hyperintensity of the lesion in the splenium of corpus Callosum (Fig. 9.2d).
E. The lesion of splenium of the corpus callosum completely disappears on follow-up axial T2WI image after 2 weeks (Fig. 9.2e).
F. The lesion of splenium of the corpus callosum completely disappears on follow-up axial DWI image after 2 weeks (Fig. 9.2f).

Discussion

Reversible compression of corpus callosum seen in reversible splenial lesion syndrome (RESLES) is a rare clinic radiological syndrome with mild clinical symptoms and good prognosis and characterized by the presence of a focal lesion often involving the central area of the splenium of the corpus callosum (SCC), followed by complete reversibility on follow-up MRI after a variable period of time [7, 8].

Although the pathogenesis of RESLES is complex and various, RESLES is most commonly associated with seizures and antiepileptic drugs. Other factors include infection, metabolic conditions, other pharmacological agents, and miscellaneous conditions. Mild encephalopathy with a reversible splenial lesion (MERS) is the most common cause of RESLES in childhood, and MERS is mainly resulted by infection, especially viruses. MERS is more common in East Asian populations, mostly Japan, and also occurs in Australian children. It is classified into two types, type I (iso-

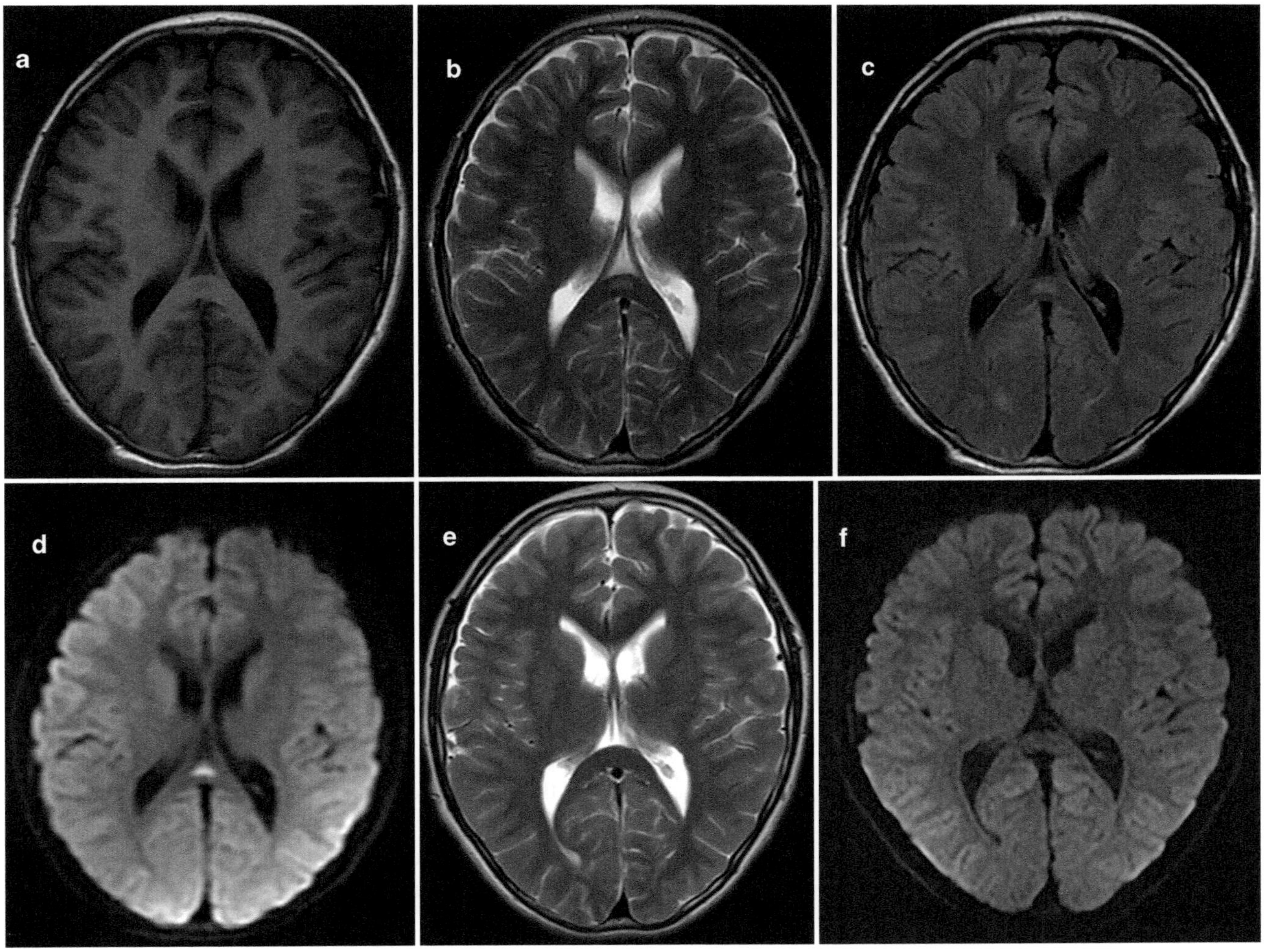

Fig. 9.2 Reversible compression of corpus callosum

lated lesion in SCC) and type II (involving SCC and other areas of the corpus callosum and adjacent periventricular white matter symmetrically). Patients of MERS mostly appear seizures, behavioral changes, altered consciousness, and motor deterioration. Sometimes EEG and CSF evaluation can be abnormal [7, 8].

MRI is the most helpful and sensitive method to identify and diagnose RESLES. There are circular or oval abnormal signal intensity in the SCC alone or also other white matter areas. The lesions show hyperintense on T2-weighted images, T2 fluid-attenuated inversion recovery (FLAIR), and diffusion-weighted imaging (DWI) sequences. They present hypointense on T1-weighted images and apparent diffusion coefficient (ADC) map, without contrast enhancement [9, 10].

RESLES should be differentiated from other leukoencephalopathies, such as acute disseminated encephalomyelitis (ADEM), reversible posterior leukoencephalopathy (RPLS), and hereditary leukoencephalopathy. Compared to RESLES, ADEM usually occurs at pediatric age and after infection. It is sustained by an autoimmune-mediated demyelination of brain and/or spinal cord, with multifocal white and gray matter lesions. Lesions can be bilateral but asymmetrical, without selectivity for the splenium or predilection for periventricular zone, and can have some enhancement without diffusion restriction, with a complete recovery in 50 ~ 60% of cases [10]. Early diagnosis of RESLES based on clinical and imaging characteristics can avoid unnecessary treatment and correctly judge prognosis [10].

Case 9.3 Arachnoid Cyst

Clinical Presentation

A 5-year-old boy presented to the emergency department (ED) for headache. His past medical, surgical, and family histories were negative. He had no recent trauma or traveling in the epidemic area.

Imaging Findings

A similar-circular cystic abnormal signal can be seen in the posterior fossa, and peripheral brain parenchyma is compressed.

- A, E. Axial T2-weightedimage and ADC image demonstrate the hyperintense (Fig. 9.3a, e).
- C, F. Axial and Sagittal T1-weighted image demonstrates the hypointense (Fig. 9.3c, f).
- B, D. Axial T2-weighted flair and DWI image demonstrate the low to intermediate signal intensity (Fig. 9.3b, d).

Discussion

Arachnoid cysts (ACs) are congenital lesions comprising 1% of all intracranial mass lesions [11]. The cyst wall is mainly composed of arachnoid membrane, glia, and pia mater. And there is cerebrospinal fluid-like cystic fluid in the cyst. ACs are more common in children and adolescents, and the incidence of left lesions is higher than that of right lesions.

Most lesions are located on the surface of the brain and do not involve the brain parenchyma. Most of them are single, while a few are multiple. ACs are mostly asymptomatic, however, the large lesions can simultaneously oppress brain tissue and skull and produce neurological symptoms and skull development changes.

According to the etiology, intracranial ACs can be divided into two types [12]: congenital or secondary to trauma, meningitis or hemorrhage. Congenital arachnoid cyst is a common type, and its pathogenesis is still unclear. The following assumptions are made: (1) During embryonic development, small arachnoid membranes fall into subarachnoid space and develop; (2) Because of the pulsation of choroid plexus, which pumps the cerebrospinal fluid, the loose perimedullary reticulum around nerve tissue can be separated to form subarachnoid space. For example, cysts can be formed in the perimedullary reticulum if the early flow of cerebrospinal fluid is abnormal; (3) Atelencephalia. Infection-induced arachnoid cysts are usually formed by local adhesion of the arachnoid membrane after infection, which is filled with cerebrospinal fluid. Most of them are multiple, and more common in children. It is common in the optic chiasma cistern, basal cistern, cerebellomedullary cistern, cisternaambiens, etc. And the cerebrospinal fluid circulation pathway is blocked. The injured arachnoid cyst is a pial cyst. The mechanism is that subarachnoid hemorrhage or adhesions around the edge of the arachnoid lead to local cerebrospinal fluid circulation disorder, and cysts are gradually formed under the constant impact of cerebral pulsation. The cyst can protrude under the scalp and compress the lower cerebral cortex. The cyst is filled with clear fluid and surrounded by scar tissue. It is common in infants and young children.

Most scholars believe that surgery is not necessary for asymptomatic patients [13]. For those with symptoms, internal decompression and cyst wall resection are needed.

Case 9.4 Rathke Cyst

Clinical Presentation

A 7-year-old female child came to the hospital for precocious puberty, and the clinicians suspect she has pituitary microadenoma, so she is advised to have a magnetic resonance (−)examination.

Imaging Findings

- A, B. There was an oval cystic signal between the adenohypophysis and the neurohypophysis (mainly located in the adenohypophysis) (Fig. 9.4a, b).
  - A. Sagittal T1-weighted image demonstrates hyperintense in the neurohypophysis,and its position was normal (Fig. 9.4a).
- B, C. The pituitary stalk shifted slightly to the left without enlargement of sellar fossa and no abnormality was found in bilateral cavernous sinus (Fig. 9.4b, c).

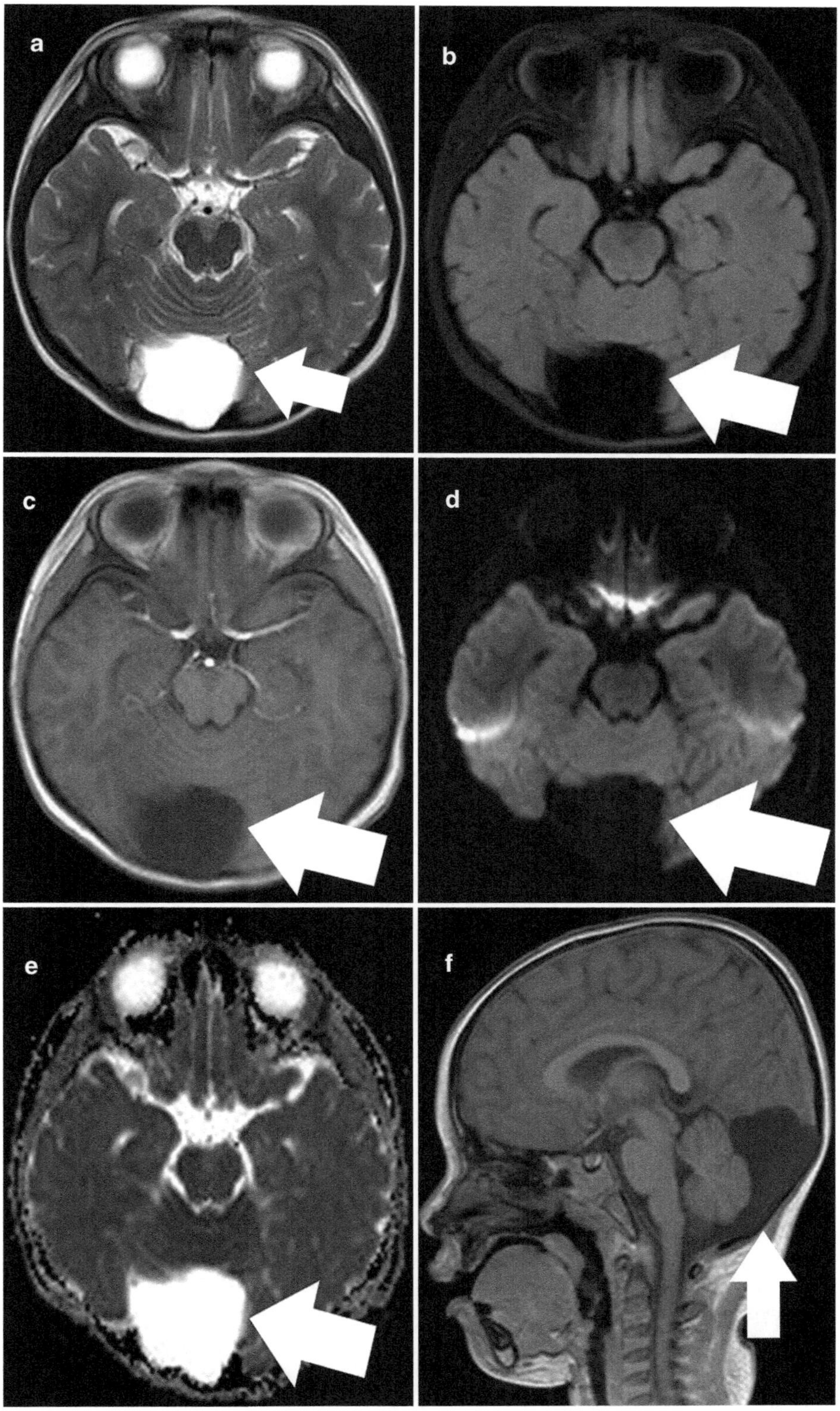

Fig. 9.3 Arachnoid cyst

Figure 9.4c–e: Dynamic contrast-enhanced scanning showed that the cystic signal was not enhanced all the time, and its boundary was clear and the size was about 7.62 mm × 3.01 mm. The remaining pituitary regions were enhanced uniformly.

Discussion

Rathke cyst often occurs in the pituitary gland, which is originated from the pituitary Rathke sac congenital dysplasia. At 4 weeks of embryo development, the buccal vesicles of digestive canal developed into a diverticula-like structure,

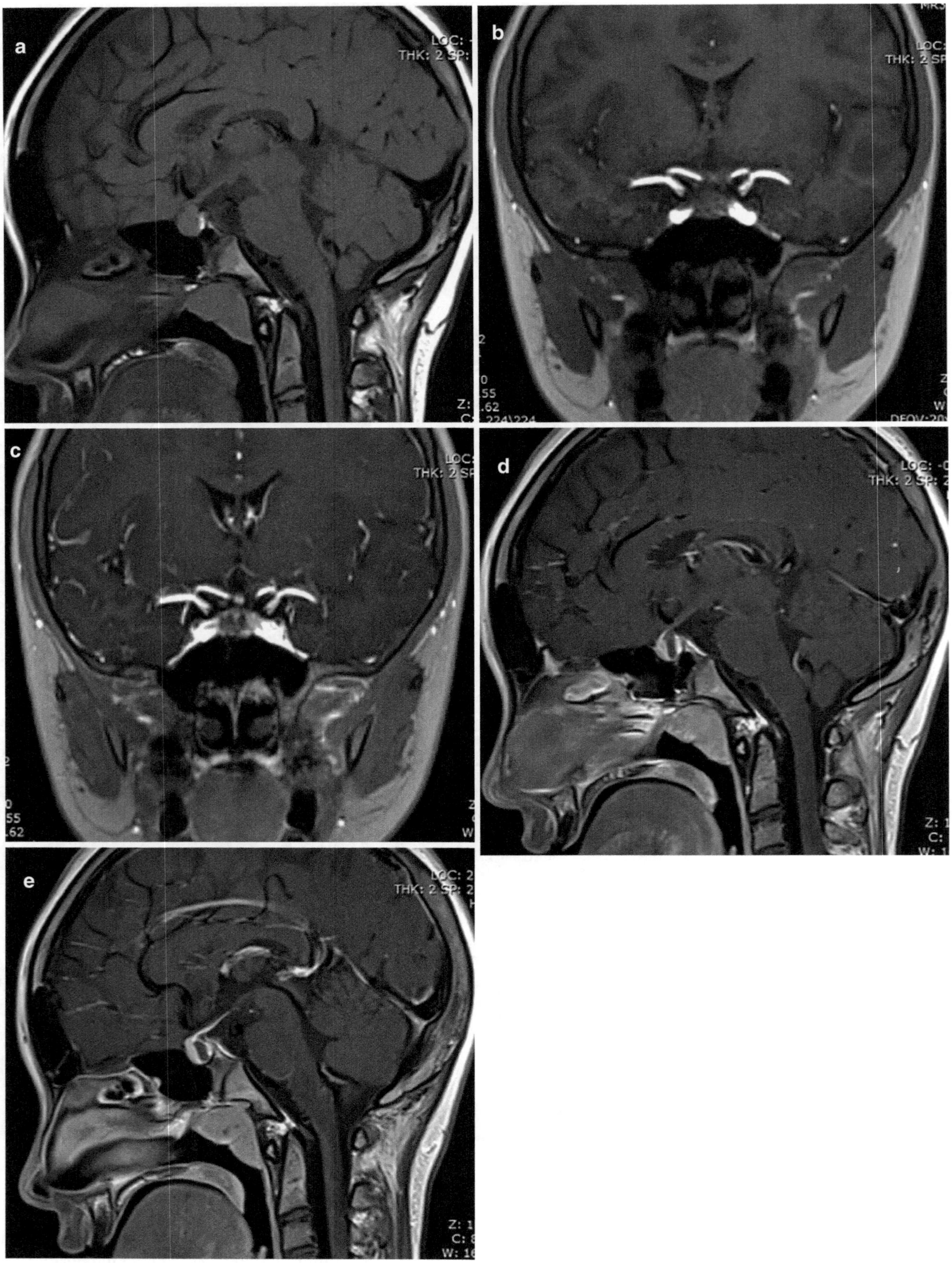

Fig. 9.4 Rathke cyst

called Rathke pouch. From week 11 to week 12, the anterior and middle pituitary gland were formed with the proliferation of anterior and posterior wall of the bag. There is a small lacuna in the middle of the pituitary gland, which is gradually filled by epithelial cells during the development of the pituitary gland. In a few people, the lacuna remains. When the secretion in the lacuna is significantly increased, the lacuna can expand to form a large cyst, that is, Rathke cyst [14, 15].

Most cysts are centered on the pituitary gland, the larger ones can pass through the diaphragma sellae to the suprasellar cistern, and the smaller ones are completely located in the sellae or the main part in the sellae [16]. Pathologically, Rathke cyst wall cells are often monolayer columnar epithelial cells, goblet epithelial cells, mucinous secretory fine cells, and a few of them are mixed with false lamellar flat epithelial cells. The contents of the cyst are mostly white myxoid or gelatinous, some of them are grass yellow or clear liquid, and the patients with bleeding can be brown and can contain cholesterol crystals [17].

The main examination methods are CT and MRI, but MRI is the first choice for this disease. CT is easy to miss diagnosis of mild lesions and does not recommend the first choice.

The smaller ones (diameter < 2 cm) were asymptomatic and most of them were found by accident. The larger ones can compress the pituitary, optic chiasma, and hypothalamus, causing symptoms.

CT findings: (1) CT findings of smaller cysts can be normal. (2) the larger ones exhibited that pituitary fossa enlarged with cystic low-density focus, and a few of them showed a slightly high-density change. (3) the tumor can develop to the suprasellar, and a few of the tumors can protrude into the sphenoid sinus at the same time.

MRI findings [18]: (1) MRI findings of Rathke cyst are varied. According to the difference of its signal, it is divided into two kinds: one is low signal intensity of T1WI, the high signal intensity of T2WI, the cystic part of which represents cerebrospinal fluid; and the other kind is that T1WI is high signal intensity and T2WI signal is different. (2) the signal of cyst characterized by low signal of T1WI and high signal of T2WI is general uniform, which is characterized by typical eccentric growth. Enhanced scan of this kind of cyst does not show enhancement. (3) the cysts with high signal intensity characteristics of T1WI were more complex, and the smaller cysts (diameter < 1 cm) had more characteristic imaging features, that is, located above the pituitary gland, the outline was smooth, regular, and adjacent to the normal pituitary tissue. However, the boundary was clear. (4) most of the cysts of medium size (1 ~ 3 cm in diameter) and larger cysts (diameter > 3 cm) were complicated with dysplasia and atrophy of pituitary, and the boundary between the typical cysts and the remaining pituitary tissues was clear. The diseases were ellipsoid in shape, and the largest diameter of that was located in the sellar, which could develop to the suprasellar while a few to the sphenoid sinus at the same time. (5) most of Rathke cysts were not enhanced, a few cyst walls could be enhanced, but the center was not enhanced. MRI can infer its pathological composition according to the various signal changes in the cyst, and if necessary, it can distinguish protein components from bleeding by adding fat suppression sequences, which has unique diagnostic value for qualitative diagnosis; Large cysts can be found by CT, but they are powerless to occur in smaller cysts in the pituitary gland.

Cysts characterized by low signal intensity (T1WI) and high signal intensity (T2WI) should be distinguished from cystic pituitary adenoma and cystic craniopharyngioma, because this type of cyst does not show enhancement on enhanced scan. However, cystic pituitary adenomas and cystic craniopharyngiomas can be enhanced to varying degrees due to the presence of residual pituitary and tumor tissue in the cyst. Therefore, enhanced scan is the only basis for distinguishing this type of cyst from other tumors. Cysts characterized by high signal intensity on T1WI need to be distinguished from cystic craniopharyngioma and pituitary adenoma stroke. Because most Rathke cysts have uniform signal intensity, this is also an important basis for differential diagnosis from other common diseases.

References

1. Malmgren K, Thom M. Hippocampal sclerosis—origins and imaging. Epilepsia. 2012;53(Suppl 4):19–33.
2. Nakayama Y, Masuda H, et al. Features of amygdala in patients with mesial temporal lobe epilepsy and hippocampal sclerosis: an MRI volumetric and histopathological study. Epilepsy Res. 2017;09(135):50–5.
3. Mingyuan H, Rui Z, Pengfei L. Study on hippocampal perfusion in patients with temporal lobe epilepsy using magnetic resonance arterial spin labeling (ASL) technique. J Med Res. 2017;46(3):82–6.
4. Yiwei Z, Hui Y, Feng F. Advances in MRI diagnosis of temporal lobe epilepsy with hippocampal sclerosis. Int J Med Radiol. 2017;40(5):528–31.
5. Cossu M, d'Orio P, et al. Focal cortical dysplasia IIIa in hippocampal sclerosis-associated epilepsy: anatomo-electro-clinical profile and surgical results from a multicentric retrospective study. Neurosurgery. 2021;88(2):384–93.
6. Tai XY, Bernhardt B, Thom M, Thompson P, et al. Review: neurodegenerative processes in temporal lobe epilepsy with hippocampal sclerosis: clinical, pathological and neuronal imaging evidence. Neuropathol Appl Neurobiol. 2018;44(1):70–90.
7. Liu J, Liu D, Yang B, et al. Reversible splenial lesion syndrome (RESLES) coinciding with cerebral venous thrombosis: a report of two cases. Ther Adv Neurol Disord. 2017;10(12):375–9. https://doi.org/10.1177/1756285617727978.
8. Feraco P, Porretti G, Marchio G, et al. Mild encephalitis/encephalopathy with reversible splenial lesion (MERS) due to cytomegalovirus: case report and review of the literature. Neuropediatrics. 2018;49(1):68–71. https://doi.org/10.1055/s-0037-1608779.
9. Chen WX, Liu HS, Yang SD, et al. Reversible splenial lesion syndrome in children: retrospective study and summary of case

series. Brain and Development. 2016;38(10):915–27. https://doi.org/10.1016/j.braindev.2016.04.011.
10. Tang Y, Zhang D, Ge J, et al. Clinical and imaging features of reversible splenial lesion syndrome with language disorder. Transl Neurosci. 2020;11(1):210–4. https://doi.org/10.1515/tnsci-2020-0126.
11. Yahal O, Katorza E, Zvi E, et al. Prenatal diagnosis of arachnoid cysts: MRI features and neurodevelopmental outcome. Eur J Radiol. 2019;113:232–7.
12. Conde Sardón R. Arachnoid cysts. Historical evolution of the concept and pathophysiological theories. Neurocirugia (Astur). 2015;26(4):192–5.
13. Ali M, Bennardo M, Almenawer SA, et al. Exploring predictors of surgery and comparing operative treatment approaches for pediatric intracranial arachnoid cysts: a case series of 83 patients. J Neurosurg Pediatr. 2015;16(3):275–82.
14. Farrash FA, Hassounah M, Helmi HA, et al. Rathke's cleft cyst presentation mimicking craniopharyngioma: case report. Int J Surg Case Rep. 2020;68:104–6.
15. Jung JE, Jin J, Jung MK, et al. Clinical manifestations of Rathke's cleft cysts and their natural progression during 2 years in children and adolescents. Ann Pediatr Endocrinol Metab. 2017;22(3):164–9.
16. Dodson V, Eloy JA, Lou JK. Chapter 40-Rathke's cleft cysts and arachnoid cyts. In: A comprehensive and interdisciplinary approach; 2021. p. 551–6.
17. Lin M, Wedemeyer MA, Bradley D, et al. Long-term surgical outcomes following transsphenoidal surgery in patients with Rathke's cleft cysts. J Neurosurg. 2018;130(3):831–7.
18. Sivaraju L, Kiran NAS, Rao AS, et al. Giant multi-compatmental suprasellar Rathke's cleft cyst with restriction on diffusion weighted images. Neuroradiol J. 2017;30(3):1–5.